THE GUIDE TO
HEALTHCARE
REFORM

Daniel B. McLaughlin, EDITOR

THE GUIDE TO
HEALTHCARE
REFORM

• • • • • •

Readings and Commentary

AUPHA

Health Administration Press, Chicago, Illinois
Association of University Programs in Health Administration, Arlington, Virginia

19   18   17   16   15   5   4   3   2   1

Library of Congress Cataloging-in-Publication Data

The guide to healthcare reform : readings and commentary / Daniel B. McLaughlin, editor.
   pages cm
Includes index.
ISBN 978-1-56793-694-0
1. National health insurance—Law and legislation—United States. 2. United States. Patient Protection and Affordable Care Act. 3. Health insurance—Law and legislation—United States. 4. Health care reform—United States. 5. Medical care—Law and legislation—United States. 6. Health services accessibility—United States. 7. Medical policy—United States. I. McLaughlin, Daniel B., 1945– editor. II. Title: Guide to healthcare reform.
   KF3605.G85 2015
   346.73'086382—dc23
                      2014030723

The paper used in this publication meets the minimum requirements of American National Standard for Information Sciences—Permanence of Paper for Printed Library Materials, ANSI Z39.48-1984. ∞™

Acquisitions editor: Janet Davis; Project manager: Amy Carlton; Cover design: Marisa Jackson; Layout: Cepheus Edmondson

Health Administration Press
A division of the Foundation of the American
   College of Healthcare Executives
One North Franklin Street, Suite 1700
Chicago, IL 60606–3529
(312) 424–2800

Association of University Programs
   in Health Administration
2000 North 14th Street
Suite 780
Arlington, VA 22201
(703) 894–0940

To my family—Sharon, Kelly, Katie, and Paul

BRIEF CONTENTS

Preface xv

Acknowledgments xix

Chapter 1 Introduction 1

Chapter 2 The Affordable Care Act 5

                 Additional Reading 16

Chapter 3 Prevention, Wellness, and Population Health 22

                 Additional Readings 31

Chapter 4 Chronic Disease Management and Primary Care 102

                 Additional Readings 112

Chapter 5 Productivity and Quality 170

                 Additional Readings 179

Chapter 6 Payment Incentives 226

        Additional Readings **240**

Chapter 7 The Safety Net... 301

        Additional Reading..**309**

Chapter 8 The Perfect Market: Health Insurance Reform 315

        Additional Reading..**326**

Chapter 9 Health Policy and Advocacy... 349

        Additional Readings **354**

Chapter 10 The Future 406

Appendix.. 415

Index.. 417

About the Contributors.. 439

About the Editor 443

DETAILED CONTENTS

Preface xv

Acknowledgments xix

Chapter 1 Introduction...1
    The Journey 1
    Purpose of This Book 1
    How the Book Is Organized..3
    Objectives 3
    Summary 4
    Applications: Discussion and Research..4
    References 4

Chapter 2 The Affordable Care Act 5
    The Groundwork Is Laid..5
    The Three Theories 6
    Legal Challenges to the ACA 13
    How to Use This Book 14
    Summary 14
    Applications: Discussion and Research..14
    References 15

Additional Reading...**16**

   Reading 2A: Legal Issues in Health Insurance and
               Health Reform (excerpt) 16
   Dean M. Harris

Chapter 3 Prevention, Wellness, and Population Health.......................... 22
   Clinical Prevention 22
   Wellness.. 25
   Community Building... 26
   Summary 28
   Applications: Discussion and Research................................. 29
   References 29

Additional Readings **31**

   Reading 3A: Introduction/Population Health Management............. 31
   Ann S. McAlearney
   Reading 3B: Population Health: Practicing Population Health
               Management and Measuring Its Success 57
   David B. Nash
   Reading 3C: Community Health: A Measurable Management
               Task.. 64
   Connie J. Evashwick
   Reading 3D: ACA Integration Initiatives That Promote
               Collaboration... 73
   Connie J. Evashwick
   Reading 3E: Population Health Improvement: A Community
               Health Business Model That Engages Partners in All Sectors 80
   David A. Kindig and George Isham

Chapter 4 Chronic Disease Management and Primary Care 102
   The Chronic Care Model 102
   The HITECH Act and Meaningful Use 104
   Policies to Support Chronic Care in the ACA 104
   Summary 109
   Notes 110
   Applications: Discussion and Research............................... 110
   References 111

Additional Readings **112**

   Reading 4A: Government Policy and Healthcare Reform 112
   Gerald L. Glandon, Detlev H. Smaltz, and Donna J. Slovensky

Reading 4B: Population Health: Coordinating Care to Provide
   Effective Population Health Management............................... 144
   Heather Jorna and Stephen A. Martin, Jr.
Reading 4C: The Patient-Centered Medical Home Solution to
   the Cost–Quality Conundrum.. 151
   Michael Ewing
Reading 4D: Primary Care.. 161
   Phoebe Lindsey Barton

Chapter 5 Productivity and Quality.. 170
   Productivity 170
   Quality.. 173
   Health Plan Quality Rating System.................................... 175
   Summary 177
   Applications: Discussion and Research............................... 177
   Note 178
   References 178

   Additional Readings **179**
   Reading 5A: How Purchasers Select and Pay for Value:
      The Movement to Value-Based Purchasing............................ 179
      François de Brantes
   Reading 5B: The Quality Improvement Landscape 194
      Kimberly D. Acquaviva and Jean E. Johnson

Chapter 6 Payment Incentives 226
   Incentives: The Carrots 228
   Penalties: The Stick 231
   Fraud and Abuse: The Big Stick 232
   The Backup Plans.. 233
   Affordability.. 234
   Structure.. 235
   Healthcare Inflation Today 235
   Summary 235
   Applications: Discussion and Research................................ 236
   References 237

   Additional Readings **240**
   Reading 6A: The Accountable Care Organization 240
      Marc Bard and Mike Nugent

Reading 6B: What Every CEO Should Know About Medicare's
Recovery Audit Contractor Program 272
Alan J. Goldberg and Linda M. Young

Reading 6C: The Quest for Affordability in Healthcare 277
Bernard J. Tyson

Reading 6D: The Medicare Hospital Payment Update 283
Daniel B. McLaughlin

Reading 6E: Post-Acute Care and Vertical Integration After
the Patient Protection and Affordable Care Act 286
Patrick D. Shay and Stephen S. Mick

Chapter 7 The Safety Net 301

Eligibility 302

Navigators 302

Dual-Eligible Beneficiaries 303

Hospitals 303

Rural Healthcare 304

Community Clinics 305

Healthcare Disparities 305

Summary 306

Notes 306

Applications: Discussion and Research 307

References 307

Additional Reading **309**

Reading 7A: Equity of Care—Eliminating Healthcare
Disparities: The Call to Action 309
Richard J. Umbdenstock

Chapter 8 The Perfect Market: Health Insurance Reform 315

Universal Coverage 315

Health Insurance Exchanges 316

Standard Benefits 320

Increased Government Regulation 321

Summary 323

Applications: Discussion and Research 323

Note 324

References 324

Additional Reading **326**

Reading 8A: Health Insurance Exchanges 326
Michael A. Morrisey

Chapter 9 Health Policy and Advocacy 349

    Health Policy Process 349

    The States 350

    Health Policy and Advocacy 350

    Summary 352

    Applications: Discussion and Research 353

    Reference 353

    Additional Readings **354**

      Reading 9A: The Context and Process of Health

          Policymaking 354

         Beaufort B. Longest, Jr.

      Reading 9B: Health Policymaking at the State and Local Levels

          and in the Private Sector 386

         Leiyu Shi

Chapter 10 The Future 406

    Making Changes: The Process 406

    Potential Targets for Change 407

    Good Ideas Likely to Remain 410

    What About a Repeal? 411

    System Changes 411

    Summary 412

    Conclusion 413

    Applications: Discussion and Research 413

    References 413

Appendix 415

Index 417

About the Contributors 439

About the Editor 443

PREFACE

I have always enjoyed health policy—as a student, teacher, and participant. For most of my career I worked for Hennepin County, which surrounds Minneapolis, Minnesota. I spent 30 years as an administrator in the Hennepin County Medical Center and the last eight of those as its CEO. I also initiated and led the Hennepin County Health Policy Center, which drafted and lobbied legislation to support the healthcare system of the county. The practical application of health policy can be frustrating, but it is essential to the success of a county-based health system.

I also had the opportunity to work on the Clinton administration's healthcare reform bill in 1992 and 1993 as a representative of the National Association of Counties. The federal process is essentially the same as that at the state level—but a lot more intense because of higher stakes.

THE ORIGINS OF LEGISLATION

Legislation arises from a strongly perceived need and is drafted by experts. These experts come from

◆ government agencies,

◆ trade associations,

◆ professional societies,

- ◆ academics,

- ◆ think tanks (usually Washington, DC–based), and

- ◆ legislative committee staff.

The legislation can seem disjointed and complex because of these multiple inputs to the process. More important, the legislation can be unclear about what new strategies need to be implemented or old strategies abandoned. The Patient Protection and Affordable Care Act—now shortened to Affordable Care Act (ACA)—is unusually confusing because the final bill never went to conference committee, where much of the logic of a bill is set.

Numerous resources clarifying the details of the law are available from consulting firms, trade associations, and advocacy groups. However, this book provides an additional and higher-level option. It provides a neutral and academically based resource designed to assist educators, students, and healthcare leaders in understanding the details and strategic implications of the ACA.

AUDIENCES

The healthcare system touches all Americans, and therefore anyone who wants to learn about this major system may wish to use this book to understand it better. However the book has been developed to meet the needs of two major groups.

HEALTHCARE MANAGEMENT STUDENTS AND INSTRUCTORS

Many programs in healthcare administration have courses that look at the broad aspects of the healthcare system (e.g., health policy, healthcare overview, health economics, capstones). These courses usually include a major textbook to provide the theoretical framework for the course. However, many instructors also want a resource to teach the application of these principles today. And students want to see practical applications to understand how these theories have been used by leading healthcare organizations. This book is intended to meet both of these needs. Because the book does contain theoretical underpinnings, it can be used as the primary textbook in a class in some cases.

Some features of this book that will be helpful to the instructor and students include

- ◆ discussion and application questions,

- ◆ URLs for current legislation and regulations (also available as links at ache. org/books/Reform2),

- ◆ instructor's resources including PowerPoint slides for each chapter,

◆   teaching notes, and

◆   a sample course syllabus.

Instructors who choose to use this book in their course may request access to its instructor resources by e-mailing hapbooks@ache.org.

HEALTH PROFESSIONALS

Health professionals are the second major audience for this book. I teach healthcare executives and professionals in our university's healthcare MBA, evening MBA, and executive development programs. I have observed that although most of our students have a high level of specific technical skills (e.g., physicians, nurses, health insurance executives, medical device developers), they do not fully understand how their work fits into the larger American healthcare system. This book can be helpful in that quest.

Planners and strategists are a subset of health professionals who also may find this book useful. Strategic analysis of the ACA is contained in another book I published with Health Administration Press, *Responding to Healthcare Reform: A Strategy Guide for Healthcare Leaders*. This new book updates *Responding to Healthcare Reform* and contains many readings that provide a useful compendium of practical strategy implementations based on many of the policies contained in the ACA.

HEALTH ADMINISTRATION PRESS AND ITS RESOURCES

Health Administration Press (HAP), the publisher of this book, is a division of the Foundation of the American College of Healthcare Executives (ACHE) and is the publishing partner of the Association of University Programs in Healthcare Administration. As a result HAP has dozens of books that are intended for the classroom and the executive suite. In addition HAP publishes periodicals intended for both audiences:

◆   *Frontiers of Health Services Management*

◆   *Journal of Healthcare Management*

Because many of these books and publications are being written with insightful and practical applications of the policies in the ACA, we determined that a useful book could be constructed that contained the basics of the ACA (written by me) and many excellent examples from other HAP publications. We additionally drew from *Futurescan 2014: Healthcare Trends and Implications 2014–2019,* a joint publication from ACHE and the Society for Healthcare Strategy and Market Development of the American Hospital

Association. Therefore, this book has been curated with the best examples from the field selected to demonstrate the principles of the ACA. We expect that future editions of this book will contain new and different readings, as HAP authors write updated books and articles.

The ACA is one of the most significant changes to American health policy since the advent of Medicare and Medicaid. Its future success is in the hands of the students of health management and today's healthcare leaders. I wish you well.

—Dan McLaughlin

ACKNOWLEDGMENTS

The legislative arena can be both challenging and exciting, and I had the opportunity to participate in it as a policy analyst and as the leader of a lobbying team.

Hennepin County is the largest county in Minnesota and surrounds Minneapolis, and I was able to lobby many proposals in the Minnesota Legislature. I want to thank Hennepin County Commissioners Randy Johnson, Mike Opat, and Peter McLaughlin (no relation) for their support and education during those years.

I also would like to thank Representatives Lee Greenfield and Tom Huntley of the Minnesota House and Senator Linda Berglin of the Minnesota Senate for their support of Hennepin County and all of the excellent healthcare legislation they enacted over the past 20 years.

At the federal level I am grateful to former Congressman Martin Sabo for his support and former Senator David Durenberger. David is a gift to Minnesota, where he taught many of our students for more than 20 years at the University of St. Thomas.

My view of the individual insurance market has been shaped by Milt and Amy Edgren. I appreciate their insights into the challenges this market presents to agents—particularly after the implementation of the ACA.

At the University of St. Thomas I am indebted to Dean Chris Puto and Associate Dean Michael Garrison of the Opus College of Business for their support of my center and work. I also am supported by faculty colleagues, professors John Militello, John Olson, and Mick Sheppeck, with whom I have ongoing discussions and debates about the future of the American healthcare system.

This collaboration with Health Administration Press has been interesting and challenging, as this is a unique textbook format and without their excellent staff support it would not have been possible. Thanks once again to Janet Davis, acquisitions director; Michael Cunningham, marketing director; Drew Baumann, editorial director; and Amy Carlton, project manager. I also want to thank all the outstanding authors of the books and articles used in this book: Dean M. Harris; Ann Scheck McAlearney; David B. Nash; Connie J. Evashwick; David A. Kindig and George Isham; Gerald L. Glandon, Detlev H. Smaltz, and Donna J. Slovensky; Heather Jorna and Stephen A. Martin Jr.; Michael Ewing; Phoebe Lindsey Barton; François de Brantes; Kimberley D. Acquaviva and Jean E. Johnson; Marc A. Bard and Mike Nugent; Alan Goldberg and Linda M. Young; Bernard J. Tyson; Patrick D. Shay and Stephen S. Mick; Richard J. Umbdenstock; Michael A. Morrisey; Beaufort B. Longest Jr.; and Leiyu Shi.

—Dan McLaughlin

CHAPTER 1

INTRODUCTION

THE JOURNEY

The term *reform* conjures images of new, massive, and permanent structures. The political storm surrounding the enactment of the Affordable Care Act (ACA) in 2010 and its subsequent implementation seemed to emphasize this permanent nature. However, to paraphrase Emerson, reform is a journey not a destination—and the ACA is another major step on this journey.

There have been many healthcare reforms in the United States—starting with a law in 1798 that levied a tax on ship owners to provide a fund for the healthcare of their seamen (Longest 2010). The last major policy change on the scale of the ACA was the enactment of Medicare and Medicaid in 1965. Exhibit 1.1 outlines selected major policy initiatives since this time.

Although these legislative policies positively affected the system in a specific manner, the ACA stands as one of the most comprehensive attempts to improve the total American healthcare system in the past 50 years. Its ambitious goals are as follows:

◆ To improve the health insurance system to achieve near-universal coverage

◆ To restrain the growth of healthcare costs

◆ To improve the quality of care and patient experience

Progress has been made since 2010 to implement many of the policies in the act; some have worked well, while others have not yet been proven to be effective. Congress and the administration will likely continue to make improvements into the future—the journey will continue.

PURPOSE OF THIS BOOK

Although the ACA provides a framework for needed improvements in the system, the law will be changed and improved over the years. This book has therefore been constructed to help the reader

1965	• The Medicare and Medicaid programs were created, making comprehensive healthcare available to millions of Americans. • The Older Americans Act created the nutritional and social programs administered by HHS Administration on Aging. • The Head Start program was created.
1966	• The Community Health Center and Migrant Health Center programs were launched.
1970	• The National Health Service Corps was created.
1971	• The National Cancer Act was signed into law.
1977	• The Health Care Financing Administration was created to manage Medicare and Medicaid separately from the Social Security Administration.
1984	• The National Organ Transplantation Act was signed into law.
1989	• The Agency for Health Care Policy and Research (now the Agency for Healthcare Research and Quality) was created.
1990	• The Ryan White Comprehensive AIDS Resource Emergency (CARE) Act began providing support for people with AIDS.
1995	• The Social Security Administration became an independent agency.
1996	• Welfare reform under the Personal Responsibility and Work Opportunity Reconciliation Act was enacted. • The Health Insurance Portability and Accountability Act (HIPAA) was enacted.
1997	• The State Children's Health Insurance Program (SCHIP) was created, enabling states to extend health coverage to more uninsured children. • Medicare Advantage (Part C) was created.
2001	• The Centers for Medicare & Medicaid Services was created, replacing the Health Care Financing Administration.
2002	• The Office of Public Health Emergency Preparedness was created to coordinate efforts against bioterrorism and other emergency health threats.
2003	• The Medicare Prescription Drug Improvement and Modernization Act was enacted; the most significant expansion of Medicare since its enactment, including a prescription drug benefit (Part D).
2008	• The Mental Health Parity and Addiction Act was passed, which provides that coverage for these conditions be more restrictive than coverage for medical/surgical conditions.
2010	• The Affordable Care Act was signed into law, putting in place comprehensive US health system and insurance reforms.

SOURCE: HHS (2014).

understand the fundamentals of the ACA and its implementation today. This book has four goals:

- ◆ Providing an understanding of the underlying models that were used to construct the ACA

- ◆ Highlighting the major elements of the ACA that are used to implement these models to achieve the law's goals

- ◆ Providing access and context for the details of the policies and their regulations

- ◆ Providing current examples of the implementation of ACA policies in leading healthcare organizations

HOW THE BOOK IS ORGANIZED

This book is organized from the perspective of the healthcare leader, not the legislator. Therefore after the first chapter on the history, structure, and theoretical framework of the ACA, chapters are organized from a broad population health perspective.

The first chapters examine the ACA from a systems perspective—how the pieces work together to achieve the desired outcomes. Next, the role of funding is explored as a major tool of the ACA incentivizing desired behaviors by providers, insurers, and patients. The theory that marketplace competition is a major part of the architecture of the ACA is explored in the chapter on health insurance changes. The book concludes with a look at the journey ahead, with a chapter on health policy development and the future.

The ACA is a massive law, with more than 2,400 pages in the original legislation. Therefore this book does not cover every detail and program in the ACA—only those that have large systemic impacts and are being actively pursued.

OBJECTIVES

This book is intended to provide the reader with the following information and skills:

➤ understanding the three theories that underlie the ACA;

➤ understanding how the ACA supports

- • population health and wellness,

- • chronic disease management,

- • improved quality and productivity,

- • a sustainable safety net,

- health insurance expansion and improvement, and
- payment policies to achieve these goals;

➤ understanding the ACA as a part of the health policy development and advocacy process; and

➤ examining the future of healthcare.

SUMMARY

The ACA is part of a long journey to improve the American healthcare system. Its goals are to improve access to health insurance, restrain costs, and improve quality. This book provides three perspectives to view and understand the ACA: systems, funds flows, and markets. The future is examined with an overview of health policy making and possible future changes to the law.

APPLICATIONS: DISCUSSION AND RESEARCH

1. What other policy options were considered during the debate on the ACA? (Use library resources and access journals such as *Health Affairs*, *Journal of the American Medical Association*, and *New England Journal of Medicine* and search on "reform.")

2. What other country's healthcare system might be a model for the future for the United States? (Use library resources and search journals for "international health" and "world health." See also Fried and Gaydos [2012].)

3. Is population health a legitimate goal of the American healthcare system? If so, why?

REFERENCES

Fried, B. J., and L. M. Gaydos. 2012. *World Health Systems: Challenges and Perspectives*, 2nd ed. Chicago: Health Administration Press.

Longest, B. 2010. "Briefly Annotated Chronological List of Selected U.S. Federal Laws Pertaining to Health." Appendix 3 in *Health Policymaking in the United States*, 5th ed. 245–92. Chicago: Health Administration Press.

US Department of Health and Human Services (HHS). 2014. "Historical Highlights." Updated June 6. www.hhs.gov/about/hhshist.html.

CHAPTER 2

THE AFFORDABLE CARE ACT

The Patient Protection and Affordable Care Act was signed into law on March 23, 2010. The title has been abbreviated to the Affordable Care Act (ACA) or, more informally, "Obamacare." The contours of healthcare's future will clearly be shaped by the ACA, and this chapter provides a foundation for understanding the theories that underlie the law. Because the ACA contains more than 400 complex sections, a straightforward reading of it is of limited use to understand its full impact. However, awareness of the theories that shaped the ACA can be useful in understanding how the law is designed to work and anticipating the future environment of the US healthcare system.

This book is organized around the three fundamental theories of the ACA. Through these theoretical viewpoints a more complete understanding of the framework for the policy changes that were eventually included in the law can be obtained:

1. *Systems.* How does each element in the system interact with and affect the other elements to achieve the desired outcomes (patient health)?

2. *Funds flow and incentives.* How can revenue and payment systems be designed to create change in behaviors to achieve desired outcomes (increased quality and patient satisfaction with lowered cost)?

3. *Markets.* How can markets be made to operate effectively to allow the "invisible hand" of capitalism to achieve the desired outcomes (provider market share and profit)?

THE GROUNDWORK IS LAID

The debate on health reform in 2009 and 2010 might lead one to conclude that the final product is simply a random collection of ideas from various interest groups, academics, and politicians. However, the ACA is the result of many years of health policy research, demonstration projects, pilots, and many of the best practices being used by leading healthcare organizations throughout the country.

Senator Max Baucus (chair of the Senate Finance Committee) released a comprehensive report on November 12, 2008, just eight days after the presidential election. "Call to Action: Health Reform 2009" (Baucus 2008) includes many of the features and architecture of the final law. This report was well researched and included more than 290 footnotes from scholarly research publications. It reports the results of many federally funded pilot projects and demonstrations. It outlined the key elements needed for reforming the US health system:

◆   Increased access to affordable healthcare

◆   Improved value by reforming the healthcare delivery system

◆   Financing changes for a more efficient system

Although the legislation passed along party lines, it includes many policies that have been recommended over the years by Republicans and Democrats alike. In addition, many of the policies were advanced by nonpartisan academics and career federal staff. Although generalization is always dangerous, the source of specific policies can be grouped as shown in Exhibit 2.1.

THE THREE THEORIES
SYSTEMS VIEW

A useful systems view of US healthcare starts with the patient–provider relationship. This is the system that is the most visible to patients and providers. The provider is frequently a physician but includes healthcare professionals such as nurses, pharmacists, chiropractors, and others.

Both the provider and the patient are influenced by other systems, and Exhibit 2.2 illustrates this relationship.

EXHIBIT 2.1
Source of Theories
Contained in the
ACA

Source	Theory
Academics, nonpartisan think tanks, and career federal officials	Systems
Liberals	Funds flow and incentives
Conservatives	Markets

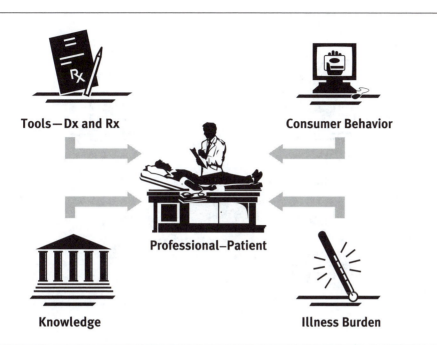

EXHIBIT 2.2
Core Elements of
the US Healthcare
System

The providers deliver the service based on the diagnostic and therapeutic tools available. The patients receive the service in the context of their own behaviors (e.g., smoking, weight control) and the burden of illness they may bear as a result of genetic makeup, their living and working environments, and other factors beyond their control.

This model can be expanded outward by examining the details of each element (Exhibit 2.3).

This expanded model has many interlocking elements. For example, the provider has an array of tools that are used for diagnosis and treatment: medical technology, facilities (e.g., hospitals, clinics), healthcare professionals, and, most recently, advanced healthcare information technology. The use of these tools is affected by financing structures (see the incentives and funds flow model in the next section).

Knowledge is another key to the effective functioning of the system. The system starts with basic research, the research is translated into practice, and then this knowledge is conveyed to practitioners through formal and informal education.

Consumers' behavior is affected by the information they gather (much of it now from the Internet), the financial constraints and incentives of their health insurance, and the information they acquire from their family, friends, and coworkers.

The final aspect of the systems view of healthcare is the underlying environmental factors that influence an individual's health, such as genetic makeup.

EXHIBIT 2.3
Second-Level
Model of the US
Healthcare System

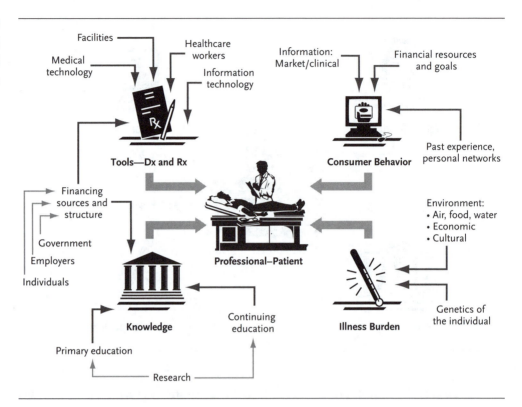

The authors of the ACA sought to improve the US healthcare system by improving almost all of the elements in the system. For example, the need for improvements in the workforce—particularly in primary care—was included in Title V: "Health Care Work-force." Healthy communities affect the disease burden on individuals, and this is addressed in the ACA in §4201, "Community Transformation Grants." The need for ongoing and comprehensive research on the effectiveness of various treatments is addressed in §6301–6302, "Patient Centered Outcomes Research."

Crosson and Tollen (2010) demonstrated that large integrated systems can deliver high-quality care cost effectively. These systems effectively manage, align, and optimize most of the elements shown in Exhibit 2.3. The designers of the ACA included many elements to encourage the growth of integrated systems.

FUNDS FLOW AND INCENTIVES VIEW

"It's not about the money—it's about the money." This quote from a leading health plan CEO provides a concise summary of the confusing financial signals currently inherent in the US healthcare system.

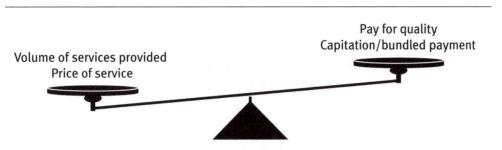

EXHIBIT 2.4
Balancing Payment
Incentives in the
ACA

Volume of services provided
Price of service

Pay for quality
Capitation/bundled payment

For example, most of the hospitals in the United States are religious and charitable institutions and maintain a nonprofit legal status, yet many of these institutions compete as aggressively as any global public for-profit company. Physicians uniformly attempt to provide optimal care but are also sometimes influenced by fee schedules and financial incentives to provide services that may be of limited value.

The designers of the ACA understood this historic conflict between organizations' desire to provide quality services and their desire to maximize revenue and profit. Exhibit 2.4 demonstrates the incentives dilemma as providers need to balance the existing fee-for-service system—which rewards volume and price—with the new elements of the ACA that reward quality and efficiency. Perhaps the greatest question of reform is whether the new incentives in the ACA are strong enough to tip this scale.

Another funds flow element of the ACA that will have a significant effect on providers is the balance between a significant reduction in uncompensated care and a reduction of Medicare base rate payment increases. Exhibit 2.5 provides an illustration of this redirected funds flow.

Funding policies and incentives in the ACA are designed to move care for an individual to its lowest cost site. Exhibit 2.6 shows a generic mapping of this movement. For example, individuals who live in healthy communities, live healthy lifestyles, and get regular preventive services are less likely to need the more expensive professional services of doctors and hospitals. Even when clinical services are required, the ACA provides

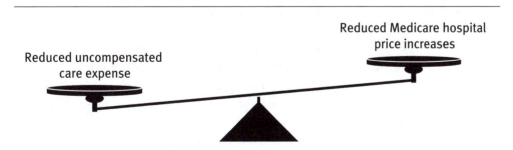

EXHIBIT 2.5
Balancing the
Newly Insured
with Reductions
in the Increase
in Medicare
Payments

Reduced uncompensated
care expense

Reduced Medicare hospital
price increases

EXHIBIT 2.6

Incentives in the
ACA Encourage
Lowest-Cost Site of
Care

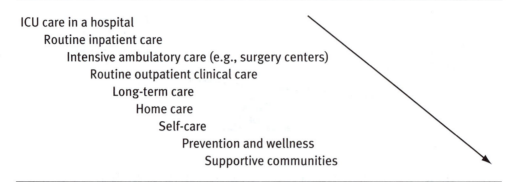

ICU care in a hospital
Routine inpatient care
Intensive ambulatory care (e.g., surgery centers)
Routine outpatient clinical care
Long-term care
Home care
Self-care
Prevention and wellness
Supportive communities

incentives for the use of the lowest cost and most effective service (e.g., home health as opposed to inpatient care).

Policymakers who believe in government-administered pricing and incentives can point to past successes. Medicare has had a relatively positive record of using administered pricing to meet policy gains. For example, the prospective payment system using diagnosis-related groups (DRGs) that was implemented in 1983 succeeded in reducing hospital length of stay significantly more than was predicted at the time of enactment. The Congressional Budget Office estimated that the DRG system would save Medicare $10 billion from 1983 to 1986. Actual savings were $21 billion (Gabel 2010).

Incentives are the carrot in the toolbox of the policymaker. Regulation is the stick. Unfortunately, regulation tends to freeze systems in place and provides limited mechanisms for innovation or needed system change. Therefore, the authors of the ACA chose incentives as their primary policy tool, but if the incentives fail, new regulations will appear. The Independent Payment Advisory Board (§3403) has been established as the vehicle for this correction to the system.

The aggregate funding for the ACA is a complex set of revenues, transferred funding, and payments made into newly created federal programs. The main sources of funding for the ACA include: reduced inflationary pay for Medicare providers, reductions in Part D payments (Medicare Advantage), taxes on health insurance plans, taxes on medical devices, and many other miscellaneous taxes, such as a 10 percent tax on indoor tanning services. This new funding goes toward the subsidies for individual buyers of health insurance, the federal portion of Medicaid (and the Children's Health Insurance Program) and its enhanced share, and many other programs that are detailed in the remainder of this book.

The impact of the ACA on the federal budget and federal deficit are always a source of intense partisan debate. The Congressional Budget Office (CBO) issues an annual report on the economy, and its April 2014 report indicated that "the ACA's coverage provisions will result in lower net costs to the federal government: The agencies currently project a net cost of $36 billion for 2014, $5 billion less than the previous projection for the year;

and $1,383 billion for the 2015–2024 period, $104 billion less than the previous projections" (CBO 2014).

A continuing question on the funds associated with the ACA is whether this new system is truly affordable. Therefore the question of affordability will be asked from a variety of perspectives. Is the new system affordable for:

- The federal government?
- A specific state government?
- Employers?
- Individuals?
- Health plans?
- Healthcare providers?
- Suppliers to the healthcare industry?

The answers to these questions will shape future changes to the ACA.

MARKETS VIEW

The healthcare system can also be conceptualized as a series of buyers and sellers of products. In this classic view of market-based capitalism, the sellers will be rewarded if their products provide high value at low prices. Although many have argued that markets do not work well in healthcare, the authors of the ACA attempted to maintain this important aspect of the system. A markets viewpoint of traditional employment-based health insurance and private healthcare delivery is illustrated in Exhibit 2.7.

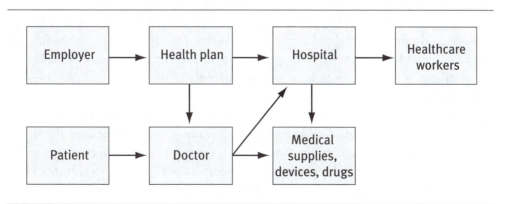

EXHIBIT 2.7
Market Perspective on Employment-Based Healthcare System

In this model the initial buyer in the system is the employer, who purchases health insurance on behalf of employees from a health plan. The employees in turn choose their providers from those available in the health plan's network.

The market is becoming more sophisticated because of the increase in high-deductible insurance plans, and because patients are beginning to pick providers based on cost and perceived quality (Robinson and Ginsburg 2009).

In the markets model, doctors (and other providers) are also buyers, as they choose the resources they need to treat the patient. Resources include everything from medical supplies to which hospital to use for a particular patient. Hospitals also purchase from other markets for their workforce and supplies. Because health plans pay for most of these items, buying and selling in this market is complex. The general economic theory of market capitalism predicts that the interactions of all of these markets should produce the greatest value at the lowest cost. The characteristics of perfect market competition are (Henderson 2002):

- many buyers and sellers,

- a standardized product,

- mobile resources, and

- buyers with access to complete and comprehensive information.

To reinforce this concept of market competition, the ACA has many competitive features, the most prominent of which are the health insurance exchanges (§1311–1313). Instead of direct regulation of health insurance rates (as is done in some European countries) the designers of the ACA expect that competition between health plans will contain costs and increase value. The law contains numerous sections in Title I: "Quality, Affordable Health Care for All Americans" that are designed to ensure a fair competitive playing field for health plans and affordability for individuals and small employers.

For health plans to be price competitive they must buy carefully from their suppliers (e.g., doctors, hospitals, pharmaceutical companies). This careful purchasing will encourage providers to improve their operations to deliver the highest value possible. The characteristics of perfect competition and the elements of the new health exchanges are compared in Exhibit 2.8.

A unique aspect of the US health system is the health savings account (HSA), which provides a direct financial incentive for consumers to purchase carefully in the healthcare market. Although many observers expected that HSAs would be eliminated in the ACA, they were preserved with only minor modifications (§9004). More than 10 million Americans use HSAs, and their use is predicted to increase (Fronstin 2010).

Perfect Competition	Affordable Care Act—Health Exchanges
Many buyers and sellers	A large number of health plans are available in the exchanges in most states. Thirty million or more individuals and small firms will buy their insurance in this market.
A standardized product	The exchanges have four different standardized benefit levels and a standardized benefit set.
Mobile resources	Health plans will be able to compete across state lines. Some healthcare organizations will become national players for both the direct provision of care (e.g., Mayo Clinic, Cleveland Clinic) and health insurance (e.g., United Health Care, Wellpoint).
Buyers with complete and comprehensive information	Healthcare.gov provides links to comprehensive data on both costs and quality. These resources will expand greatly in the future.

EXHIBIT 2.8
Perfect Market Competition and the ACA

Other competitive bidding opportunities exist for durable medical equipment suppliers (§6407) and healthcare systems that wish to participate in the national pilot project for bundled inpatient care payments (§3023).

Relying entirely on market forces to constrain costs in the US health system has not proved effective. However, market competition is an underlying philosophy and important part of the law. If market forces fail to restrain healthcare inflation after the full enactment of the ACA, the next round of legislative action will include much stronger direct federal regulation of all of the financial aspects of the system.

LEGAL CHALLENGES TO THE ACA

Twenty-six states challenged the ACA's constitutionality, and in June 2012 the US Supreme Court held that the individual mandate is valid under Congress's power to tax. It also held that the mandate for states to expand Medicaid was optional. **Reading 2A** at the end of this chapter provides a detailed analysis of the legal issues surrounding the ACA.

How to Use This Book

The ACA was originally more than 2,400 pages long, and it is accompanied by the final reconciliation bill, which is 200 pages long. Although numerous summaries are available, considering the specific legislative language is useful. This can be accomplished by opening the bill (available in a link on this book's companion website at ache.org/books/reform). This book contains many references to specific sections of the ACA as it was enacted by Congress. They are preceded by the section symbol (*signum sectionis*) §. The congressional act has been codified as Public Law 111-148 and is integrated into the Code of Federal Regulations—predominately in Titles 42 and 45. This book will use the original congressional sectional notation.

The congressional research summary is here: bit.ly/Reform2_2.

The full text of the ACA and the Supreme Court decision is here: bit.ly/Reform2_3.

SUMMARY

The ACA contains policies that will initiate the largest change in the US healthcare system since the enactment of Medicare and Medicaid. To develop successful strategies in this new environment, healthcare leaders should understand the three theories that underlie these policies.

The first theory is based on a systems perspective. This theory advances the concept that because all elements of the healthcare system are connected, strategic changes to individual elements can have widespread effects. The second theory is based on funds flow and incentives. Many Medicare programs have succeeded with administered pricing, which includes incentives to change provider behavior. Because of this history, these types of tools are also part of the ACA. The funding sources and uses for the ACA will remain controversial as healthcare stakeholders evaluate their impact. Finally, US capitalism and a markets view of the healthcare industry is also a part of the ACA—most prominently on display in the health insurance exchanges.

APPLICATIONS: DISCUSSION AND RESEARCH

1. What other national policies outside of healthcare are based on

    a. Systems theory?

    b. Funds flow?

    c. Markets?

(Consider these federal systems and do library or Internet research: the military, federal highways, securities regulations, the US Food and Drug Administration, the US Department of Education [e.g., No Child Left Behind], the Commerce Department, the Environmental Protection Agency.)

2. Which theory is the most powerful in moving a healthcare organization's strategy? Why? (Interview healthcare executives and ask them which theory is more important to their strategy development.)

3. Where do states fit into the implementation of the ACA? (Access the National Conference of State Legislatures and search on ACA: bit.ly/Reform2_4.)

REFERENCES

Baucus, M. 2008. "Call to Action: Health Reform 2009." US Senate Finance Committee, Nov. 12.

Congressional Budget Office (CBO). 2014. "Updated Estimates of the Effects of the Insurance Coverage Provisions of the Affordable Care Act, April 2014." Accessed July 15. www.cbo.gov/publication/45231.

Crosson, F. J., and L. A. Tollen. 2010. *Partners in Health: How Physicians and Hospitals Can Be Accountable Together.* San Francisco: Jossey-Bass.

Fronstin, P. 2010. "Health Savings Accounts and Health Reimbursement Arrangements: Assets, Account Balances, and Rollovers, 2006–2009." *EBRI Issue Brief* 343.

Gabel, J. R. 2010. "Does the Congressional Budget Office Underestimate Savings from Reform? A Review of the Historical Record." *Commonwealth Fund Issue Brief* 76: 1–10.

Henderson, J. W. 2002. *Health Economics and Policy.* Mason, OH: South-Western/Thomson Learning.

Robinson, J. C., and P. B. Ginsburg. 2009. "Consumer-Driven Health Care: Promise and Performance." *Health Affairs* 28 (2): w272–w281.

READING 2A

LEGAL ISSUES IN HEALTH INSURANCE AND HEALTH REFORM (EXCERPT)

Dean M. Harris

From *Contemporary Issues in Healthcare Law and Ethics,* 4th ed. (2014), Chapter 15, 380–401. Chicago: Health Administration Press.

THE 2010 FEDERAL AFFORDABLE CARE ACT

ENACTMENT OF THE 2010 FEDERAL LAW

In Congress, serious disagreements arose about several issues. Some members of Congress wanted to create a public health insurance plan similar to Medicare as an option for the general public, but others were strongly opposed to that idea. In addition, members of Congress disagreed about the cost of health reform and how we should pay for it. Conflicts also occurred about using government funds to help people buy health insurance that would cover abortion. In many ways, the legislation that was finally enacted represented a compromise among conflicting views.

The legislation was enacted in two parts. First, Congress enacted HR 3590 as the Patient Protection and Affordable Care Act (PPACA),[1] which was signed by President Obama on March 23, 2010. A few days later, Congress resolved some outstanding issues by enacting HR 4872 as the Health Care and Education Reconciliation Act of 2010,[2] which the president signed on March 30, 2010. For convenience, the two parts of that legislation are often referred to collectively as the Affordable Care Act or the ACA.

Some critics have argued that the ACA is an example of excessive government intervention in the healthcare system. However, it is important to recognize what the ACA does *not* do. The ACA does not establish a Canadian-style single-payer system or a United Kingdom-style national health system. The ACA continues the system in which millions of people obtain coverage through their place of employment. It continues to allow the sale of private health insurance policies in a competitive market, and it does not establish a public option for all residents of the country.

Before enactment of the ACA, the U.S. system of healthcare financing was fragmented, with different sources of coverage for different groups of people, such as participants in Medicare, Medicaid, employer-based health plans, and private health insurance plans. After enactment of the ACA, healthcare financing remains fragmented, with different sources of coverage for different groups of people. As one commentator has noted, "[U]nlike Medicare or Social Security, the ACA is not a single program. Rather, it is a collection of mandates, public insurance expansions, subsidies, and regulations that affect different groups of Americans in different ways and at different times."[3] Therefore, analyzing the ways in which the ACA affects these different groups of people is useful.

Medicare: The ACA made some improvements in coverage for beneficiaries. For example, the ACA provided for the reduction and eventual elimination of the "doughnut hole," which was the gap in coverage under Medicare prescription drug plans after the beneficiary exhausts the standard amount of coverage and before she qualifies for catastrophic coverage. In addition, the ACA includes many initiatives to reduce costs, improve efficiency, and increase the quality of care for Medicare beneficiaries. As one example, the ACA promotes the development of accountable care organizations (ACOs) under the Shared Savings Program, in which groups of healthcare providers deliver quality care to Medicare patients in a coordinated manner and share the cost savings resulting from those efforts. In addition, the ACA makes some adjustments to Medicare payment on the basis of quality by reducing the level of payment to hospitals that have a high rate of hospital-acquired conditions and an excessive rate of readmissions.

The ACA also provides for an Independent Payment Advisory Board (IPAB) to be established in 2014 to review excessive Medicare spending and submit legislative proposals for cutting spending. Some critics of the IPAB have argued that it would evaluate decisions about treatment options as a sort of "death panel." However, the ACA explicitly limits the power of the IPAB by providing that its proposals "shall not include any recommendation to ration health care, raise revenues or Medicare beneficiary premiums . . . increase Medicare beneficiary cost-sharing (including deductibles, coinsurance, and copayments), or otherwise restrict benefits or modify eligibility criteria."[4]

Medicaid: The ACA expands the Medicaid program by providing coverage for many poor adults under age 65 who have no dependent children and who had been unable to qualify for Medicare or Medicaid. However, as discussed in Chapter 8, the U.S. Supreme Court held in 2012 that the federal government cannot withdraw existing Medicaid funds from states that decline to participate in the ACA's expansion of Medicaid.[5] Thus, expansion of Medicaid is optional for the states. As of this writing, some state governments have decided to expand their Medicaid programs, while others have refused to participate in the expansion.

Employer-based coverage: Under the ACA, employers may continue to provide health insurance benefits for their employees. The ACA does not explicitly require employers to provide health insurance for their employees. However, employers that have at least 50 employees must pay penalties if any of their employees obtain subsidized insurance through an exchange, as discussed later. That requirement was delayed until 2015.[6]

The ACA also imposes requirements in regard to coverage and benefits in health insurance plans, including the health insurance plans that employers provide for their employees. One of the most controversial requirements is the mandate for most employers to provide insurance coverage for contraceptives, as one type of preventive service, with no copayment or deductible. This requirement does not apply to employees of churches, but it does apply to employees of some church-affiliated organizations, such as universities and hospitals. This requirement also applies to private, for-profit businesses that are owned by religious individuals. At the time of this writing, legal challenges to this mandate were pending in federal courts, and courts have disagreed among themselves about the legal issues.

Individual coverage: The ACA establishes new exchanges where individuals may purchase health insurance regardless of their current health status. For some individuals, government subsidies are available on the basis of income. Under the ACA, each state may choose to operate its own exchange, partner with the federal government in operating the exchange, or let the federal government operate it alone. Many states have refused to establish an exchange, and, therefore, the federal government will operate the exchange in those states.

Some opponents of the ACA argue that, under the statutory language, federal subsidies may not be provided for coverage purchased through a federally operated exchange. However, the IRS, which is responsible for implementing the health insurance premium tax credits under the ACA, takes the position that subsidies are indeed available.[7] As of this writing, the issue is subject to litigation in federal courts.[8] Because this is an issue of statutory interpretation rather than constitutional law, most courts would be likely to give deference to the interpretation of the IRS as the agency responsible for implementing the statute.

The ACA also increases the regulation of health insurance companies and prohibits specific practices that have an adverse effect on consumers. For example, health insurance companies may not "rescind" (cancel) a health insurance policy because a person becomes sick. Health insurance companies may not refuse to cover people who have preexisting medical conditions or charge higher rates to people who are sick or have preexisting medical conditions.

Finally, the ACA provides that most individuals will be required to pay a penalty if they do not have health insurance. The individual mandate to have insurance—and the penalty for failure to do so—provided the basis for legal challenges to the ACA and a ruling by the Supreme Court in 2012 on the law's constitutionality.

LEGAL CHALLENGES AND THE SUPREME COURT'S DECISION

Together with some private parties, state officials from 26 states challenged the federal government's authority to adopt the ACA, including the individual mandate to obtain health insurance and the penalty for failing to have insurance. On June 28, 2012, the U.S.

Supreme Court held in *National Federation of Independent Business v. Sebelius* that the individual mandate to buy health insurance is not a valid regulation of interstate commerce, but the penalty for failure to do so is valid under Congress' power to tax.[9]

The individual mandate from Congress to buy health insurance is *not* analogous to requiring owners of automobiles to buy insurance because automobile insurance mandates are state laws. State governments have police power to protect the public.[10] Thus, state governments clearly have the power to require their residents to buy health insurance, as the state of Massachusetts has done. In contrast, a dispute arose over whether Congress has the power to require individuals to buy health insurance under its constitutional power to regulate interstate commerce.

Parties challenging the ACA argued that refusing to buy health insurance is merely "inactivity," and, therefore, cannot be regulated as conduct affecting interstate commerce. Supporters of the ACA argued that refusing to buy insurance is really an "activity" of imposing one's inevitable healthcare costs on other people, and, therefore, can be regulated as conduct affecting interstate commerce. Parties challenging the ACA responded that, if the federal government could require people to buy health insurance, Congress could also require people to buy broccoli or other healthy foods.[11]

The Supreme Court agreed with those challenging the ACA that Congress may not regulate inactivity under its constitutional power to regulate interstate commerce. However, the court also held that Congress may use its constitutional taxing power to impose taxes on those individuals who remain inactive by refusing to buy health insurance.

The debate over health reform and the constitutionality of the ACA was often viewed in partisan terms as a dispute between Democrats and Republicans or between liberals and conservatives. Yet the deciding vote at the Supreme Court to uphold most of the ACA was provided by Chief Justice John Roberts, who is widely regarded as a conservative. The reason for this apparent anomaly is that conservative jurisprudence includes a profound respect for decisions that were made by the legislative branch of government.

In making predictions about the outcome of that litigation, some people had emphasized the tendency of conservative justices to limit federal authority vis-à-vis the authority of the states. That is accurate, but it is not the only principle of conservative legal analysis. Another important conservative principle is to defer to decisions of the people's elected representatives in Congress.

From a political perspective, many people had viewed the litigation over constitutionality of the ACA as a judgment on the work of President Barack Obama and his administration. From a constitutional perspective, however, the ACA was not simply the work of President Obama and his appointees, even though he signed the law and provided the leadership for its enactment. Rather, the ACA was an act of the United States Congress. That was the basis on which the Supreme Court reviewed the law, and that was the basis for the deference which was given to the law by the majority of justices.

The Supreme Court reasoned that the individual mandate was not a valid exercise of Congress' power to regulate interstate commerce because the law attempted to regulate inactivity rather than activity. If Congress could require inactive individuals to enter commerce and buy insurance, what else could Congress require individuals to buy?

When one party to litigation argues for a particular interpretation of a law, the other party often tries to point out the harmful consequences that would occur if that argument were to be taken to its logical extreme. Then, the party arguing in favor of that interpretation bears the burden of demonstrating how its proposed rule could be limited in a reasonable and practical manner.

In the dispute over the individual mandate, parties challenging the law argued that, if the federal government could make people buy health insurance, that principle would also allow the federal government to make people buy broccoli. Supporters of the ACA were not able to articulate a logical and practical limit to their interpretation of the Constitution's Commerce Clause. Instead, supporters were forced to insist that health insurance is simply unique, but the Supreme Court was not persuaded by that argument. The inability to identify and articulate a limit was a major reason for holding that the individual mandate was not a valid regulation of interstate commerce.

Nevertheless, the court reasoned that the penalty for failure to buy health insurance was a valid exercise of Congress' constitutional power to impose taxes. In that part of its opinion, the court relied on longstanding conservative principles, such as providing significant deference to acts of Congress.

Moreover, when a statute enacted by Congress can be interpreted in two different ways, courts should interpret the statute in the way that makes it constitutional. In this case, the federal government argued that the penalty provision in the ACA could be interpreted as a tax, in which case it would be constitutional. Although the ACA could be interpreted in other ways, the court concluded that the financial penalty could reasonably be described as a tax. That was sufficient to uphold the constitutionality of the penalty under conservative legal principles.

Significantly, the Supreme Court did *not* hold that Congress lacked the power to require individuals to participate in a health insurance system. The court merely held that Congress could not rely on its power to regulate interstate commerce as the basis for requiring individuals to buy insurance. As one possible alternative, Congress could use its taxing power to establish a new tax-supported health insurance system for the entire country or expand the existing, tax-supported Medicare program to cover all residents of the United States. In 1937, the Supreme Court held that, because Congress has the power to tax and spend, it may require individuals to contribute to the federal Social Security system.[12] On the same basis, Congress would have the power to establish a government health insurance system for all residents of the country and could require all individuals to pay taxes in support of that system.

As another possible alternative, Congress could use its conditional spending power to provide federal funding to those states that are willing to impose an individual mandate or adopt other reforms that would expand health insurance coverage in a particular state. Congress has the power to impose conditions on the use of specific federal funds, but it may not impose conditions that relate to the use of other federal funds. In another part of its opinion, the Supreme Court explained that "[n]othing in our opinion precludes Congress from offering funds under the Affordable Care Act to expand the availability of health care, and requiring that States accepting such funds comply with the conditions on their use."[13] In fact, beginning in 2017, the ACA will provide an option for states to implement their own systems to expand insurance coverage and receive federal funds for state systems that meet ACA requirements.

NOTES

1. Pub. L. No. 111-148 (2010).

2. Pub. L. No. 111-152 (2010).

3. J. Oberlander (2010). "Beyond Repeal—The Future of Health Care Reform." *New England Journal of Medicine* 363 (24): 2277–79.

4. Pub. L. No. 111-148, § 3403 (c)(2)(A)(ii), 10320(b) (changing the name of the board).

5. *National Federation of Independent Business v. Sebelius*, 132 S. Ct. 2566 (2012).

6. U.S. Department of the Treasury, "Continuing to Implement the ACA in a Careful, Thoughtful Manner" (July 2, 2013). www.treasury.gov/connect/blog/pages/continuing-to-implement-the-aca-in-a-careful-thoughtful-manner.aspx.

7. 77 Fed. Reg. 30377 (May 23, 2012) (final regulations), at 30378.

8. See, e.g., *Halbig v. Sebelius*, 2014 U.S. Dist. LEXIS 4853 (D.D.C. 2014).

9. 132 S. Ct. 2566 (2012).

10. *Jacobson v. Massachusetts*, 197 U.S. 11, 25 (1905).

11. See, e.g., W. K. Mariner, G. J. Annas, and L. H. Glantz, "Can Congress Make You Buy Broccoli? And Why That's a Hard Question," *New England Journal of Medicine* (2011), 364 (3): 201–203.

12. *Helvering v. Davis*, 301 U.S. 619 (1937) (upholding mandatory Social Security contributions under the taxing power).

13. 132 S. Ct. at 2607.

PREVENTION, WELLNESS, AND POPULATION HEALTH

Prevention and programs to promote wellness have always been a part of healthcare in the United States. In some cases, these programs have been successful (e.g., in the eradication of smallpox). However, historically these efforts have been fragmented within federal and state government departments and disconnected from the US healthcare delivery system.

A broader concept that includes these activities is now being advanced to improve the broad spectrum of the healthcare continuum—population health. McAlearney (2003) provides a framework to understand population health management (see page 38). In her diagram she identifies five management strategies that can be applied to defined populations: lifestyle, care demand, disease, catastrophic care, and disability. **Reading 3A** explains the concept of population health.

This chapter examines the many new policies contained in the Affordable Care Act (ACA) that address *lifestyle management* and *demand management*, including the following:

1. *Clinical prevention*—the routine provision of tests and services (e.g., immunizations) to prevent disease or to uncover and treat it in its early stages (demand management)

2. *Individual wellness*—the maintenance of a healthy lifestyle, including diet, exercise, and the avoidance of risky behaviors (lifestyle management)

3. *Community building*—creating communities that encourage healthy living and strong personal relationships and caring (lifestyle management)

Exhibit 3.1 illustrates how these policies fit into the systems view of health reform.

CLINICAL PREVENTION

Prevention of disease is a laudable goal—prevention helps individuals live longer and more vital lives and saves money in the system by avoiding the demand for unneeded clinical services (e.g.,

Exhibit 3.1
Systems View
of Prevention,
Wellness, and
Community

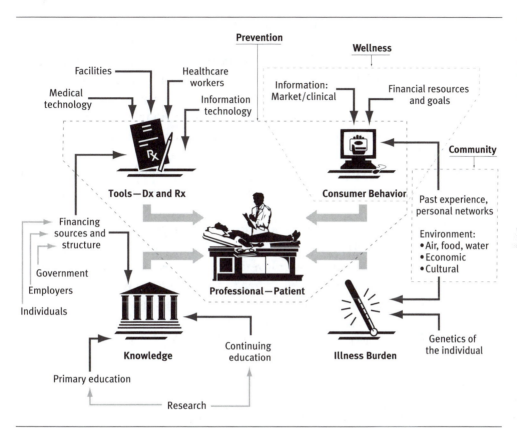

hospitalization for the flu). The savings accrued from prevention can be significant and could reduce cost throughout the system (Maciosek et al. 2010).

Prevention activities are not yet as widespread as they should be. A recent survey of nearly 1,300 primary care physicians in the United States found that only about 20 percent of them recommend colorectal cancer screening tests to their patients in accordance with current practice guidelines. About 40 percent of the doctors followed some of the practice guidelines, while the remaining 40 percent ignored practice guidelines (Yabroff et al. 2010).

COORDINATION

Clinical prevention is delivered through a mix of public and private healthcare organizations. Public health departments are responsible for broad prevention activities (e.g., restaurant inspection) and specific programs (e.g., Ryan White CARE Act funding for HIV/AIDS prevention).

Most primary care practices adhere to the recommendations of the US Preventive Services Task Force (2011). However, its list of preventive services is long (more than 100 services), and some clinicians may not recall an appropriate test or treatment. This challenge is one of the important reasons to install health information technology (HIT) in primary care practices. Almost all HIT systems contain clinical decision support modules that make preventive services recommendations to clinicians at each patient visit.

Title IV of the ACA is solely devoted to prevention and public health. The ACA establishes the National Prevention, Health Promotion, and Public Health Council (§4001) to coordinate federal activities, including substantial new funding. The Preventive Services Task Force continues §4003 but is augmented with the Community Preventive Services Task Force (§4003), which focuses on population health in addition to the individual needs of each patient.

The work of the National Prevention Council can be found at bit.ly/Reform3_1. Recommendations from the Preventative Services Task Force can be found at bit.ly/Reform3_2.

Title IV also includes a variety of other strategies to improve public health, including school-based clinics (§4101) and oral health programs (§4102). Title IV adds a Medicare benefit for an annual wellness visit to create a personalized prevention plan (§4103) and removes coinsurance and deductible payments for preventive services. Preventive services for Medicaid recipients are also increased in §4106 and §4107. The elimination of cost sharing for preventive services in private insurance is contained in §4104. The list of covered preventive services is contained here: bit.ly/Reform3_3.

EDUCATION

Public education regarding preventive services is enhanced by a federal education and outreach campaign. The campaign "(1) describes the importance of utilizing preventive services to promote wellness, reduce health disparities, and mitigate chronic disease; (2) promotes the use of preventive services recommended by the United States Preventive Services Task Force and the Community Preventive Services Task Force; (3) encourages healthy behaviors linked to the prevention of chronic diseases" (§4004).

An additional policy to inform the public about health issues is contained in §4205, which requires restaurants with more than 20 locations to post the nutritional content of their standard menu items. This section was supported by national restaurant chains because many states and localities were beginning to enact similar requirements, but each with different standards. Under the ACA, one federal standard will be established.

The support for school-based clinics is increased in §4101. In 2009 the Institute of Medicine released a report on "comparative effectiveness research prioritization" that listed 100 clinical services that IOM felt should be studied soon because of the variability of their application and results. One of these priorities is to "compare the effectiveness of school-based interventions involving meal programs, vending machines, and physical education, at different levels of intensity, in preventing and treating overweight and obesity in children and adolescents" (IOM 2009). Because of this new emphasis in the ACA, the school may become one of the most effective delivery sites for prevention and wellness education.

WELLNESS

In contrast to clinical prevention, wellness programs are self-directed, and most individuals in the United States are aware of the key elements of wellness:

◆ An active engagement in routine exercise

◆ A healthy diet

◆ Maintenance of a healthy weight

◆ Avoidance of risky behaviors (e.g., smoking, alcohol or drug abuse, driving without seatbelts)

Unfortunately, many residents of the United States have become sedentary and overweight. The ACA promotes wellness though a number of tools.

Employers have been leaders in wellness promotion, with programs to encourage employees to adopt more healthy lifestyles, such as diet counseling, smoking cessation programs, and fitness club memberships. Unfortunately, these voluntary programs have had only limited success (Probart et al. 2010; Schmidt, Voigt, and Wikler 2010). Safeway, Inc., has been a leader in biometric wellness programs, with a new approach that focuses on measurable outcomes such as body mass index, blood pressure, and cholesterol levels. If employees meet specified goals, a substantial portion of their health insurance premium is returned to them as a reward. Safeway had no increase in its health insurance premiums from 2003 to 2008 (no later data have been published) (Burd 2009). UnitedHealth Group has implemented a similar system for its 70,000 employees; employees were eligible for a reward of up to $900 in 2011 (Migliori 2010). However recent research raises concerns about the cost-effectiveness of employer-based biometric programs (Horwitz, Kelly, and DiNardo 2013). In spite of these concerns, these types of programs continue to be refined and implemented by employers.

The ACA supports this policy in §2705, which allows employers to reward employees who meet goals a refund of up to 30 percent of their premium costs. The secretary of HHS can raise this limit to 50 percent in the future. However, some critics have argued that these systems discriminate against individuals who have preexisting conditions and are physiologically unable to achieve the goals. Therefore this wellness rewards program is a part of §1201/2705 titled "Prohibiting discrimination against individual and beneficiaries based on health status." The remainder of §2705 contains language that prohibits insurance companies from denying coverage to individuals because of preexisting conditions—one of the key goals of health reform.

Medicaid also provides incentives for wellness in §4108. States can establish programs that provide financial rewards to Medicaid beneficiaries for achieving one or more of the following:

◆   Ceasing use of tobacco products

◆   Controlling or reducing their weight

◆   Lowering their cholesterol

◆   Lowering their blood pressure

◆   Avoiding the onset of diabetes or, in the case of a person with diabetes, improving the management of that condition

COMMUNITY BUILDING

One of the most accurate predictors of an individual's health status is her zip code. Community and public health leaders have long advocated for community building—particularly in those communities challenged by poverty, crime, and poor housing. The ACA accepts this challenge in §4201 with a new program of community transformation grants. The purpose of these grants is to:

◆   create healthier school environments, including increasing healthy food options, physical activity opportunities, promotion of healthy lifestyle, emotional wellness programs, prevention curricula, and activities to prevent chronic diseases;

◆   create the infrastructure to support active living and access to nutritious foods in a safe environment;

◆   develop and promote programs targeting a variety of age levels to increase access to nutrition, increase physical activity, encourage smoking cessation, improve social and emotional wellness, and enhance safety in the community;

◆   assess and implement work-site wellness programming and incentives;

◆   work to highlight healthy options at restaurants and other food venues;

◆   prioritize strategies to reduce racial and ethnic disparities, including social, economic, and geographic determinants of health; and

◆   address special population needs, including all age groups and individuals with disabilities, and individuals in urban, rural, and frontier areas.

Exhibit 3.2 details examples of these projects.

Although these activities may seem far removed from the healthcare delivery system, they actually may be a new market for many providers.

The status of Community Transformation Grants can be found at bit.ly/Reform3_4.

EXHIBIT 3.2
Community Transformation Grant Examples

	Oklahoma County, Oklahoma	Pierce County, Washington	Iowa
The Challenge	Oklahoma ranks forty-eighth nationally in smoking prevalence and has one of the highest rates of smoking-related deaths in the nation.	An estimated 31 percent of adults in Pierce County are obese, more than the national and state prevalence levels.	Twenty-six rural Iowa counties have been identified as having high stroke mortality rates. High stroke mortality is especially concentrated in an area in southeast Iowa.
The Goal	By September 2016, 700,000 people who work and reside in Oklahoma County will have access to completely tobacco-free or smoke-free environments.	By September 2016, 229,500 residents of Pierce County will have improved access to healthy food and beverage options.	By September 2016, Iowa will increase the number of dental practices having systems in place for blood pressure and tobacco use screening and referral.
Current Activities	Oklahoma County is establishing smoke-free multi-unit housing for more than 80,000 units in the community, reducing exposure to secondhand smoke for thousands of individuals. Additionally, the county is partnering with the largest employers to implement tobacco-free worksites, helping to reduce exposure to secondhand smoke for approximately 60,000 residents and others.	Pierce County is working to improve the availability of nutritious foods and beverages by strengthening institutional and organizational food procurement practices. This will provide residents with the opportunity to have access to healthy foods; Pierce County has already seen success toward this goal. More than 11,000 students and 1,500 staff within the Clover Park School District now have access to vending machines that offer healthy options that meet the USDA's sodium and sugar guidelines.	The state of Iowa is building on a previous strategy (2009–2011 Iowa Dental Pilot) in asking dental practices throughout southeast Iowa counties to voluntarily participate in blood pressure and tobacco use screening and referral training. This activity may help to ensure that more than 300,000 individuals are screened for risk factors and referred to necessary resources. In addition, this training will be offered to community health dental clinics to ensure these activities are extended to reach low income and uninsured populations.

SOURCE: Data from CDC (2013).

A survey of current practices by leading healthcare systems in providing effective population health management is contained in **Reading 3B**.

COMMUNITY BENEFIT

Almost all nonprofit hospitals claim to have a significant role in community building. However, some members of Congress have questioned this role because of their perception of the limited charitable activities and high executive salaries of some nonprofit healthcare systems In response to this concern §9007 of the ACA requires tax-exempt charitable hospitals to: (1) conduct a community health needs assessment every two years; (2) adopt a written financial assistance policy for patients who require financial assistance for hospital care; and (3) refrain from taking extraordinary collection actions against a patient until the hospital has made reasonable efforts to determine whether the patient is eligible for financial assistance.

The challenge and opportunity in developing and implementing a community benefit plan are provided in **Reading 3C**. The direct connection of community benefit to the ACA is outlined in **Reading 3D**.

The scientific basis for broad, community-based intervention is still being developed, and the business case for building healthy communities is uncertain. However, two leaders in this field provide a comprehensive road map for the creation of effective mechanisms for broad population health in **Reading 3E**.

SUMMARY

Two of the major causes of the high cost of the US healthcare system are preventable diseases and unhealthy lifestyles. The ACA addresses these problems with improved programs of clinical prevention including the requirement that preventive services be offered in all health insurance programs with no cost-sharing requirements. Public education regarding prevention is significantly expanded.

Employer-based wellness programs that reward specific health outcomes have shown success and are carefully supported in the ACA. Requirements are included to ensure that employees are not discriminated against because of preexisting conditions. A similar pilot program is available to Medicaid beneficiaries.

In addition, policies to improve community health are supported through community transformation grants and the demonstration of community benefit by nonprofit healthcare organizations.

APPLICATIONS: DISCUSSION AND RESEARCH

1. Review the Preventive Service Task Force list of services. Find three services you think would have difficulty being widely adopted. What are the reasons for these difficulties?

2. Identify local restaurants that have posted the nutritional content of their menus. Which entrees are the healthiest? The least healthy? What is the restaurant doing to promote the healthy entrees?

3. What are the challenges to biometric-based wellness programs? How can they be overcome? (Interview the benefits manager of a large company in your town and ask her if the company has a biometric-based wellness program. If not, why not? If so, what is her perspective is on how well it is working? This will illuminate the challenges of these programs.)

4. What are the most important elements of a health system's community benefit plan? Why? (Interview the director of the local public health department in your city or county. Ask him what the most important elements of the local hospital or health system's community benefit plan should be and if they are meeting this need.)

REFERENCES

Burd, S. A. 2009. "How Safeway Is Cutting Health-Care Costs." *Wall Street Journal*. Published June 12. http://online.wsj.com/article/SB124476804026308603.html.

Centers for Disease Control and Prevention (CDC). 2013. "Community Transformation Grants: Accomplishments." Updated October 25. www.cdc.gov/nccdphp/dch/programs/communitytransformation/accomplishments/index.htm.

Horwitz, J. R., B. D. Kelly, and J. E. DiNardo. 2013. "Wellness Incentives in the Workplace: Cost Savings Through Cost Shifting to Unhealthy Workers." *Health Affairs* 32 (3): 468–76.

Institute of Medicine (IOM). 2009. "Initial National Priorities for Comparative Effectiveness Research Report Brief." www.iom.edu/~/media/Files/Report%20Files/2009/ComparativeEffectivenessResearchPriorities/CER%20report% 20brief%2008-13-09.ashx.

Maciosek, M. V., A. B. Coffield, T. J. Flottemesch, N. M. Edwards, and L. I. Solberg. 2010. "Greater Use of Preventive Services in U.S. Health Care Could Save Lives at Little or No Cost." *Health Affairs* 29 (9): 1656.

McAlearney, A. S. 2003. *Population Health Management: Strategies to Improve Outcomes*. Chicago: Health Administration Press.

Migliori, R. 2010. Keynote speaker at Midwest Healthcare Business Intelligence Summit, October 19.

Probart, C., E. T. McDonnell, L. Jomaa, and V. Fekete. 2010. "Lessons from Pennsylvania's Mixed Response to Federal School Wellness Law." *Health Affairs* 29 (3): 447.

Schmidt, H., K. Voigt, and D. Wikler. 2010. "Carrots, Sticks, and Health Care Reform—Problems with Wellness Incentives." *New England Journal of Medicine* 362 (2).

US Preventive Services Task Force. 2011. "Recommendations." Accessed January 7. www. uspreventiveservicestaskforce.org/recommendations.htm.

Yabroff, K. R., C. N. Klabunde, G. Yuan, T. S. McNeel, M. L. Brown, D. Casciotti, D. W. Buckman, and S. Taplan. 2010. "Are Physicians' Recommendations for Colorectal Cancer Screening Guideline-Consistent?" *Journal of General Internal Medicine* 26 (2): 177–84.

CHAPTER 3

ADDITIONAL READINGS

READING 3A
INTRODUCTION/POPULATION HEALTH MANAGEMENT
Ann S. McAlearney
From *Population Health Management: Strategies to Improve Outcomes* (2003),
Chapters 1 and 2, 3–11. Chicago: Health Administration Press.

Strategies designed to improve the health and well-being of the public are increasing in both visibility and importance. *Population health management* is a term used to describe a variety of approaches developed to foster health and quality of care improvements while managing costs. Health services organizations faced with the challenge of managing financial risk for a defined population are challenged to find ways to more efficiently and effectively serve that population, and population health management strategies can help.

Strategies for health and care management that strive to improve quality as well as reduce the cost of medical care are appealing to payers, providers, and patients. As long as patient care needs are not subsumed by financial considerations, the potential for population health management programs to foster health improvements in a patient-centered and clinically responsive environment is undeniably attractive.

When managing health for a specific population, the characteristics of the defined population establish the parameters for what types of health improvement and management strategies will be appropriate. For instance, in a population with a high proportion of Native Americans, diabetes services may be more of a priority than in a population with more Caucasians. Similarly, an elderly population may need more attention to chronic disease management services while a younger population may be an appropriate target for maternal and child wellness programs or workplace injury reduction initiatives. Taking the characteristics of the target population into account when designing and implementing health management approaches is critical to ensure that such programs succeed in meeting appropriate and achievable health improvement goals.

Population health management strategies include many different initiatives. *Lifestyle management* approaches use the techniques of health behavior change in a health promotion or prevention context to improve individuals' health habits and reduce health risks. *Demand management* programs typically use remote patient management to direct individuals toward appropriate utilization of medical care services. *Disease management* strategies focus on a particular disease and attempt to provide medical and care management services related to the needs of patients with that condition. As another disease management model, *catastrophic care management* programs concentrate on providing the spectrum of services required by individuals who suffer from catastrophic illnesses or injuries that are typically defined by either condition or expensive claims. *Disability management* programs are usually developed from an employer perspective and try to bridge the gap between healthcare management and disability management to reduce lost worker productivity due to illness or injury. Finally, an *integrated population health management* model promotes comprehensive consideration of the health and well-being of each member of a population by coordinating different health and care management strategies. Each of these approaches is designed with specific goals and objectives in mind and makes patients' healthcare needs central to program development. By concentrating on the needs of individuals as they access the healthcare system or make decisions about their health behaviors, population health management programs hope to promote health and wellness among their defined populations and strive to manage healthcare costs without compromising the quality of healthcare provided.

Examples of population health management programs can be found in multiple settings. Employers may sponsor demand management programs while medical groups or health plans have interest in the potential of disease management to help improve health and reduce costs for their chronically ill patients. Disability management programs are being adopted by large employers, and catastrophic care management approaches may be offered through insurance carriers, employers, or dedicated vendor companies.

Population health management strategies are particularly common in managed care. A managed care organization (MCO) is typically trying to manage healthcare services for their defined population of members, keeping in mind both cost and quality of care. This defined MCO membership may be further segregated into subpopulations based on the managed care product lines that are offered. These subpopulations may include a commercial population, a Medicare population, or a Medicaid population, depending on the membership served. Developing health management strategies that address the needs of its membership can help both patients and the MCO by focusing on health improvements and trying to manage the costs of medical care.

The need to focus on service and health improvements for defined populations is increasingly important from both payer and provider perspectives. Methods to identify and care for segments of the population that are utilizers of health services leverage the capabilities of information technologies to obtain timely information about individuals and their care progress. New provider types such as care managers are working to respond to patient care and care coordination needs. Population health management programs with the potential to integrate quality improvement goals with cost-saving goals can have a tremendous impact on care delivery and outcomes.

A CASE FOR POPULATION HEALTH MANAGEMENT

Shifting demographics, the tremendous burden of chronic illness and disability, and the problem of fragmentation in the U.S. healthcare system are three major factors increasing the visibility and need for population health management solutions. The challenges presented by these issues can be addressed by population health management solutions as health services organizations attempt to focus on both service and health improvements.

DEMOGRAPHICS

One of the reasons population health management is increasing in importance is the shifting demographics of the U.S. population. By 2000, almost 13 percent of the U.S. population, or 35 million individuals, were age 65 or older. This proportion has increased over ten-fold since 1900 when persons over 65 represented only 4 percent of the U.S. population. By 2030, one in five Americans are projected to be age 65 or older as this population segment doubles to 70 million persons. Individuals age 85 and older represent the fastest growing older population segment. While 4 million persons, or 2 percent of the U.S. population, were estimated to be age 85 and older in 2000, this number is projected to increase by 5 percent to 19 million individuals by 2050 (Federal 2000).

With the average age of the population increasing and life expectancies extending as well, users of medical care services will be older. These shifts in age are also associated with an increase in the number of persons suffering from chronic conditions. Elderly persons experience a greater proportion of chronic illnesses, with 47 percent of older adults suffering from arthritis, 37 percent from hypertension, 29 percent from heart disease, and 17 percent from orthopedic impairments (Haber 1994). Elderly persons tend to need more medical care services than younger persons, and the population segment age 85 and older tends to be in the poorest health, requiring the most services among the elderly population overall (Federal 2000). Chronic illnesses and poor health are clearly associated with a greater need for medical care services, and these services can be expensive, difficult to access, and largely uncoordinated.

Additional shifts in U.S. demographics indicate increasing proportions of women, minorities, and poor people who will need healthcare services in most communities. Because population health management programs must begin by defining target populations, these shifting demographics will undoubtedly have implications for program development. Among the elderly, women were estimated to represent 58 percent of the U.S. population age 65 and over in 2000, and 70 percent of the age 85 and over population (Federal 2000). Disease management programs, for example, can focus on conditions that specifically target women or particular minority groups. A women's wellness program may be designed to serve a population of women past childbearing age who are starting to deal with menopause. Similarly, a disease management program that targets diabetes may be a priority program development area for a population with more low-income and minority persons for which uncontrolled diabetes and diabetes-related morbidity have been shown to be major problems (U.S. Department of Health and Human Services 1999). Keeping these demographic issues in mind helps establish a framework for population health management approaches as they are implemented for individuals.

CHRONIC DISEASE AND DISABILITY

Chronic illness is a major problem in the United States where, as of 2000, almost half of all Americans were found to be living with some form of chronic disease. Among these 125 million individuals, around 60 million have multiple chronic conditions, and over 3 million live with 5 chronic conditions (Partnership for Solutions 2001). According to the Institute for Health and Aging (1996), approximately 40 million persons experience definite limitations in their activities of daily living because of their chronic conditions.

Unfortunately, the numbers of disabilities and limitations due to chronic conditions are on the rise. Since 1991, the proportion of individuals who report experiencing a limitation in a major activity because of a chronic condition has been increasing for all population groups (U.S. Department of Health and Human Services 1999). The number of Americans projected to have at least one chronic condition by 2020 is almost 157 million individuals (Partnership for Solutions 2001).

Considering expenses, the cost of chronic illness is staggering. In fact, the Institute for Health and Aging of the University of California at San Francisco estimated that the medical care costs for people with chronic diseases were responsible for over 60 percent of U.S. medical care costs (The Robert Wood Johnson Foundation 1996). Partnership for Solutions is an initiative led by Johns Hopkins University and The Robert Wood Johnson Foundation designed to improve care and the quality of life for Americans with chronic health conditions. They estimate that the direct medical costs associated with chronic conditions reached $510 billion by 2000, and they project that these costs will increase to $1.07 trillion by 2020 (Partnership for Solutions 2001). Annual out-of-pocket medical care costs for individuals with chronic conditions are estimated to be about $369, almost double those of persons without such conditions. Total medical expenditures for those with chronic conditions are over five times greater than for healthy individuals, at $6,032 per year compared to $1,105 per year (Partnership for Solutions 2001).

The cost of disability attributable to chronic conditions in the United States is also overwhelming. For employers alone, the cost of lost productivity from both illness and injury represents 74 percent of their total employee benefit costs (Integrated Benefits Institute 2001). Individuals who have functional limitations or disabilities in addition to chronic conditions are estimated to have medical expenditures over twice as high as those with chronic conditions alone. These expenses are calculated as $10,908 per year for those with a disability in addition to a chronic condition, and $16,245 per year for those with functional limitations as well as a chronic condition (Partnership for Solutions 2001).

Another major issue associated with chronic diseases is the problems that may result from untreated primary illnesses (Suber 2001). If such conditions are not managed well, many chronic diseases will result in secondary conditions (Pope and Tarlow 1991) caused by the existing condition. As an example, diabetes is a chronic disease that can result in multiple disabling complications including heart disease, stroke, blindness, and amputations. Analysis of data from 1997 showed that over half of the 67,000 limb amputations in the United States could have been prevented if diabetics had managed their chronic illness better through routine foot exams ("Get a Foothold" 1998).

Given the high prevalence of and cost associated with chronic conditions in the United States, it would make sense that care provision for these illnesses would be a focus. However, the U.S. medical care system has tended to focus on acute care services. Even when treatment for acute exacerbations of chronic illnesses is provided, such care is rarely coordinated with other services that a patient is receiving or needs. Most care for chronic conditions is disorganized and difficult to obtain, with many services provided that are inappropriate or duplicative (Robert Wood Johnson Foundation 1996).

When properly designed and implemented, population health management programs can help to improve the care of persons with chronic conditions by both improving patient health and well-being and reducing medical care costs. In fact, the goal of chronic care is not necessarily to cure patients but to help individuals maintain their independence and functionality at high levels (Robert Wood Johnson Foundation 1996). By defining target populations and then designing health management programs to address the care requirements for individuals in those populations, comprehensive programs can be effectively introduced into an otherwise disjointed system of care.

FRAGMENTATION

Organization and delivery of medical care services in the United States is extremely fragmented. Due in large part to the foundations of the medical care system as a decentralized cottage industry that has not emphasized coordination or continuity of care (Starr 1982), the present healthcare system is very disorganized. In general, the health of the U.S. population as a whole has not improved as rapidly as might have been predicted based on advances in medical care and technology (U.S. Department of Health and Human Services 1990). Instead, indicators of health leave much room for system improvement, whether measured on the basis of life expectancy, childhood mortality, health-adjusted life expectancy (Kindig 1998), or disability-adjusted life expectancy (World Health Organization 2000).

Fragmentation is problematic in multiple levels of the healthcare system, including patient care, provider, organization, financing, and overall health policy (Shortell et al. 1996). Multiple providers involved in patient care, complex organizational and financial structures, and health policy issues such as access, insurance coverage, costs, and quality all complicate healthcare management and delivery (McAlearney 2002). This uncoordinated service provision presents a major opportunity for population health management programs that can be designed to organize and integrate services across institutions, among providers, and along the continuum of care.

POPULATION HEALTH MANAGEMENT FRAMEWORK

Population health management strategies fit into an overall framework for population health management that is illustrated in Figure 1. As shown in this figure, the first step in population health management is to target the specific program. This targeting process involves determining the perspective of the program and the concerns of the sponsoring organization, defining the population that will be managed, developing approaches to target individuals for health and care management strategies, and classifying those individuals for population health management interventions.

After targeting populations and individuals within those populations for health management interventions, the next stage in this process is to determine the appropriate strategies for population health management. In this text, five strategic options are described: lifestyle management, demand management, disease management, catastrophic care management, and disability management. Depending on the strategy selected, implementation issues such as design, development, and management of the program will vary. Issues around planning and organization, staffing, physician relations, organizational change, program evaluation, and strategic control of the process are all important.

Critical issues in program design, development, and implementation must be resolved to ensure that a population health management program is effective. Areas such as incentive alignment, program focus, and physician involvement should all be addressed to maximize the likelihood of program success. Program staff must be recruited and trained, and investments must be made in appropriate information technologies.

Clearly, given the debilitating fragmentation and lack of coordination in the U.S. healthcare system, better management of population health is needed. Population health management strategies provide an opportunity to improve the delivery and outcomes of medical care in the context of the existing U.S. healthcare system.

FIGURE 1

Framework for Population Health Management

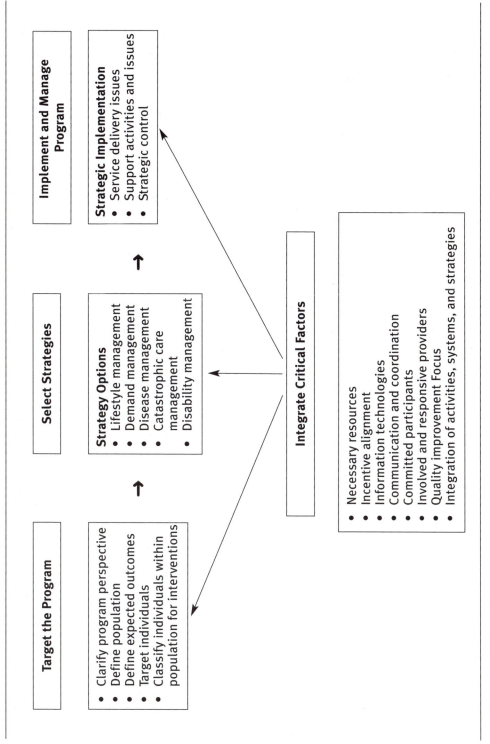

SOURCE: McAlearney (2003).

REFERENCES

Federal Interagency Forum on Aging-Related Statistics. 2000. *Older Americans 2000: Key Indicators of Well-Being*. Washington, DC: Federal Interagency Forum on Aging-Related Statistics, U.S. Government Printing Office.

"Get a Foothold on the Cost of Diabetes Complications." 1998. *Healthcare Demand and Disease Management* 4 (5): 65–69.

Haber, D. 1994. *Health Promotion and Aging*. New York: Springer Publishing Company.

Integrated Benefits Institute. 2001. [Online article or information; retrieved 3/14/01.] http://www.ibiweb.org/breaking-news/index.shtml.

Kindig, D. A. 1998. "Purchasing Population Health: Aligning Financial Incentives to Improve Health Outcomes." *Health Services Research* 33 (2): 223–42.

McAlearney, A. S. 2002. "Population Health Management in Theory and Practice." In *Advances in Health Care Management* (Volume 3), edited by G. T. Savage, J. Blair, and M. Fottler. New York: JAI Press/Elsevier Science, Ltd.

Partnership for Solutions. 2001. *Prevalence and Cost of Chronic Conditions*.

Baltimore, MD: Partnership for Solutions. [Online article or information; retrieved 2/6/02.] http://www.chronicnet.org/statistics/issue_briefs. htm; http://www.chronicnet.org/statistics/prevalence.htm.

Pope, A. M., and A. R. Tarlow. 1991. *Disability in America: Toward a National Agenda for Prevention*. Washington, DC: National Academy Press.

Shortell, S. M., R. R. Gillies, and D. A. Anderson. 1996. *Remaking Health Care in America: Building Organized Delivery Systems*. San Francisco: Jossey-Bass Publishers.

Starr, P. 1982. *The Social Transformation of American Medicine*. New York: Basic Books.

Suber, R. M. 2001. "Total Health Management: Prevention and Management of Chronic Disease." In *The Continuum of Long-Term Care*, edited by C. Evashwick. Albany, NY: Delmar Publishers.

The Robert Wood Johnson Foundation. 1996. *Chronic Care in America: A 21st Century Challenge*. Princeton, NJ: The Robert Wood Johnson Foundation.

U.S. Department of Health and Human Services. 1990. *Healthy People 2000: National Health Promotion and Disease Prevention Objectives*. Publication No. (PHS) 91-50213. Washington, DC: U.S. Department of Health and Human Services.

U.S. Department of Health and Human Services. *Healthy People 2000 Review 1998–99*. 1999. Publication No. (PHS) 96-1256. Washington, DC: U.S. Department of Health and Human Services.

World Health Organization. 2000. *World Health Report*. Geneva, Switzerland: World Health Organization. [Online article or information; retrieved 3/14/01.] http://www.who.int/whr/2000/en/report.htm.

CHAPTER 2: POPULATION HEALTH MANAGEMENT

Ann S. McAlearney

A book about population health management must begin by clarifying what is meant by population health management. This chapter poses the following four questions:

1. *What* is to be managed in population health management?

2. *Who* is to be managed?

3. *Where* can population health management occur?

4. *Why* does population health need to be managed?

Answers to these four questions will help establish a context for individual population health management strategies, as well as build support for their practical importance in the U.S. healthcare system. The remainder of the book will then attempt to explain *how* population health management can occur.

WHAT IS TO BE MANAGED?

Considering the issue of population health management, one of the first questions that arises is what is meant by *health*? Definitions of health and well-being have been put forth by a number of entities. Best known is the definition used by the World Health

Organization (WHO) that states, "Health is a state of complete physical, mental, and social well-being and not merely the absence of disease or infirmity" (WHO 1948). This definition is effective in the context of population health as well, because the goals of preventing disease, improving well-being, and promoting healthy behaviors are all integral parts of population health management.

Another definitional issue surrounds the concept of *management*. When used in the context of a business, management is defined as an operational process. Management is geared towards achieving the objectives of that business, whether those objectives are focused on maximizing revenues, value to shareholders, or benefit to society. In the context of healthcare, management can again be viewed as an operational process designed to achieve specific objectives. However, within the realm of health services, the objectives of healthcare management are geared towards attaining, maximizing, or improving health, as health is defined above. In population health management, the objective of management is to maximize the health of a population.

This leads to the third part of the term population health management: *population*. Why is it important to consider health management within a population separate from health management in general? The goal of managing health within a defined population has become a critical issue for many. Whether the population specified is that of a health plan's membership, a hospital's patients, an employer's employees, or a community's citizens, the issue of describing that population and determining the needs of individuals as members of that group is central. By specifying a population group, a health management program can be initiated that responds to the needs of that group. This perspective helps establish boundaries for a health management program by defining a population of concern.

The broadest definitions of populations are, of course, national or global. Considering the goals of the World Health Organization, the global population is the population of interest, and programs are designed to help improve the health and well-being of the world's residents. However, beyond acknowledging the health needs of the world's population, even WHO effectively defines and segments populations when it designs specific health programs. An initiative to control the spread of tuberculosis in less developed countries will not be targeted to reach residents in U.S. suburbs. Similarly, messages about reducing the spread of HIV and AIDS may be substantially different depending on whether the target audience consists of intravenous drug users in urban areas or sex workers in less developed countries. Defining a population for a health management program allows such initiatives to concentrate resources and tailor messages in ways that will be most effective for that population.

Multiple forces influence health. In addition to the medical care system, nonmedical factors such as socioeconomic status (Adler et al. 1994), education (Pappas et al. 1993), income (Kaplan et al. 1996), individual behaviors (McGinnis and Foege 1993), social support, genetics, and the physical environment can all affect individual health (Kindig 1998). Figure 2.1 illustrates how these various factors can affect both personal outcomes,

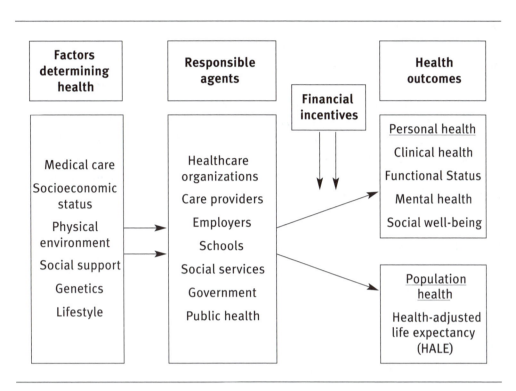

FIGURE 2.1
Influencing Health

SOURCE: Kindig, D. A. 1998. "Purchasing Population Health: Aligning Financial Incentives to Improve Health Outcomes." Health Services Research 33 (2): 223–42.

including clinical health and functional status, and population health outcomes, such as health-adjusted life expectancy (Kindig 1998; 1997), as they are moderated by the roles played by intervening agents including healthcare organizations, care providers, and the government. (See 2.1 "Measuring Population Health Outcomes" at www.ache.org/pubs/ mcalearney/ start.cfm.)

For the United States, the management and improvement of health is a major financial, political, and social issue. The Healthy People initiative was designed as a national, cooperative effort by the government, in partnership with both voluntary and professional organizations, to try to improve the health of Americans. Objectives for health were established and progress toward the achievement of those objectives is measured (Suber 2001). Healthy People 2000 included three broad goals covering 300 specific objectives across 22 priority health areas: 1) to increase the span of healthy life; 2) to reduce health disparities; and 3) to achieve access to preventive services (U.S. Department of Health and Human Services 1990).

Prevention and health promotion goals for the U.S. were updated as 2000 approached, and Healthy People 2010 now includes 467 objectives covering 28 focus areas. Main goals were also refined for Healthy People 2010 and these are: (1) to increase quality and years of healthy life; and (2) to eliminate health disparities, including disparities due to race, ethnicity, gender, income, and insurance status. In addition to health goals and objectives, 10 leading health indicators were developed to focus the attention of the nation on needed health promotion and disease prevention strategies. These health indicators for 2010 are: (1) physical activity; (2) overweight and obesity; (3) tobacco use; (4) substance abuse; (5) responsible sexual behavior; (6) mental health; (7) injury and violence; (8) environmental quality; (9) immunization; and (10) access to healthcare (Centers for Disease Control and Prevention 2001). Health goals and health indicators for 2010 are displayed in Table 2.1. Healthy People 2010 now provides perspective about the many facets of health and well-being that can be managed and improved for Americans using population health management strategies.

Who Is to Be Managed?

In addition to the issue of what will be managed is the consideration of who will be managed in a population health framework. Indeed, defining a particular population whose

TABLE 2.1
National Health Goals and Health Indicators for 2010

Health Goals

1. To increase quality and years of healthy life

2. To eliminate health disparities, including disparities due to race, ethnicity, gender, income, and insurance status

Health Indicators

1. Physical activity

2. Overweight and obesity

3. Tobacco use

4. Substance abuse

5. Responsible sexual behavior

6. Mental health

7. Injury and violence

8. Environmental quality

9. Immunization

10. Access to healthcare

SOURCE: Kindig, D. A. 1998. "Purchasing Population Health: Aligning Financial Incentives to Improve Health Outcomes." Health Services Research 33 (2): 223–42.

health is to be managed is the first step in determining how to manage that population's health. As described above, populations can be defined in many different ways, and individuals may be members of different population groups. Membership in these different population groups will affect individuals as programs are designed and implemented to help them manage their own health, as well as that of their peers within the population group.

As an example, a 50-year-old woman employed by a major bank in a metropolitan area who has health insurance can be considered a member of three distinct population subgroups: she is an employee of the bank, a citizen of that community, and a member of the particular health insurance plan that provides her coverage. Each of these three populations has a vested interest in managing her health, both for her own benefit and the benefit of these groups (the bank, the community, the health plan) that have a social and/ or financial interest in her health and well-being.

First, this woman's employer wants her to remain healthy so that she will be a productive employee, miss few days of work, and perform her job on a regular basis. To that end, the employer may have a health promotion program in place to encourage her to quit smoking, maintain a healthy weight, and reduce stress. The employer may also offer an Employee Assistance Program (EAP) designed to help her if she has any personal problems such as grief, alcohol dependence, or legal concerns that might interfere with her ability to perform her job.

As a member of the second population group, her community, this woman may be part of community-wide projects that have been developed to improve her individual health and personal well-being. Her community may participate in a project designed to facilitate data sharing among healthcare institutions throughout the city. For example, medical record data may be shared among healthcare facilities making it easier for all healthcare providers to offer coordinated care to individual patients regardless of practice setting. Similarly, there may be a statewide initiative in place to reduce smoking by making smoking illegal in public places. Her membership in this community population enables her to take advantage of such health improvement initiatives, either knowingly or unwittingly, as they affect her daily life.

Finally, as an insured member of a health plan, the woman is a member of a third population whose specific interest is also to oversee and manage her health. A health plan may offer a demand management program designed to support health plan members as they make decisions about appropriate healthcare utilization. Furthermore, if this woman has a chronic disease such as diabetes, she may be enrolled in a disease management program that has been developed to help her manage her condition and avoid costly and dangerous complications of the disease. Other programs such as reminders to get a mammogram or an initiative to encourage her to get an annual immunization against influenza may also be in place to help this woman and others like her receive preventive services on an appropriate schedule.

A population health management framework relies upon the notion of defining a population in order to assess the health and medical care needs of the individuals of concern. Chapter 3 provides an extended discussion of this topic to clarify the issues raised by population definition.

WHERE CAN MANAGEMENT HAPPEN?

Given the variety of population health management programs that can be developed, such strategies are appropriate in a number of settings. Employers, communities, and health plans all provide settings in which programs can be implemented to address the needs of distinct populations. Which programs are selected depends on the characteristics of the population to be managed, as well as how easily the individuals in that population can be reached and influenced to change their health behaviors. The federal government, for example, may be interested in having all its citizens eat five servings of fruits and vegetables each day, but it can do little to mandate this personal health behavior. Instead, a state-level initiative may concentrate on those health issues that it can legislate, such as developing mandatory seatbelt and helmet laws, enforcing mandatory speed limits, and prohibiting smoking in public places. Similarly, a community-wide initiative may be developed to publicize quality and accreditation information about healthcare facilities and adult day care centers to inform local citizens about such facilities. Entities with this broad level of concern but limited control over individual behaviors may need to concentrate health management initiatives on particular subpopulations or on strategies such as education and legislation appropriate for the entire population.

Employer-level initiatives, in contrast to governmental initiatives, are often developed to take advantage of the employer's access to the employee population. This immediate access may also be associated with the potential ability of an employer to have more influence over employees' lives than a state or community may have. An employer concerned about getting employees to quit smoking may prohibit smoking on its premises, offer a financial incentive in health insurance premiums for nonsmokers, and provide complete insurance coverage for smoking cessation programs and nicotine patches to encourage all employees to quit. Beyond smoking cessation, lifestyle management programs may be put in place that are designed to increase employee knowledge about healthy behaviors by providing health information and incentives such as discounted health club memberships. Depending on the needs of the employee population, employers may contract with health plans or independent businesses to provide specific population health management services that meet both employee needs and their own needs as employers try to maintain a productive workforce and contain their healthcare premium costs.

Population health management initiatives are also developed at the level of institutions such as health insurance plans and healthcare facilities. Demand management and disease management programs may be offered at the health plan level to facilitate self-care management and appropriate utilization. Comprehensive strategies designed to coordinate care or help with disease management and catastrophic care management are increasingly available within both the health plan setting and at the individual provider level for those providers who have the incentives to manage and improve patients' health.

Considering the needs of the target population as well as the organization developing or paying for the health management program will help ensure that programs are designed and implemented in settings appropriate to achieve desired outcomes. As an example, for a demand management programs where remote care management is the primary form of patient contact, geographic location is less important than for programs such as disease management or catastrophic care management initiatives that incorporate face-to-face contacts with their participants. Structuring programs to focus specifically on attaining defined outcomes such as clinical improvements, functional status improvements, or less time lost from work will also help inform the *where* of the program location decision by establishing parameters for participant contact and expected provider communications.

WHY DOES POPULATION HEALTH NEED TO BE MANAGED?

The issue of why population health needs to be managed involves the concept of scarce resources. Healthcare resources are finite, and healthcare expenditures continue to increase. The United States spent $1.3 trillion in national healthcare expenditures in 2000, a 6.9 percent increase over 1999 (Levit et al. 2002; CMS 2002). With approximately 14 percent of the United States' gross domestic product (GDP) dedicated to healthcare spending, the U.S. ranks first among all nations in health expenditures.

Average health spending per person in the United States was $4,637 in 2000 (Levit et al. 2002). However, this expenditure level does not guarantee health for all Americans. Data from a recent comparison of 13 countries showed that the United States actually ranks an average of 12th on a variety of health indicators, including ranking 11th in life expectancy for females at age 1, and 12th for males at age 1 (Starfield 2000). Using different indicators of health such as disability-adjusted life expectancy, child survival to age 5, and other metrics, the World Health Organization ranked the United States as 15th among 25 industrialized countries in 2000 (World Health Organization 2000).

Managing the health of a defined population must include the health policy considerations of access, cost, and quality. First, in defining the population served, access to healthcare services is a major issue, and access problems and disparities should be addressed as much as possible. Similarly, the cost of providing healthcare services to support that population must be taken into consideration. Depending on the organization or government funding or providing services, the cost of including population health management services must also be accounted for within a program budget. Limits on the available budget may determine what type of strategies for population health management are feasible for that population. Finally, the issue of the quality of healthcare services must also be taken into account. The actual quality of healthcare services must be monitored, health outcomes must be tracked, and the quality of healthcare management services must be assessed. By keeping these health policy issues in the forefront of considerations about population health management programs, the likelihood of improvements in health for individual participants and financial health for payers will be increased.

ACCESS

Access to healthcare and health insurance is not well-established in the United States. In fact, the United States is the only developed country that does not provide guaranteed insurance coverage for all citizens and thereby does not ensure access to health services. By the end of the twentieth century, over 42 million Americans lacked health insurance, or 16 percent of the U.S. population (U.S. Census Bureau 2000). For children, the statistics are just as grim; studies revealed 11 million uninsured children in 1996, 90 percent of whom lived in households with at least one working adult.

The lack of universal coverage in the United States fundamentally contributes to the problem of controlling healthcare costs because poor, sick, and uninsured people have considerable difficulty seeking and receiving preventive services. In addition, the fragmented healthcare financing system requires that a safety net remain in place for those poor and uninsured. This partial solution is expensive and creates further problems by encouraging cost shifting for healthcare services as providers subsidize un-reimbursed care with fees obtained from insured patients (Anderson et al. 1996).

From a population health management perspective, access is a critical issue. In general, access to most health management programs is associated with some sort of private or government insurance coverage. Health plans like health maintenance organizations (HMOs) may offer options such as disease management programs to their members, while employers contract with demand management companies to help improve their employees' health and wellness. State Medicaid programs consider disease management programs to help manage their chronic illness costs, and hospitals, insurance companies, and provider groups work with catastrophic care management programs to limit their losses from catastrophic medical events.

Traditionally, employers have shared health insurance premiums with their employees through employee benefit packages so that employees are not fully responsible for the actual costs of their insurance or their medical care. However, when firms elect not to provide health insurance coverage or when individuals are unemployed, health insurance coverage may be prohibitively expensive for individual purchase. Government insurance coverage options such as Medicaid and Medicare are available to members of certain populations of individuals; however, if disability, income, or age criteria are not met, these individuals can remain uninsured.

Individuals who lack health insurance coverage do not have access to the health and wellness benefits of many population health management programs. Instead of being members of defined population groups targeted for health management, uninsured adults and children face a myriad of potential health and disability problems. Being uninsured is often associated with poorer health status, lack of a usual source of care, and abysmal rates for preventive health screenings such as immunizations, pap smears, and mammograms. Although in an ideal world this disenfranchised group should be a perfect target for population health management, their lack of insurance means that no sponsor exists to pay for the program, regardless of the potential benefits.

Optimally, while access to health management services is usually tied to health insurance coverage, opportunities may exist to leverage the value of such programs in ways that support uninsured and underinsured individuals. Programs that succeed in lowering medical care costs for covered individuals may be able to divert saved resources to provide care for the underserved. Health management programs that save providers time may succeed in supporting initiatives to use that time to provide services to uninsured or underinsured individuals in need of care but unable to pay. More specifically, developing a disease management program under the auspices of a particular insurance plan but extending the reach of the program to individuals who are uninsured or underinsured could be effective. (See 2.2 "Health Reform to Expand Access to Care Benefits from Population Health Management" at www.ache.org/pubs/mcalearney/start.cfm.)

For the employer dedicated to community improvement and to supporting employees in their community service efforts, health management programs may present another opportunity to provide such service. Offering access to a lifestyle management or demand management program for members of an underserved community may be a valuable contribution to that community. For health plans and vendors providing health management services, dedicating a portion of company proceeds or time to providing services to underserved individuals is a very effective way of showing support for the community and for the goals of health improvement. Applying creativity in the development and implementation of health management initiatives can help promote the values of access to care and health services in the broader population as more individuals are included in defined population groups that can benefit from health management services.

COST

As noted above, healthcare spending in the United States far exceeds expenditures in all other developed countries. Yet even at this expenditure level, medical care services are unaffordable for many Americans. Increases in technology and expertise have led to amazing success in the clinical treatment of disease. New technologies have made early diagnosis possible, and new treatments have extended as far as permitting surgical intervention on fetuses in the womb, and the identification and treatment of genetic anomalies. However, even with increased technology and high costs, health indicators for Americans are not as good as for residents of many other countries.

Containing healthcare costs has been a major goal of U.S. healthcare reform efforts. As described by Thomas Rice, conceptually, there are two categories of cost containment methods: methods based on fee-for-service reimbursement, and methods based on capitation (Anderson et al. 1996). Because population health management programs can be applied in either financial environment, attempts to contain costs under both systems will be briefly discussed. The importance of the concept of financial risk is also described, as is the overall perspective of using population health management strategies to reduce healthcare costs.

Fee-for-Service Systems

Cost containment strategies based on fee-for-service fall into three groups: price controls, volume controls, and expenditure controls (Rice 1996). Among these groups, the literature shows many examples of cost containment strategies including diagnosis-related groups and hospital rate-setting programs as examples of price controls; certificate-of-need programs, utilization review programs, and practice guidelines as examples of volume controls; and global budgets and Medicare's Volume Performance Standards as examples of expenditure controls (Rice 1996). Each of these strategies has met with limited success, but cost-control mechanisms under a fee-for-service system have not been reliable or consistent.

Many population health management strategies are consistent with the volume and expenditure control approaches to cost containment. Demand and disease management programs provide new opportunities to control volume by reviewing demand for utilization prospectively, as with demand management, and by guiding appropriate utilization through disease management. Overall, an environment with expenditure controls such as global budgets may value a population health management strategy because resources will be more tightly managed within the defined budget available.

Capitation Systems

Controlling expenditures under a capitation system requires that costs per person be controlled, the number of persons be monitored, and the shifting of costs between payers be managed (Rice 1996). Two main strategies for capitation-based cost control include the use of HMOs and managed competition. HMOs are paid on the basis of capitation, receiving a fixed payment to provide care for an enrollee for a specific amount of time. Payments are unrelated to how much money is actually spent by the HMO; therefore, if expenditures are lower for a given population of enrollees, the HMO can keep more money from the prepayments (Rice 1996). Population health management strategies are appealing to HMOs because they offer the promise of lowering expenditures for this defined population of enrollees, thereby permitting the HMO to retain more money as a business.

As Rice describes, the managed competition model acknowledges that the market for healthcare services is unlike other markets that support pure competition, and instead allows competition to flourish among players who must conform to certain rules (Rice 1996). These rules include conditions such as providing a minimum benefit package, establishing premium payment limits for employers, and even taxing health plans. The managed competition model might be enacted by the development of health insurance purchasing cooperatives or health alliances that would help establish rules and monitor progress. Although this managed competition model has not been widely tested, proponents argue that costs can be controlled under this approach and highlight success by the California Public Employees Retirement System (CalPERS) purchasing consortium of public employers in California. Opponents, however, argue that managed competition by itself is not likely to contain healthcare costs and suggest that including limits on insurance premiums within a managed competition framework may better increase the chance of success (Rice 1996). Depending on the model developed, incorporation of population health management strategies could be established as part of the rules for interested players with the intent of lowering costs and improving the quality of care for all covered individuals.

Financial Risk

Payment systems for medical care are often described in terms of financial risk. As an example, HMOs accept prepayment for medical services their enrollees may need and are then at risk to cover the costs of that medical care. This notion of financial risk in healthcare is associated with all types of insurance coverage. Insurance coverage provides protection for the insured individual against the downside risk of expensive medical care costs. Financially, insurance is offered for a price, or premium, that is collected, and care is provided up to the limits of policy coverage. Premiums are established based on actuarial estimates of past medical care utilization, which is a very good predictor of future utilization. When predictions about actual utilization are incorrect, the risk-bearing entity either benefits from lower utilization than expected or must cover the actual cost of care for higher utilization levels.

Because many population health management programs have emerged out of the desire to better manage financial risk, health management programs are often linked to risk-bearing entities. Even the level of personal financial risk may be affected when population health management strategies change care-seeking behaviors and the need for medical care. Under such circumstances, the amount of money consumers must pay in copayments, deductibles, and coinsurance rates may be reduced by better health and by better health and care management. Whether fee-for-service or capitation payment systems are in place, there is considerable financial benefit for the entity at risk, as well as for patients, if healthcare expenditures are reduced by better population health management.

Reducing Healthcare Costs

Regardless of type, population health management program development requires an investment of resources and managerial commitment. Justification of this investment is unlikely if financial savings are not expected from a program. Whether a program is developed by a hospital, a health plan, the government, or an employer, one of the primary goals of the program is to better manage health to reduce costs while hopefully improving health and healthcare services. Unfortunately, given the financial structure of most programs, it is unlikely for a program to emerge from the purely altruistic goals of helping improve patient health and well-being in the absence of cost considerations.

Program development is often justified on the basis of multiple goals and multiple potentially beneficial outcomes. However, the high costs of medical care for chronic and catastrophic illnesses are of particular concern for payers. Population health management strategies are attractive to these payers because of a demonstrated commitment to healthcare cost containment that is consistent with their interest in improving health outcomes and the quality of care provided.

Quality

The third major issue in health policy debates is that of quality. With increasing healthcare expenditures, the expectation of concurrent increases in quality has not been realized. As noted by McGlynn and Brook (2001), failures in quality of care result in premature death and needless suffering for patients in all parts of the healthcare system. The Institute of Medicine has presented a definition of quality of care that is accepted by many: "the degree to which health services for individual populations increase the likelihood of desired health outcomes and are consistent with current professional knowledge" (Lohr 1990). Health management strategies benefit by considering this definition as they define populations and desired outcomes for the targeted individuals.

Measuring actual quality in healthcare, however, is fraught with problems. Agreement about which indicators of healthcare quality to measure and deciding how frequently measurements should be undertaken is part of the program development process for many health management initiatives. In addition, defining quality improvement goals for programs and designing a program environment that provides incentives to attain such goals is an important component of program development. Consideration of the different issues in quality assessment and the special problem of medical errors helps to conclude this discussion about why population health management is important.

Quality Assessment

As described by McGlynn and Brook, quality monitoring occurs when one examines different dimensions of the healthcare system and assesses their quality. Performance quality is assessed by either a systems strategy such as total quality management or continuous quality improvement, or by a clinical strategy that focuses on specific health conditions or ser vices (McGlynn and Brook 1996).

Both quality assessment frameworks are important in the context of population health management. Population health management strategies are consistent with a systems approach to quality assessment because they consider the structures, processes, and outcomes of care as they attempt to improve the health and well-being of individuals. Programs are often developed with specific system improvement objectives such as improving care coordination and communication among providers. Also important for many health management programs is consideration of clinical quality. Program objectives such as improving patient health status or improving the care delivered to a particular population of patients are very common. The use of practice guidelines, treatment algorithms, and patient care protocols in many population health management programs is consistent with this quality assessment approach and helps ensure that the care delivered is both appropriate and high-quality.

Another aspect of quality monitoring is the contrast between internal and external quality assessment (McGlynn and Brook 1996). Internal quality assessment involves monitoring quality for an individual institution or program with the intention of assuring and improving its own quality. Population health management programs that define goals and objectives for both clinical and systems improvements can monitor progress and measure success according to those established targets. By comparison, external quality assessment involves comparing quality among several different entities or programs and making the information available for evaluation and decision making (McGlynn and Brook 1996). Benchmarking data, institutional report cards, and accreditation reviews are all examples of external quality assessment processes that affect healthcare organizations. For population health management programs, efforts to compare program outcomes and to evaluate program achievements in comparison to alternative approaches to cost containment or health improvement may be a part of the quality assessment process. It is critical that such programs maintain high internal standards for quality so that programmatic success will be viewed favorably by external observers as well.

Medical Errors

The devastating impact of medical errors highlights the need for improvement in the American healthcare system. The Institute of Medicine's (IOM) report, *To Err is Human,* documents that approximately 44,000 to 98,000 individuals die each year as a result of medical errors (Kohn et al. 1999). Additional studies have shown that as many as 20 to

30 percent of patients in the United States receive care that is contraindicated for their conditions (Starfield 2000; Schuster et al. 1998).

Many adverse effects of medical care itself can also be considered problems of medical quality (Starfield 2000). Errors and adverse effects that occur because of hospital care are reflected in the following estimates:

◆   12,000 deaths per year from unnecessary surgery (Leape 1992)

◆   7,000 deaths per year due to medication errors in hospitals (Lazarou et al. 1998)

◆   106,000 deaths per year due to adverse effects from medications that were not considered errors (Lazarou et al. 1998)

Outpatient care is also associated with multiple adverse effects. One study developed a probability model and estimated that drug-related adverse effects including morbidity and mortality affected between 4 and 18 percent of consecutive patients presenting for outpatient care. These adverse events resulted in 116 million extra visits to physicians, 77 million extra prescriptions, 17 million visits to the emergency department, 8 million hospitalizations, and 3 million admissions for long-term care facilities, at an added cost of $77 billion to the healthcare system (Johnson and Bootman 1995).

Population health management programs have the potential to reduce the number of medical errors and adverse effects associated with use of the healthcare system in a variety of ways. As suggested by Becher and Chassin (2001), part of improving quality and minimizing error must include systems and care processes designed to minimize human error. Strategies that employ care managers to oversee a group of patients can help avoid problems such as unnecessary utilization and medication errors by providing consistent care monitoring, access to care guidelines, and coordination. Most population health management programs are, in fact, designed to address the problem of inappropriate utilization, and thus program success could be credited with reductions in these adverse effects. Additional opportunities to reduce the frequency of medical errors may be realized by having new participants in the care management arena. By having dedicated providers and care managers helping to address issues such as transitions between and among providers and sites of care, the number of errors and problems associated with these situations may be decreased.

Attempting to Cross the Quality Chasm

As described in the Institute of Medicine's report, *Crossing the Quality Chasm* the challenge of the healthcare system in the 21st century is "to improve the American healthcare delivery system as a whole, in all its quality dimensions, for all Americans." Presenting an agenda for redesigning the healthcare system, two of the five topic areas to improve the system are directly related to the potential of population heath management programs (IOM 2001):

◆   "That healthcare organizations design and implement more effective organizational support processes to make change in the delivery of care possible.

◆   That purchasers, regulators, health professions, educational institutions, and the Department of Health and Human Services create an environment that fosters and rewards improvement by (1) creating an infrastructure to support evidence-based practice; (2) facilitating the use of information technology; (3) aligning payment incentives; and (4) preparing the workforce to better serve patients in a world of expanding knowledge and rapid change."

Population health management programs can help to achieve these goals by providing strategies that encourage changes in care delivery as well as promoting an environment focused on improvement. As emphasized by Shortell and Selberg (2002), much of the hope for improving quality in the American healthcare system is to work differently, not merely harder. Population health management strategies benefit from the application of evidence-based knowledge, encourage and rely on the use of information technology, promote the alignment of financial incentives, and help to focus the goals of care provision and healthcare service on improved service and outcomes enhancement.

A further overview of the IOM quality agenda focuses on six factors that the committee notes address key areas for improvement: safe, effective, patient-centered, timely, efficient, and equitable (IOM 2001). Population health management strategies are best designed for success when they also include such considerations, focusing on the goals of improving health and healthcare for defined populations. By attempting to coordinate care and services and focusing on quality overall, population health management strategies can try to do their part in bridging the quality chasm in the U.S. healthcare system.

CONCLUSION

Population health management strategies are desperately needed in the United States. Even given unequal access to health insurance and health management programs, the potential for such programs to better allocate healthcare resources makes them an important component of well-designed healthcare systems. These strategies enable governments and institutions to address the three major components of healthcare policy: access, cost, and quality. By defining a population to be served, access and quality can be measured, monitored, and improved at a given cost level. Furthermore, by managing health for that population, a system can be put into place that helps individuals maintain healthy behaviors and helps institutions to promote appropriate utilization of healthcare services.

REFERENCES

Adler, N. E., T. Boyce, and M. Chesney. 1994. "Socioeconomic Status and Health: the Challenge of the Gradient." *American Psychologist* 49 (1): 15–24.

Anderson, R. M., T. H. Rice, and G. F. Kominski. 1996. *Changing the U.S. Health Care System*. San Francisco: Jossey-Bass Publishers.

Becher, E. C., and M. R. Chassin. 2001. "Improving Quality, Minimizing Error: Making it Happen." *Health Affairs* 20 (3): 68–81.

Centers for Disease Control and Prevention. 2001. *Healthy People 2010.*

Washington DC: National Center for Health Statistics. [Online information; retrieved 3/1/01.] http://www.cdc.gov/nchs/about/otheract/ hpdata2010/abouthp.htm.

Centers for Medicare and Medicaid Services. 2002. *National Health Expenditures Aggregate 2002.* [Online information; retrieved 3/4/02.] http://www. hcfa.gov/stats/NHE-OAct/ tables/t1.htm.

Institute of Medicine, Committee on Quality of Health Care in America. 2001.

Crossing the Quality Chasm: A New Health System for the 21st Century. Washington, DC: National Academy Press.

Johnson, J. A., and J. L. Bootman. 1995. "Drug-related Morbidity and Mortality: A Cost-of-illness Model." *Archives of Internal Medicine* 155 (18): 1949–56.

Kaplan, G. A., E. Pamuk, J. Lynch, R. Cohen, and J. Balfour. 1996. "Inequality in Income and Mortality in the United States: An Analysis of Mortality and Potential Pathways." *British Medical Journal* 312 (7037): 999–1003.

Kindig, D. A. 1998. "Purchasing Population Health: Aligning Financial Incentives to Improve Health Outcomes." *Health Services Research* 33 (2): 223–42.

Kindig, D. A. 1997. *Purchasing Population Health: Paying for Results.* Ann Arbor: University of Michigan Press.

Kohn, L., J. Corrigan, and M. Donaldson. 1999. *To Err is Human: Building a Safer Health System.* Washington, DC: National Academy Press.

Lazarou, J., B. Pomeranz, and P. Corey. 1998. "Incidence of Adverse Drug Reactions in Hospitalized Patients." *Journal of the American Medical Association* 279:1200–05.

Leape, L. L. 1992. "Unnecessary Surgery." *Annual Review of Public Health* 13: 363–83.

Levit, K., C. Smith, C. Cowan, H. Lazenby, and A. Martin. 2002. "Inflation Spurs Health Spending in 2000." *Health Affairs* 21 (1): 172–81.

Lohr, K. N. 1990. *Medicare: A Strategy for Quality Assurance,* Vol. 1. Washington, DC: National Academy Press.

McGinnis, J. M., and W. H. Foege. 1993. "Actual Causes of Death in the United States." *Journal of the American Medical Association* 270 (18): 2207–12.

McGlynn, E. A., and R. H. Brook. 1996. "Ensuring Quality of Care." In *Changing the U.S. Health Care System* edited by R. M. Anderson, T. H. Rice, and G. F. Kominski. San Francisco: Jossey-Bass Publishers.

McGlynn, E.A., and R. H. Brook. 2001. "Keeping Quality on the Policy Agenda." *Health Affairs* 20 (3): 82–90.

Mills, R. J. *Health Insurance Coverage: 1999. Current Population Report.*

Washington, DC: U.S. Census Bureau. September 2000. [Online information; retrieved 8/7/01.] http://www.census.gov/hhes/www/ hlthin99.html.

Pappas, G., S. Queens, M. Hadden, and G. Fisher. 1993. "The Increasing Disparity in Mortality Between Socioeconomic Groups in the United States: 1960 and 1964." *The New England Journal of Medicine* 329 (2): 103–09.

Rice, T. H. 1996. "Containing Healthcare Costs." In *Changing the U.S. Health Care System* edited by R. M. Anderson, T. H. Rice, and G. F. Kominski. San Francisco: Jossey-Bass Publishers.

Schuster, M., E. McGlynn, and R. Brook. 1998. "How Good is the Quality of Healthcare in the United States? *Milbank Quarterly* 76: 517–63.

Shortell, S. M., and J. Selberg. 2002. "Working Differently: The IOM's Call to Action." *Healthcare Executive* (15) 1: 6–10.

Starfield, B. 2000. "Is U.S. Health Really the Best in the World?" *Journal of the American Medical Association* 284 (4): 483–85.

Suber, R. M. 2001. "Total Management: Prevention and Management of Chronic Disease." In *Continuum of Long-Term Care*, edited by C. Evashwick. Albany, NY: Delmar Publishing.

U.S. Census Bureau. 2000. *Health Insurance Coverage: 1999. Current Population Survey.* Washington, DC: U.S. Census Bureau.

U.S. Department of Health and Human Services. 1990. *Healthy People 2000: National Health Promotion and Disease Prevention Objectives*. Publication No. (PHS) 91-50213. Washington, DC: DHHS.

World Health Organization. 1948. *World Health Organization Constitution.* (Ratified 1948). *Geneva, Switzerland: World Health Organization.* [Online information; retrieved 8/7/01.] http://www.who.int/aboutwho/en/definition.html.

World Health Organization. 2000. *World Health Report.* Geneva, Switzerland: World Health Organization. [Online information; retrieved 3/14/01.] http://www.who.int/whr/2000/en/report.htm.

READING 3B

POPULATION HEALTH: PRACTICING POPULATION HEALTH MANAGEMENT AND MEASURING ITS SUCCESS

David B. Nash

From *Futurescan 2014: Healthcare Trends and Implications 2014–2019* (2014), Chapter 2, 11–16. Chicago: Society for Healthcare Strategy & Market Development of the American Hospital Association and Health Administration Press, a division of the Foundation of the American College of Healthcare Executives.

Americans are dying younger and living with a greater burden of disease than are residents of Slovenia and other less prosperous countries (Fineberg 2013; U.S. Burden of Disease Collaborators 2013).

Can the United States achieve improvements in the health of its population through reform provisions in the Affordable Care Act (ACA)? What is population health? What does it mean to "practice" population-based healthcare, and how do we measure its success? Finally, where is the movement toward population health going in the next five years?

DEFINING POPULATION HEALTH

The lack of agreement on any single operational definition of population health presents difficulties in interpreting current survey data and predicting the future. Population health can refer to "health outcomes and their distribution in a population. These outcomes are achieved by patterns of health determinants (such as medical care, public health, socioeconomic status, physical environment, individual behavior, and genetics) over the life course produced by policies and interventions at the individual and population levels" (Kindig 2007). This definition has been in our lexicon for at least three decades. Population health may also be viewed as the "aggregate health outcome of health-adjusted life expectancy (quantity and quality) of a group of individuals, in an economic framework that balances the relative marginal returns from the multiple determinants of health" (Kindig and Stoddart 2003). Others believe that population health is a sophisticated care delivery model that involves a systematic effort to assess the health needs of a target population and proactively provide services to maintain and improve the health of that population.

POPULATION HEALTH AND REFORM

Healthcare reform, through the ACA, features the implementation of two innovations in the delivery system to promote population health: patient-centered medical homes (PCMHs) and accountable care organizations (ACOs).

The PCMH model rests on the ability of a defined team to focus on the needs of the patient or family by coordinating a range of medical and social services. Among

Futurescan Survey Results: Population Health

How likely is it that the following will be seen in your hospital's area by 2019?

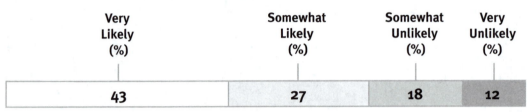

Very Likely (%)	Somewhat Likely (%)	Somewhat Unlikely (%)	Very Unlikely (%)
43	27	18	12

Your hospital or health system **will control** a complete continuum of care in your service area through a variety of relationships.

21	32	29	19

Your hospital or health system will be a **noncontrolling** participant in a complete continuum of care in your service area through a variety of relationships.

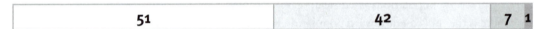

51	42	7 1

Formal mechanisms will be in place in your service area to ensure seamless coordination across the care continuum (e.g., documented handoff processes for transition management, integrated health information portal).

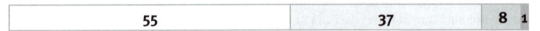

55	37	8 1

A formal communication structure will be established between your hospital or system and community partners to promote population health (e.g., regular meetings, representation of community partners on board or planning committees).

NOTE: Percentages may not total to exactly 100% due to rounding.

What Practitioners Predict

Hospitals or health systems will participate in a continuum of care in their service area. A majority (70 percent) of survey respondents report that by 2019 it is likely that their hospital or health system will be in control of a complete continuum of care in their service area. Approximately half of the CEOs in the survey believe that their hospital or health system will be a noncontrolling partner in a care continuum by that time.

Formal mechanisms will ensure coordination across the continuum of care. Of CEOs surveyed, nearly 93 percent predict that mechanisms such as documented handoff processes and an integrated health information portal will be in place to ensure seamless coordination across the care continuum in their area by 2019.

Hospitals or health systems will work with community partners to promote population health. Almost all (92 percent) of the CEOs surveyed report it is likely that by 2019 a formal structure of communications, including regular meetings, will be

(continued)

Futurescan Survey Results: Population Health

How likely is it that the following will be seen in <u>your hospital</u> by 2019?

	Very Likely (%)	Somewhat Likely (%)	Somewhat Unlikely (%)	Very Unlikely (%)
	76		22	2 ◊

Your hospital will be partnering with community organizations to support population health management initiatives (e.g., community needs assessments, chronic disease management).

	80		17	3 1

Your hospital will be participating in a health information exchange (HIE), which allows electronic sharing of health information among provider organizations.

12	42	31	15	

Your hospital will require that its governing board have at least one member with population health expertise.

43	49		7	1

Your hospital will have effective measures of "population health" to support the community health improvement mandate.

Note: Percentages may not total to exactly 100% due to rounding.

◊ Less than 0.5%

(continued from previous page)

established between their hospital or health system and community partners to promote population health. Ninety-eight percent believe their organizations will work with community partners to promote population health management initiatives, such as community needs assessments or chronic disease management, by that time.

Hospitals or health systems will participate in a health information exchange (HIE). Almost all (97 percent) of the survey respondents predict that their organization will participate in an HIE that allows sharing of health information among providers by 2019.

Practitioners are divided about population health expertise on boards. Just over half of CEOs in the survey report it is likely that their hospital or health system will require that its governing board include at least one population health expert.

Population health measures will be established. Almost all CEOs surveyed (92 percent) predict that their hospitals or health systems will have effective measures of "population health" in place to support the community health mandate by 2019.

the challenges facing the PCMH movement is the fact that the evidentiary basis for the model's potential success does not yet exist! Work by leading investigators (e.g., Alexander et al. 2013) indicates that turning a typical primary care practice into a PCMH-designated center will require transformational change and a great deal of resources and organizational support that currently are not readily available.

ACOs, the other core reform component, rely on effective partnering among healthcare providers of all shapes and sizes—health systems, hospitals, clinics, physician practices, urgent care centers—to share responsibility for the health of a population and accountability for the cost of their care.

PRACTICING POPULATION-BASED MEDICINE

Practicing population health management is very different from the work of most health systems today. According to one industry analyst (Sg2 2013):

> Organizations involved in population health must be concerned with all the determinants of health—environmental, social, economic and individual. Most of these factors fall outside the realm of traditional medicine, and there is no organization with the administrative, financial, and clinical resources to address them all. Therefore, PHM [population health management] must occur across a system of care—a broad network of alliances, partners and complementary organizations.

The essential components of such a comprehensive program might include, at a minimum, a care delivery infrastructure with advanced workforce models, innovative care delivery models (such as a PCMH), and a robust primary care network. Another key component is a technology infrastructure that will enable providers to risk-stratify the patients within a population and readily share information about both processes and outcomes. Finally, practicing population health management requires a culture of innovation, effective physician leadership, and risk-contracting payment models (Sg2 2013).

FUTURESCAN SURVEY RESULTS

Let's examine the current *Futurescan* survey results in light of the challenges in defining, organizing, and implementing systems to support population health management.

Notably, a majority (70 percent) of survey respondents report that in the next five years their hospital or health system will likely be in control of a complete continuum of care in their service area. Personally, I find this prediction implausible because of all of the inherent challenges in managing a coordinated continuum of care. Another surprising result is that, of the CEOs surveyed, nearly 93 percent predict that mechanisms, such as documented handoff processes and integrated health information portals, will be in place to ensure seamless coordination of care across the continuum in the next five years. All of the available evidence indicates that implementation of such mechanisms will be a nearly insurmountable challenge (DesRoches et al. 2013).

I was heartened to learn that 92 percent of the CEOs surveyed believe that, within the next five years, they will create a formal structure of communication, including regular meetings between their hospitals and local community partners, to promote population health.

Finally, practitioners remain sharply divided on population health expertise at the governance level. I was surprised that more than half of CEOs in the survey report that their hospital will likely require at least one population health expert on its governance board. Where will this expertise come from, and how will boards find these persons and bring them into the fold? As the dean of the only school of population health in the nation, I certainly hope that some of our emerging leaders will fill this role!

MEASURING SUCCESS

How will we measure the success of the population health movement? Here, I am in complete agreement with the majority of CEOs who predict that hospitals and health systems will have effective measures of population health in place to support the community health mandate by 2019.

Let's take a broader look at measuring population health. Some experts (e.g., Stiefel and Nolan 2013) believe that greater attention to achieving the so-called Triple Aim of the Institute for Healthcare Improvement (health of the population, individual experience of care, and per capita cost) will advance our ability to measure the health of the population.

As organizations move from strategy to execution, they will need better measures for each dimension of the Triple Aim. Population health measures might include years of potential life lost, life expectancy, and standardized mortality rates. For measuring the experience of care, Consumer Assessment of Healthcare Providers and Systems (CAHPS) data might provide benchmarks. Finally, for per capita cost, measures such as the total cost per population member per month and certain hospital and emergency department utilization rates might be appropriate.

In a recent report, the Institute of Medicine made recommendations about quality measures for population health (IOM 2013). This watershed report links major public health outcomes, such as the Leading Health Indicators (selected key objectives of the Healthy People 2020 agenda), to population health outcomes, such as better care coordination and reduction in waste. Perhaps the IOM report, combined with work on the Triple Aim, might help formulate measures of population health in the near future.

IMPLICATIONS FOR HOSPITAL LEADERS

Stepping into population health management will present a series of challenges to most hospitals and health systems. These challenges can be addressed in several stages (Sg2 2013). The first stage builds the basic foundation for population health management by focusing on traditional cost and quality measures, such as unnecessary emergency department visits or readmission rates by disease and source of admission. Potentially avoidable admission rates or admissions per 1,000 measures of a defined population could be other first-stage measures. This first stage can be implemented right now.

The second stage might deploy available first-generation population health metrics, such as those for diabetic adults with a hemoglobin A1C level greater than 8 percent or adults with a body mass index greater than 25 who have a documented follow-up plan. How about screening rates for colorectal and breast cancer, tobacco use, and depression? We can experiment and begin an early organizational transformation using some of these off-the-shelf population health metrics.

The next stage might focus on our ability to deploy core population health management capabilities and to master longitudinal metrics, such as managing a population in a per-member per-month payment scheme or obtaining detailed information about out-of-network utilization and true resource utilization in both the inpatient and outpatient settings. We should study how much we are really spending on certain chronic conditions and where that spending occurs (in the hospital versus in the ambulatory setting). And then we might be ready for the final stage, which would be to refine population-wide quality-of-life and functional assessments and customized measures of the effectiveness of certain interventions.

We need to create a checklist for population health management (Nash et al. 2011), which would include

- ◆ implementing health risk assessments,

- ◆ promoting prevention and wellness programs,

- ◆ building PCMHs,

- ◆ linking with local retail clinics or building our own,

- ◆ partnering with managed care companies,

- ◆ establishing true electronic registries so that we can track patient populations, and

- ◆ implementing physician leadership training in all areas relevant to population health management.

In the end, we must have a parallel strategy for keeping healthy people healthy and for managing the small percentage of patients who drive the vast majority of total costs in each of our local systems.

Some vexing questions remain that we will have to answer in the next five years. For example, who owns the patient? Is it the attending physician, the ACO, the multispecialty group practice? Who is the real driver in improving the health of the population? Will this improvement all occur at the local, regional, or national level? How will we measure our success? Will the Triple Aim be relevant in five years, or will the Leading Health Indicators become the front-runner?

There is no excuse for Americans dying younger and living with more illness than the residents of other nations. For a country that spends more on healthcare than any other country on the planet (Kumar and Nash 2011), we all should demand better!

REFERENCES

Alexander, J. A., G. R. Cohen, C. G. Wise, and L. A. Green. 2013. "The Policy Context of Patient Centered Medical Homes: Perspectives of Primary Care Providers." *Journal of General Internal Medicine* 28 (1): 147–53.

DesRoches, C. M., A. M. Audet, M. Painter, and K. Donelan. 2013. "Meeting Meaningful Use Criteria and Managing Patient Populations: A National Survey of Practicing Physicians." *Annals of Internal Medicine* 158 (11): 791–99.

Fineberg, H.V. 2013. "The State of Health in the United States." *Journal of the American Medical Association* 310 (6): 585–86.

Institute of Medicine (IOM). 2013. *Toward Quality Measures for Population Health and the Leading Health Indicators*. Washington, DC: National Academies Press.

Kindig, D. A. 2007. "Understanding Population Health Terminology." *Milbank Quarterly* 85 (1): 139–61.

Kindig, D. A., and G. Stoddart. 2003. "What Is Population Health?" *American Journal of Public Health* 93 (3): 380–83.

Kumar S., and D. B. Nash. 2011. *Demand Better! Revive Our Broken Healthcare System*. Bozeman, MT: Second River Healthcare Press.

Nash, D. B., J. Reifsnyder, R. Fabius, and V. P. Pracilio. 2011. *Population Health: Creating a Culture of Wellness*. Sudbury, MA: Jones & Bartlett Learning.

Sg2. 2013. *Population Health Management*. White paper. Skokie, IL: Sg2. www.sg2.com.

Stiefel, M., and K. Nolan. 2013. "Measuring the Triple Aim: A Call for Action." *Population Health Management* 16 (4): 219–20.

U.S. Burden of Disease Collaborators. "The State of US Health, 1990–2010: Burden of Diseases, Injuries, and Risk Factors." *Journal of the American Medical Association* 310 (6): 591–608.

READING 3C

COMMUNITY HEALTH: A MEASURABLE MANAGEMENT TASK

Connie J. Evashwick
From *Hospitals and Community Benefit* (2013), Chapter 2, 8–17. Chicago: Health Administration Press.

One challenge to community engagement is that it can be perceived as a "soft" activity, with amorphous borders and no measurable outcomes. This is not the case. To appreciate why hospitals must pay attention to the community and to know how to do so effectively, hospital leaders must understand how community health is conducted today and how it can be used to help accomplish the hospital's mission. An evidence-based approach to management is as applicable to community health as it is to any of the other management tasks of the hospital. The relationship of community health to the formal discipline of public health is particularly important.

DEFINITIONS

Community benefit (CB) is a term used by the Internal Revenue Service (IRS) to refer to specific actions that allow a nonprofit hospital to maintain its tax exemption (IRS 2012a). This book uses CB with this specific definition rather than as a generic term.

Community health is an amorphous concept and a term whose meaning lacks consensus. This lack of clarity is made worse by the IRS allowing each hospital to define its own community and indeed to declare that it serves several communities. For the purposes of this book, we will refer to *community health* as measurable by indicators of community health status and *community health activities* as those activities intended to improve the health of the community on a discrete and measurable dimension. A hospital might serve multiple communities, some of which are the focus of its formal CB activities while others are served for its mission without regard to IRS reporting or tax consequences. In using the term *community health*, the community of reference should be made explicit, not assumed.

Public health is a broad and potentially all-encompassing field of practice, as well as academic discipline. It is defined by the Institute of Medicine (2002) as "any activities undertaken to improve the health and well-being of the greater community." It places a great emphasis on prevention of healthcare problems. The Centers for Disease Control and Prevention (CDC 2012a) has identified ten essential public health functions—the practical tasks done by government public health departments (see Exhibit 2.1). These same functions are the basis for the new accreditation available to local and state health departments through the Public Health Accreditation Board (PHAB 2012). As an academic

EXHIBIT 2.1
Ten Essential
Public Health
Functions

1. Monitor health status to identify community problems.

2. Diagnose and investigate health problems and hazards.

3. Inform, educate, and empower people about health issues.

4. Mobilize community partnerships.

5. Develop policies and plans.

6. Enforce laws and regulations.

7. Provide personal healthcare services when unavailable.

8. Ensure a competent public and personal health workforce.

9. Evaluate effectiveness, accessibility, and quality.

10. Research innovative solutions to health problems.

SOURCE: CDC (2012a).

discipline, public health is taught in schools of public health, medicine, nursing, and other health professions universities as well as in burgeoning undergraduate programs offered by liberal arts colleges. Academic graduate training in public health typically includes the subjects of epidemiology, biostatistics, behavioral health, environmental health, and health management and policy. Some would argue that nutrition is also a core element of public health.

Population health is another general term with multiple interpretations. It is "used to describe different strategies that can be developed and implemented to improve health and the quality of care while also managing costs" (McAlearney 2003). Population health overlaps with public health but has different connotations. The term is a bit of a misnomer in that it is applied to programs that target segments of the population rather than the entire population. Physicians and the medical profession use the term to refer to how disease states are approached on a populationwide rather than on an individual patient level.

Hospitals, like physicians, have realized that treating individual patients alone cannot prevent communitywide disasters. Preventing a negative occurrence at a community level is more cost-effective for the hospital than having one occur for which the hospital loses money on dozens or even hundreds of individual patients. The cost–benefit of preventing a negative health occurrence rather than remediating it is clear in many instances, but some elusive conditions avoid measurement. The challenge is often to persuade a single institution, such as a hospital, that investing in a population-wide activity, such as vaccination, that reaches many individuals beyond its own patients is in its best financial interest. Activities for which the cause-and-effect has not been demonstrated incontrovertibly or those with a long time lag between action and impact present similar challenges.

Board commitment and an understanding of public and population health are essential in these situations.

EPIDEMIOLOGY 101

Epidemiology is the best example of the intersection of public health and population health—and their relevance to the hospital. Modern epidemiology was propelled by Dr. John Snow's 1854 discovery that the incidence of fatalities from a London cholera epidemic congregated around the water pump at Broad Street. The science of epidemiology has now advanced to employ sophisticated measures of the incidence and prevalence of disease, including trends over time. GPS and electronic media have added to the timeliness of such measures.

Epidemiology is relevant to hospital engagement with the community because it provides well-established measures to use in planning and evaluating hospital performance (Fleming 2008). The CDC is the nation's leading government public health agency. Directly and indirectly, the CDC has contributed to the emergence of public health as a measurable discipline. This enables hospitals to move community activity from "random acts of kindness" to a highly precise activity with a community impact that can be measured for process performance as well as short-term and long-term outcomes. Logic models (Exhibit 2.2) are widely employed by public health experts to show the relationships between external factors and inputs for achieving short-term and long-term outcomes in ameliorating diseases and chronic conditions (Frechtling 2007). An entire field of public health informatics has emerged (AMIA 2012). As public health has become an evidence-based field, it has enabled other healthcare entities, including hospitals, to take advantage of measurement science to identify, select, and evaluate the activities that are likely to have the greatest impact on the health status of the community (Brownson et al. 2011; IOM 2011).

Epidemiology also enables hospitals to analyze the health problems of their communities in great detail. Describing one's community using disease-specific aggregate data

EXHIBIT 2.2
Logic Model
Framework

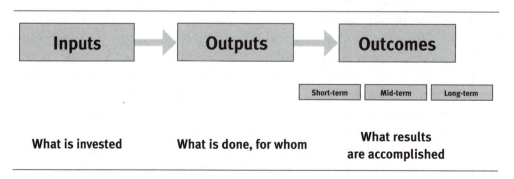

based on time-lagged information reported to the state or decennial census data is no longer acceptable.

MEASURES OF COMMUNITY HEALTH STATUS

Sophisticated ways to measure the health status of a community are emerging, which then facilitate measuring the impact of different interventions and comparing their relative effectiveness.

One example of applying public health science to hospital activities is in the area of screenings. The CDC operates the Community Guide (www.thecommunityguide.org), a website that compares the evidence-based effectiveness of a long list of screenings for many specific subpopulations. For hospitals that regularly engage in community health fairs and offer free or reduced-price screenings, this website is invaluable for pinpointing screenings that will be appropriate for the target population and those that will be a waste of time and money. For example, the Community Guide (CDC 2012b) uses the evidence available from high-quality research studies to compare and rate different types of cancer screenings—as they apply to defined subgroups—as "recommended," "recommended against," or "insufficient evidence" (Exhibit 2.3). For those screenings found to be effective, the Community Guide includes evaluations of their economic efficiency (costs).

The CDC has compiled a broader list of frequently recommended health outcomes and determinants (CDC 2013). Starting with a logic model of factors influencing health status, the CDC analyzed ten seminal sources of meta-analyses that analyzed 42 factors (determinants) that either directly affect morbidity and mortality or affect factors known to affect morbidity and mortality. The result is a highly condensed guide to activities targeted at either communities or individuals that will improve overall community health status. Using such data-based studies can help hospitals allocate scarce resources to achieve the greatest effectiveness. A classic example is the emergency department that treats a child successfully for acute asthma attacks but neither asks about nor follows up to address home conditions and behaviors that will prevent future emergencies. The CDC determinants guide is one resource for identifying initiatives in the community that would have a significant return in community health improvement.

The Agency for Healthcare Research and Quality (AHRQ) has supported and examined extensive data on the measurement and effectiveness of various prevention and treatment methods. These data have been compiled into accessible, searchable databases, including the National Quality Measures Clearinghouse (www.qualitymeasures.ahrq.gov) and the National Guideline Clearinghouse (http://guideline.gov) for evidence-based clinical practice guidelines (AHRQ 2012). The Substance Abuse and Mental Health Services Administration (SAMHSA 2012) has cataloged treatments that are effective for those with behavioral problems in the National Registry of Evidence-based Programs and Practices (www.nrepp.samhsa.gov).

EXHIBIT 2.3

Excerpt from The
Community Guide:
Interventions
Related to Cancer
Prevention and
Control

Interventions for clients either provide education to increase cancer screening or make it easier for clients to be screened. Results are reported separately for breast, cervical, and colorectal cancer screening because routine screening recommendations differ by age and sex.

Task Force Recommendations and Findings
This table lists interventions reviewed by The Community Guide, with Task Force findings for each.

Interventions	Breast Cancer	Cervical Cancer	Colorectal Cancer
Client Reminders	Recommended July 2010	Recommended July 2010	Recommended July 2010
Client Incentives	Insufficient Evidence July 2010	Insufficient Evidence July 2010	Insufficient Evidence July 2010
Small Media	Recommended December 2005	Recommended December 2005	Recommended December 2005
Mass Media	Insufficient Evidence October 2009	Insufficient Evidence October 2009	Insufficient Evidence October 2009
Group Education	Recommended October 2009	Insufficient Evidence October 2009	Insufficient Evidence October 2009
One-on-One Education	Recommended March 2010	Recommended March 2010	Recommended March 2010
Reducing Structural Barriers	Recommended March 2010	Insufficient Evidence March 2010	Recommended March 2010
Reducing Client Out-of-Pocket Costs	Recommended October 2009	Insufficient Evidence October 2009	Insufficient Evidence October 2009

SOURCE: CDC (2012c).

Healthy People is another major government initiative, supported by many private healthcare and public health organizations, to determine the status of the nation's health conditions and to set priorities for the future (HHS 2012). Healthy People began in the 1980s with its first national goals set for 2000. The goals—which include 42 major topic areas, 600 objectives, and 1,200 measures—are revised each decade; the 2010 goals are now past, and goals for 2020 are in place. The objectives set target rates of incidence or prevalence, based on current statistics and realistic programs for achieving change. The large list has been narrowed to leading health indicators to create a pared-down set of 26 indicators pertaining to 12 topics. For example, within the major topic of Nutrition and Weight Status, Objective NW5-9 is "Reduce the proportion of adults who are obese" from 34 percent to 30.6 percent, a 10 percent decrease. The Healthy People website (www.healthypeople.gov) includes targets, data sources for each condition, and a link to research studies pertaining to the condition and its remediation. Although most public health professionals are well aware of the Healthy People program and its goals, many of those working in hospitals, physician practices, and other clinically oriented organizations are not familiar with this initiative and how it can be used to guide and measure hospital activities with the community.

The collective activities of the CDC, the National Institutes of Health, the US Department of Health & Human Services, many state governments, and private initiatives have produced numerous sources of free yet detailed and current data that can be used to assess the health of a community (Exhibit 2.4). County Health Rankings (www .countyhealthrankings.org) is one example of a nationwide database that measures and ranks each county in the United States on characteristics that are known to affect health status. The Health Indicators Warehouse (http://healthindicators.gov) compiles many of these data sets and facilitates easy access to data on a given topic. Hospitals can tap into these data sets, add hospital-specific data, and establish realistic and measurable goals for improving community health status while engaging in programs that are consistent with the hospital's mission and resources.

State and local governments and private sources also gather useful data relevant to community health status, much of which is available at no charge. The National

---

Census data: http://quickfacts.census.gov

County data: www.countyhealthrankings.org

National Cancer Institute: www.cancer.gov

Health Indicators Warehouse: http://healthindicators.gov

Behavioral Risk Factor Surveillance System: www.cdc.gov/brfss

Mental health and substance abuse: www.nrepp.samhsa.gov

Community Guide: www.thecommunityguide.org

Agency for Healthcare Research and Quality National Quality Measures Clearinghouse: www.qualitymeasures.ahrq.gov

Healthy People: www.healthypeople.gov

EXHIBIT 2.4
Free National Data Sources That Include Local Data

Association of County and City Health Officials (NACCHO 2013) engages in a range of programs that often include data collection about community health status as well as workforce and local surveillance trends. The Healthy Communities Institute (2012) in Northern California has created a sophisticated dashboard for tracking changes in community health status based on automatic input of county-level data. This dashboard is used by a consortium of organizations so that the individual and collective contributions to community targets can be measured over time. Dignity Health, in partnership with Truven Health, has created its own data system, the Community Need Index, for measuring community health for its member institutions (Barsi 2009). These measures are incorporated into the strategic plan for each institution, and progress is tracked and reported annually as part of the performance report of individual healthcare executives as well as reported to each community. The top-level data and community mapping are available for free at www.dignityhealth.org/cni.

REALISTIC EXPECTATIONS

One caveat is that changing the health of an entire community requires time. A hospital—and its community partners—must allow time for changes to take place. This process includes educating the public, changing individual and institutional behaviors, implementing monitoring systems, and tracking trends over time. Some changes, such as vaccination rates and the diseases they prevent, can be measured immediately and the impact projected with relative accuracy. Other activities, such as sun protection, are more difficult to measure. Moreover, since skin cancer can take 30 years to develop, outcome measures are less precise or require a realistic expectation of the length of time required for the disease pattern to change.

A second consideration is that the attribution of results to collaborative versus individual efforts is often challenged. Where direct impact cannot clearly be ascribed to the actions of an individual institution, having the hospital select evidence-based activities for which outcomes can be measured is all the more important.

ACTIONS FOR HEALTHCARE EXECUTIVES

◆ Become familiar with the measures available for monitoring the health status of the community.

◆ Define the demographic and health status of the community or communities the hospital serves in detail using current data, including a bigger picture than just the patients served by the hospital.

◆ Apply the principles of evidence-based healthcare management to selecting and prioritizing the hospital's activities with each community it serves.

◆ Set realistic but measurable goals and objectives for the hospital's community engagement.

◆ Tap into data sources from public health and other national databases to analyze the health of the hospital's community and to evaluate the hospital's role.

REFERENCES

Agency for Healthcare Research and Quality (AHRQ). 2012. "National Quality Measures Clearinghouse." Accessed November 1. www.qualitymeasures.ahrq.gov.

American Medical Informatics Association (AMIA). 2012. "Public Health Informatics." Accessed October 24. www.amia.org/programs/working-groups/public-health-informatics.

Barsi, E. 2009. "Community Benefit: Moving Forward with Evidence-Based Policy and Practice." Presentation at the preconference to the Annual Research Meeting of Academy Health, Chicago, June 27.

Brownson, R., E. Baker, T. Leet, K. Gillespie, and W. True. 2011. *Evidence-Based Public Health,* 2nd ed. New York: Oxford University Press, Inc.

Fleming, S. 2008. *Managerial Epidemiology,* 2nd ed. Chicago: Health Administration Press.

Frechtling, J. 2007. *Logic Modeling Methods in Program Evaluation.* San Francisco: Jossey-Bass.

Healthy Communities Institute. 2012. "Home Page." Accessed November 2. www.healthy communitiesinstitute.com.

Institute of Medicine (IOM). 2011. *For the Public's Health: The Role of Measurement in Action and Accountability.* Washington, DC: The National Academies Press.

———. 2002. *Who Will Keep the Public Healthy? Educating Public Health Professionals for the 21st Century.* Washington, DC: The National Academies Press.

Internal Revenue Service (IRS). 2012a. "Form 990." Accessed December 11. www.irs.gov/form990.

McAlearney, A. 2003. *Population Health Management: Strategies to Improve Outcomes.* Chicago: Health Administration Press.

National Association of County and City Health Officials (NACCHO). 2013. "Toolkit." Accessed January 22. www.naccho.org/toolbox/veritysearch/search.cfm?keywords=Data&p=ALL&st=ALL&jurisdiction=ALL&x=63&y=13.

Public Health Accreditation Board (PHAB). 2012. "Standards and Measures." Accessed August 8. www.phaboard.org/accreditation-process/public-health-department-standards-and-measures/.

Substance Abuse and Mental Health Services Agency (SAMHSA). 2012. "National Registry of Evidence-Based Programs and Practices." Accessed November 29. www.nrepp.samhsa.gov.

US Centers for Disease Control and Prevention (CDC). 2013. *Community Assessment for Population Health Improvement: Resource of Frequently Recommended Health Outcomes and Determinants.* Atlanta, GA: Office of Surveillance, Epidemiology, and Laboratory Services.

————. 2012a. "10 Essential Public Health Services." Accessed October 24. www.cdc.gov/nphpsp/essentialServices.html.

————. 2012b. "The Community Guide." Accessed August 6. www.thecommunityguide.org.

————. 2012c. "The Community Guide: Cancer Prevention and Control: Client-Oriented Interventions to Increase Breast, Cervical, and Colorectal Cancer Screening." Accessed January 10, 2013. www.thecommunityguide.org/cancer/screening/client-oriented/index.html.

US Department of Health and Human Services (HHS). 2012. "Healthy People 2020." Accessed August 24. www.healthypeople.gov.

READING 3D
ACA INTEGRATION INITIATIVES THAT PROMOTE COLLABORATION

Connie J. Evashwick

From *Hospitals and Community Benefit* (2013), Chapter 5, 44–52. Chicago: Health Administration Press.

Other elements of the Patient Protection and Affordable Care Act (ACA) have implications for partnerships between hospitals and healthcare systems and community organizations. Whereas community health needs assessments (CHNAs) and community health implementation plans (CHIPs) focus on hospital–community coordination at the population level, several aspects of the ACA deal with collaboration between hospitals and other organizations in serving the community primarily for prevention or clinical care at the individual level. The majority of these initiatives address the financing of care, and they focus on Medicare and Medicaid patients—two groups that the hospital might ordinarily seek to minimize because of poor payment.

Most of the ACA initiatives are being tested through demonstrations managed by the Centers for Medicare & Medicaid Services' (CMS) Innovation Center (CMS 2012). Consensus on the definitive direction for any of these initiatives has not yet emerged, and universal regulations are not likely to be enacted for several years while the innovative programs are tested. Moreover, how the ACA evolves over time remains to be determined. However, to the extent that the programs promoted by the ACA deal with the integration of clinical care across settings and over time, strive for high quality with lower costs, and emphasize prevention and the management of chronic illness, these integration initiatives are worthwhile long-term efforts that could well be sustained regardless of federal laws and regulations.

This chapter highlights the ACA provisions that have potential implications for hospital organizational arrangements with other community entities, then it delineates principles of collaboration relevant to multi-entity coordinated clinical care. Regardless of the outcome of the demonstrations or subsequent modifications of the law, hospitals can examine the potential to improve their internal operations by working with external entities more effectively. The lessons learned will have valuable applications for the future.

ACA PROGRAMS

This book makes no pretense of capturing all of the ACA provisions that potentially affect hospitals. It does not address changes in payment mechanisms, quality, or access. However, this section, summarized in Exhibit 5.1, identifies ACA initiatives of particular relevance to the theme of this book: opportunities for hospitals to collaborate with community entities and the organizational processes and structures that facilitate such collaboration. To the extent that ACA initiatives are tested, modified, and eventually incorporated into Medicare or Medicaid conditions of participation or payment mechanisms, the hospitals that have willingly engaged in efforts to achieve successful integration will be ahead of their competitors in market domination, financial stability, and patient and community loyalty. (Further details of the ACA initiatives can be found on the CMS website for the Innovation Center at innovations.cms.gov.)

Partnership for Patients. This umbrella term covers a variety of initiatives. CMS (2012) describes it as "a nationwide public–private partnership that aims to reduce [preventable] errors in hospitals by 40 percent and reduce hospital readmissions by 20 percent." By partnering with community-based and institutional long-term care providers as well as patients and families, hospitals can employ a variety of tested techniques to reduce readmissions.

Community-Based Care Transitions Program. Hospitals contract with community-based organizations (CBOs) to coordinate support service upon patient discharge. These partnerships help improve the transitions of high-risk Medicare patients from the hospital to other care settings, improve quality of care, reduce readmissions, and document measurable savings to Medicare. Criteria for CBOs are specified by CMS (2012): "Interested CBOs must provide care transition services across the continuum of care and have formal relationships with acute care hospitals and other providers along the continuum of care. An interested CBO must be physically located in the community it proposes to serve,

---

EXHIBIT 5.1

CMS Innovation
Initiatives, 2012

Partnerships for Patients

Community-Based Care Transitions

Accountable Care Organizations

Bundled Payments for Care Improvement

Reduce Avoidable Hospitalizations Among Nursing Facility Residents

Independence at Home

Comprehensive Primary Care

Federally Qualified Health Center Advanced Primary Care Practice

Multipayer Advanced Primary Care Practice Demonstration (medical homes)

Medicaid Incentives Program for the Prevention of Chronic Diseases

---

SOURCES: CMS (2012, 2011).

must be a legal entity that can accept payment for services, and have a governing body with representation from multiple healthcare stakeholders including consumers. . . . CBOs will be paid an all-inclusive rate per eligible discharge based on the cost of care transition services provided at the patient level and of implementing systemic changes at the hospital and community levels."

Accountable Care Organizations (ACOs). Provider organizations accept the financial risk for improving quality—including more efficient care coordination—and lowering costs for all of their Medicare patients. CMS (2012) defines ACOs as "groups of doctors, hospitals, and other healthcare providers, who come together voluntarily to give coordinated high-quality care to the Medicare patients they serve. Coordinated care helps ensure that patients, especially the chronically ill, get the right care at the right time, with the goal of avoiding unnecessary duplication of services and preventing medical errors." Several ACO models have been developed, with hospitals, medical groups, and payment mechanisms at the heart of most of them. Other community providers and support organizations are often involved as well. ACOs are one of several CMS initiatives to which the concept of the patient-centered medical home applies.

Bundled Payments for Care Improvement. This initiative tests several methods for bundling payment for all services rendered to patients during a single episode of care. For the hospital to succeed at bundled payment, relationships between acute and post-acute providers must be efficient and effective at producing high-quality care outcomes. The goal for this initiative is to develop ways to align the financial incentives for hospitals, physicians, and post-acute payers to improve coordination of care and thereby improve quality with lower costs.

Reduce Avoidable Hospitalizations Among Nursing Facility Residents. This initiative supports organizations that partner with nursing facilities to implement evidence-based interventions to both improve care and lower costs. The initiative focuses on long-stay nursing facility residents who are enrolled in Medicare and Medicaid. As evident in the name, the goal is to reduce avoidable inpatient hospitalizations. Hospitals can partner with nursing facilities to share evidence-based practices, staff expertise, medical records, and other techniques that benefit both the hospital and the nursing facility in preventing unnecessary hospital admissions.

Independence at Home Demonstration. This demonstration supplements standard benefits by "providing chronically ill patients with a complete range of primary care services in the home setting. Medical practices led by physicians or nurse practitioners will provide primary care home visits tailored to the needs of beneficiaries with multiple chronic conditions and functional limitations" (CMS 2012). The initiative "will test whether home-based care can reduce the need for hospitalization, improve patient and caregiver satisfaction, and lead to better health and lower costs to Medicare" (CMS 2012). Hospitals, as well as hospital-sponsored medical groups, have been among those awarded grants to test this care-at-home model.

Comprehensive Primary Care. This initiative supports clinicians in managing and coordinating comprehensive care for their patients, particularly those with serious or chronic diseases. Comprehensive Primary Care "supports collaboration between public and private payers and primary care practices that agree to give patients 24-hour access to care, create personalized care plans, and coordinate with other providers to ensure patients get well and stay healthy" (CMS 2012). The concept of a patient-centered medical home applies here. CMS is working with state-sponsored and commercial health insurance plans to offer extra payments to primary care doctors who are better able to coordinate care for their patients. The goal is to improve access to primary care. Hospitals can be involved to the extent that they offer primary care clinics, subsidize clinics in the community, or work with primary care providers to coordinate specialty or emergency services for those patients who have a primary care provider.

Federally Qualified Health Center (FQHC) Advanced Primary Care Practice. This initiative demonstrates how FQHCs can "act as patient-centered medical homes to improve coordination and quality of care to Medicare patients as well as others. This demonstration project…will test the effectiveness of doctors and other health professionals working in teams to coordinate and improve care for Medicare patients.… Participating FQHCs are expected to achieve Level 3 patient-centered medical home recognition, help patients manage chronic conditions and … adopt care coordination practices that are recognized by the National Committee for Quality Assurance (NCQA)" (CMS 2012). This initiative includes specific use of the *patient-centered medical home* terminology.

For any of these demonstration initiatives to succeed, hospitals must partner with other organizations in the community. Some relationships—such as those with nursing homes and medical groups—will have a long history. Where agreements are new, senior leaders can contribute by giving guidance in selecting community partners, shaping effective contracts to formalize collaboration, and managing a portfolio of relationships.

LESSONS LEARNED ABOUT INTEGRATION

The US healthcare system has a considerable history of constructing integrated systems to provide a continuum of care. The 1980s and 1990s saw a wave of initiatives that brought together hospitals, physicians, long-term care, managed care, and various other stakeholders. Truly integrated systems, such as Kaiser Permanente, have demonstrated cost savings and superior quality. The ACA's contributions include providing financial incentives to promote integration and applying those incentives on an ongoing basis to large segments of the population through Medicare and Medicaid. The move toward electronic medical records predates the ACA but is an essential foundation for integrated care that has been lacking until recent federal mandates. The combination of electronic medical records and financial incentives to provide comprehensive and quality care may turn out to be the tipping point that moves the United States away from the fragmented care that exists currently.

Management lessons have been learned about integration from both successes and aborted efforts (Evashwick and Weiss 1987; Evashwick 1997; National Chronic Care Consortium 2001; Shortell et al. 1996; Shortell, Gillies, and Anderson 2000; Weil, Bogue, and Morton 2001; Zuckerman 2010; AHA 2012a). This wealth of knowledge can be applied to advancing hospital efforts today. Selected recommendations include the following:

- Choose community partners for long-term strategies, not short-term demonstrations. In the rush to be out front in testing new models (and applying for CMS grants), hospitals should be wary of quick marriages. Long-term relationships between organizations are based on shared values, shared vision, compatible cultures, harmonious leadership, and a solid business case for each organization.

- Articulate partnership terms in writing (including formal contracts), especially for partnerships that involve payment arrangements. When arrangements are put into precise words, seeing if all parties can agree is much easier. Clearly articulated purposes can then be translated into measurable goals and objectives in the accompanying business plan, thereby giving all parties objective criteria to assess whether the agreement is working as expected.

- Allow for a mutually agreeable escape clause. Just as with vendor contracts, having a cancellation clause is important. Maintaining positive relationships with the community and community organizations is much easier if the reasons for cancellation are agreed on up front rather than after a program has launched.

- Gain board approval. The board should represent the range of hospital stakeholders, including the community. Relationships should be approved by the board in advance of implementing a new program, especially if the activity or the partnerships might be controversial.

- Allow sufficient time to build infrastructure, especially for community organizations that might not have the magnitude of operational processes and resources as the hospital. Hospitals, medical groups, and managed care companies are typically the largest entities in the healthcare system of any community. Community agencies want to be players in the partnerships but are likely to be well aware of the difference in resource base. Hospitals walk a fine line in sharing responsibility while balancing appropriate resource contribution. There is no right formula, only issues to be considered.

- Assess the status of partners' information management systems—both for patients and for operations. Because of federal government mandates, hospitals and physician groups are well set up to develop electronic medical records. Other providers are less so. If the hospital expects to track patient utilization across settings, monitor outcomes, share revenue and expenses, and achieve efficiencies of operations, the information management systems of its partners will be critical. Evaluating the status of each organization's information management system and allowing for the time and costs of achieving interoperability or other means of data sharing are critical to the long-term success of a collaboration that goes beyond being superficial.

◆ Consider relationships from the community residents' standpoint. Relationships made with one partner that require patients and families, as well as referring providers, to use a specific provider might meet with resistance if this runs counter to a well-established utilization pattern. Educating patients, families, and providers and explaining the relationships to them are essential to gain acceptance of new providers. Community residents may treasure preferred providers who provide information on quality and cost.

◆ Expect resistance to change as formal relationships replace informal patterns. As with changes in patients' customary use patterns, changes that require staff to engage with different organizational partners could well be met with resistance and distrust. Providing information and explanation for staff may be necessary to gain their cooperation.

◆ Educate the hospital staff and the community partners about the processes and procedures for collaborating on patient empowerment and education. Terminology alone can be a barrier to success if the hospital staff use one set of acronyms and a community agency uses another. Legal requirements might vary or simply be implemented differently. Corporate cultures, if not incompatible, could still vary. Even when willing to make a change, frontline staff of all partner entities should be given the attention and education essential to making future operations smooth.

◆ Consider formal relationships for a given program within the greater context of multiple relationships. As efforts to coordinate care expand, a hospital might find itself involved with more than one communitywide collaborative or internal care coordination program. Senior leadership might be the only place with a broad enough view or span of control to be aware of all that the organization is doing. Competing or conflicting relationships must be sorted out so that the formal initiatives pursued by the hospital are compatible with one another. Need for resources—including the intangible but essential staff commitment—must also be adjudicated at the highest levels of the hospital leadership or board.

ACTIONS FOR HEALTHCARE EXECUTIVES

◆ Assign someone at a senior level to monitor the successes (and failures) of current national demonstrations, including lessons learned, and to serve as the planning and organizational liaison with new community-based programs.

◆ Approach partnerships with community organizations with the same business rigor as the hospital would a merger or acquisition.

◆ Maintain transparency with the board and close communication with internal and external stakeholders. Both are vital for long-term success even though solidifying the terms of an agreement might require discretion and confidentiality.

◆ Monitor the actions of competitors and collaborators to assess relationships that might affect the hospital's market.

◆ Keep the hospital's mission and community in the forefront while positioning the hospital for eventual changes. The ultimate goal of the CMS innovation demonstrations is to test new ways to control the costs and improve quality and access to Medicare and Medicaid.

REFERENCES

American Hospital Association (AHA). 2012a. "Community Connections Project." Accessed December 6. www.caringforcommunities.org.

Centers for Medicare & Medicaid Services (CMS). 2013. "Nursing Home Compare." Accessed January 23. www.medicare.gov/NursingHomeCompare/.

———. 2012. "CMS Innovation Center." Accessed December 13. www.innovations.cms.gov.

Evashwick, C. J. 1997. *Seamless Connections.* Chicago: American Hospital Association.

Evashwick, C. J. and L. Weiss. 1987. *Managing the Continuum of Care.* Rockville, MD: Aspen Publishers.

National Chronic Care Consortium. 2001. "Self-Assessment for Systems Integration Tool." Accessed November 16, 2012. www.nccconline.org/SASI/SASi_Objectives.pdf.

Shortell, S., R. Gillies, and D. Anderson. 2000. *Remaking Health Care in America: The Evolution of Organized Delivery Systems*, 2nd ed. San Francisco: Jossey-Bass.

Shortell, S., R. Gillies, D. Anderson, K. Erickson, and J. Mitchell. 1996. *Remaking Health Care in America: Building Organized Delivery Systems,* 1st ed. San Francisco: Jossey-Bass.

Weil, P., R. Bogue, and R. Morton. 2001. *Achieving Success Through Community Leadership.* Chicago: Health Administration Press.

Zuckerman, A. 2010. *Leading Your Healthcare Organization Through a Merger or Acquisition.* Chicago: Health Administration Press.

READING 3E

POPULATION HEALTH IMPROVEMENT: A COMMUNITY HEALTH BUSINESS MODEL THAT ENGAGES PARTNERS IN ALL SECTORS

David A. Kindig and George Isham
From *Frontiers of Health Services Management* 30 (4): 3–20.

SUMMARY

Because population health improvement requires action on multiple determinants—including medical care, health behaviors, and the social and physical environments—no single entity can be held accountable for achieving improved outcomes. Medical organizations, government, schools, businesses, and community organizations all need to make substantial changes in how they approach health and how they allocate resources.

To this end, we suggest the development of multisectoral community health business partnership models. Such collaborative efforts are needed by sectors and actors not accustomed to working together. Healthcare executives can play important leadership roles in fostering or supporting such partnerships in local and national arenas where they have influence.

In this article, we develop the following components of this argument: defining a community health business model; defining population health and the Triple Aim concept; reaching beyond core mission to help create the model; discussing the shift for care delivery beyond healthcare organizations to other community sectors; examining who should lead in developing the community business model; discussing where the resources for a community business model might come from; identifying that better evidence is needed to inform where to make cost-effective investments; and proposing some next steps.

The approach we have outlined is a departure from much current policy and management practice. But new models are needed as a road map to drive action—not just thinking—to address the enormous challenge of improving population health. While we applaud continuing calls to improve health and reduce disparities, progress will require more robust incentives, strategies, and action than have been in practice to date. Our hope is that the ideas presented here will help to catalyze a collective, multisectoral response to this critical social and economic challenge.

INTRODUCTION

Increasing attention is being given to improving health in all communities across the United States. As a nation, in terms of our health outcomes, we lag most developed countries by a wide margin, despite spending substantially more (IOM 2013). In addition, significant geographic variation is seen in health outcomes within the United States (County Health Rankings 2011), including unacceptable disparities in morbidity, mortality, and risk factors. Absolute worsening of mortality rates in many US counties has been noted over the last several years (Kulkarni et al. 2011; Kindig and Cheng 2013).

It is one thing to highlight this poor performance; it is another to motivate sustained improvement. As shown in Exhibit 1, from the University of Wisconsin County Health Rankings model, health outcomes are produced by multiple factors, or health

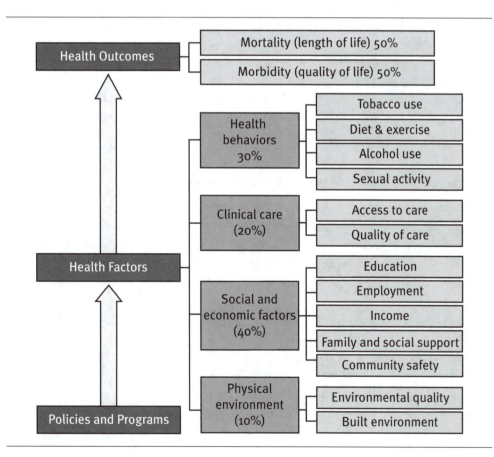

EXHIBIT 1

County Health Rankings Model, 2012

SOURCE: University of Wisconsin Population Health Institute. County Health Rankings 2013. Accessible at www.countyhealthrankings.org. Used with permission.

determinants—including medical care, health behaviors, and the social and physical environments (County Health Rankings 2013a). Furthermore, the contribution of healthcare to health is modest—only 20 percent—a fact that many healthcare leaders may find surprising.

In light of these factors, no single entity can be held accountable for achieving the goals of improved population health. Collective effort is needed by sectors not accustomed to working together and by stakeholders who may not be aware of how their actions affect population health. In addition, incentives and new public and private resources (both knowledge and funding) must be created to ensure that plans are implemented.

In this article we call for a new generation of multisectoral partnerships, organized using the elements of a community health business model, to accomplish these goals. The issue is not that such efforts have not been tried in the past or do not exist today. The Healthy Community movement of the 1980s was a significant effort, but it was not sustained or supported (Pittman 2010). In many communities, public health leaders have been developing relationships with healthcare and business organizations, often supported by foundation or federal grants or community philanthropy. National bodies such as the Institute of Medicine (2011b) have called for more robust multisectoral partnerships at the local level.

So the idea is not new, but its robust and sustained implementation would be. It is time to move beyond grants and isolated efforts to partnerships with substantial structures, incentives, and financing. Using one example from the healthcare sector, we advocate here for community-level partnerships built on a community health business model to achieve goals heretofore not achieved.

DEFINING A COMMUNITY HEALTH BUSINESS MODEL

Population health improvement cannot be the responsibility of a single sector. Essential contributions must also come from those that have secondary influence on health outcomes, such as business, education, state and local government, community development, and philanthropy. We argue that efforts must be made to form partnerships drawn from all sectors and that those partnerships be integrated using a community health business model.

A business model describes how an organization creates, delivers, and captures economic, social, or other forms of value. Business models represent the core aspects of a business, including its purpose, offerings, strategies, infrastructure, organizational structure, trading practices, and operational processes and policies (Johnson, Christensen, and Henning 2011). While such models are usually developed by individual firms in the corporate sector, some that are suitable for application in the health business arena are available from entities in business, government, and the nonprofit sector. This idea is related to the concept of social entrepreneurship or collective impact (Kania and Kramer 2011), in which innovative, social value–creating activity occurs both within and across the nonprofit, government, and business sectors. Harvard Business School Professor Michael E. Porter, PhD, recently observed that the "solution lies in the principle of shared value, which involves creating economic value in a way that *also* creates value for society by addressing its needs and challenges" (Porter and Kramer 2011).

We believe the business model concept, if adapted for use by communities, may provide a platform for the more robust and sustained implementation effort that is required to accelerate and sustain population health improvement in communities across the United States. A community health business model would have to go beyond narrow interests to involve many sectors and organizations that can command sufficient resources or control over the actions required for improving health outcomes. An Institute of Medicine (2011b) report suggests a framework for measuring accountability of different actors in producing better public health processes as well as potential joint accountability for health in communities. The report identifies government, education, healthcare, business, and community organizations as among those that can allocate resources toward achieving results.

To adapt the business model concept for use by multisectoral partnerships in communities, we propose that the following elements of a community health business model be designed and implemented in each community across the country:

1. All stakeholders from relevant sectors that can affect the population's health must be engaged in the process, as no single stakeholder has the resources to achieve, or can be accountable for, improved health in communities.

2. The community health business model must operate in a transparent manner and engage and report its progress to the general public.

3. A leadership structure needs to be designed and implemented.

4. Common purpose needs to be established. To do so, the benefits of improved health to the community must be identified and aligned with the benefit to be gained by individual stakeholders. Common purpose for these partnerships would address improved health for the community and depend on the identification of effective strategies that get to that overall goal. Those strategies would need to consider the particular state of health and availability of resources in each community.

5. Resources, including required skills, financial resources, and infrastructures, need to be identified.

6. Collective and in-kind evidence-based interventions that are directed at the overall purpose of improving community health and that are consistent with

the identified community health improvement strategies must be established and implemented collectively and in each sector by the partners.

7. Economic incentives need to be identified to shape collective and individual stakeholder actions that are consistent with the overall purpose of improved community health and with the identified community health improvement strategies.

8. The state of health in each community needs to be assessed and monitored on an ongoing basis to inform the efforts of the community health partnership. The effectiveness of the community health improvement strategies and the progress of the evidence-informed interventions need to be measured and assessed.

9. The lessons learned from each cycle of effort must be incorporated into the continuous redesign and improvement of the community business model for health improvement.

Successful community health business models across the country will also require the commitment, supportive policies, and infrastructures of state, regional, and federal levels of government to assign the appropriate national context to the importance of health improvement, provide incentives for that improvement in communities, and provide information against which a community may evaluate its success relative to other communities.

POPULATION HEALTH DEFINED, AND THE TRIPLE AIM

While healthcare organizations have as their core responsibility to improve population health through the delivery of clinical services, they can also work beyond this core mission to address other determinants of health. The past five years have seen the evolution of the Triple Aim, first articulated by Donald M. Berwick, MD; Thomas W. Nolan, PhD; and John Whittington when Berwick was CEO of the Institute for Healthcare Improvement (Berwick, Nolan, and Whittington 2008) and later adapted for the National Quality Strategy when Berwick was administrator of the Centers for Medicare & Medicaid Services (HHS 2011). (The main difference between the two versions is that the Triple Aim proposes that improvement initiatives pursue a broad system of linked goals—the improvement of individual experience of care, the improvement of the health of populations, and the reduction of per capita cost of care for populations—whereas the three aims of the National Quality Strategy are better care, healthy people and communities, and affordable care.)

The Triple Aim is one of the leading contemporary forces for population health change in the United States. Not only does it motivate healthcare systems to focus on the two healthcare goals of reduced costs and improved care experience, but it also includes improved population health as the third leg of the triangle. However, this third aim is far from fully understood or developed, either conceptually or in practice.

Most healthcare leaders are fully occupied with the more familiar goals of improving the experience of healthcare and reducing per capita cost of healthcare. Indeed, it would be foolish to diminish the importance of the model's clinical goals, which may represent our best short-term strategy to mobilize resources for improvement in the broader determinants of health. But the reality is that even major progress in these two areas over the next decade will not help us achieve our goals related to robust life expectancy and disparity reduction without explicit attention to improving health.

To achieve our broad population health goals, we need to understand and intervene across the whole spectrum of determinants, not just healthcare. However, this requirement is not clearly communicated by the Triple Aim model. Exhibit 2 compares the Triple Aim model with a broader model of population health taken from the MATCH/County Health Rankings project at the University of Wisconsin–Madison School of Medicine and Public Health (Kindig 2011b).

As the exhibit shows, the two lightly shaded legs of the Triple Aim stool (bottom of triangle) relate only to a single determinant, healthcare. The third component is titled "population health," but it is not clearly defined. We think it is important that the population health part of the Triple Aim model be clarified to convey that population health outcomes (among populations or individuals) are influenced by multiple determinants,

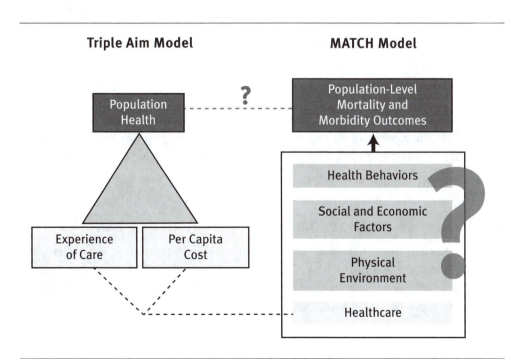

Triple Aim Model   **MATCH Model**

EXHIBIT 2
Comparison of the Triple Aim and MATCH Models

most of which are beyond the scope of healthcare delivery (the boxes on the right-hand side of Exhibit 2 accompanied by the large question mark).

The Institute of Medicine's (IOM) Roundtable on Population Health Improvement, which we co-chair (IOM 2011a), uses the following definition of *population health* to guide its work: "the health outcomes of a group of individuals, including the distribution of such outcomes within the group" (Kindig and Stoddart 2003). While not a part of the definition itself, it is understood that such population health outcomes are the product of multiple determinants of health, including medical care, public health, genetics, behaviors, social factors, and environmental factors.

The Roundtable definition goes on to say the following:

> [W]e recognize that this term is currently being used by some health care organizations to describe the clinical, often chronic disease, outcomes of patients enrolled in a given health plan. Certainly an enrolled patient group can be thought of and managed as a population, but defining population health solely in terms of clinical populations can draw attention away from the critical role that non-clinical factors such as education and income play in producing health.

Jacobson and Teutsch (2013) recommend that "current use of the abbreviated phrase *population health* should be abandoned and replaced by the phrase *total population health.*" They state that "this will avoid confusion as the clinical care system moves rather swiftly toward measuring the health of the subpopulations they serve. Geopolitical areas rather than simply geographic areas are recommended when measuring total population health since funding decisions and regulations are inherently political in nature" (Jacobson and Teutsch 2013).

The IOM Roundtable further observes that (IOM 2011a)

> at the current time there is variation in which concept or definition Triple Aim practices use. . . . [W]hile many embrace a population health or population medicine perspective, a few are striving towards a geographic regional emphasis moving towards a population health definition.

REACHING BEYOND CORE MISSION: A HEALTHCARE EXAMPLE

Stakeholders need to evaluate their capabilities and opportunities in order to form partnerships in addressing a broad array of health determinants. Gaining experience within their own organization prepares stakeholders for eventual participation in fully established community partnerships based on the community health business model.

One healthcare stakeholder serves as an example by engaging in population health improvement in an expanded way, going beyond its core mission of healthcare delivery and, in partnership with others, addresses additional determinants of health.

HealthPartners, a 1.4 million member, consumer-governed, nonprofit integrated health system in Minnesota, began to discuss such partnerships during its 2010 formal strategic planning as goals and objectives were being established for 2014 (Isham et al. 2013). Through these initial preparations, the HealthPartners board of directors became aware that to achieve its mission—"To improve health and well-being in partnership with our members, patients and community"—much more than excellent clinical care would be required. Using the population health model from the University of Wisconsin (which estimates that clinical care contributes 20 percent of the total impact on health outcomes, health behaviors 30 percent, social and economic factors 40 percent, and the physical environment 10 percent; see Exhibit 1), one of us (GI) worked with HealthPartners' staff and board members to define the relationship of various determinant categories to the organization's mission, existing capabilities, and degree of control over outcomes.

The HealthPartners board understood that all four categories were important to its stated overall mission. However, its members recognized that HealthPartners' existing capabilities and degree of control were more robust in clinical care, it shared control with public health for health behaviors, and it had less robust capabilities and control compared to those of other actors for socioeconomic and environmental factors. It followed that HealthPartners would have to execute well in clinical care, partner effectively with public health in modifying health behaviors, and be an effective partner with other stakeholders in community efforts to address socioeconomic and environmental determinants of health. This paradigm was new territory for some HealthPartners board members; they observed during this process that "we are not the public health department" and we "can't be everything to everyone," and directed that HealthPartners "find our niche" given the organization's capabilities and priorities and find ways to partner with others in the community to improve health.

The board and staff then arrayed the existing HealthPartners community initiatives in the four determinant categories (Exhibit 3) for the purpose of setting priorities among existing and new activities for 2010–2014.

A group of internal experts in public health was convened and interviews were conducted with community leaders to learn more about needs and opportunities. As a result, for example, HealthPartners created a set of materials and tools to promote healthy eating for schools, workplaces, and individual consumers. It was determined that these existing assets could be deployed more broadly in partnership with community-based organizations and schools. State and public health data were also reviewed, and HealthPartners staff participated in many local and state planning activities, obtaining a sound knowledge of

EXHIBIT 3
HealthPartners
Health Driver
Program

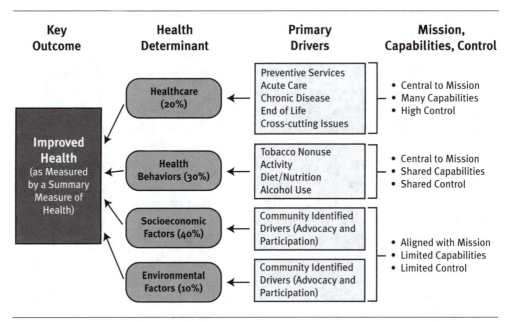

SOURCE: Adapted from G. Isham and D. Zimmerman, presentation, HealthPartners Board of Directors Retreat, October 2010.

community health priorities. Areas were prioritized for consideration by matching the best assets of HealthPartners with the highest need.

BEYOND HEALTHCARE ORGANIZATIONS TO OTHER COMMUNITY SECTORS

Which organizations should lead in developing the community business model? A collection of background essays on population health partnerships published in a special issue of *Preventing Chronic Disease* (Shortell 2010; Bailey 2010) indicated that, in some communities, leadership may come from the healthcare sector, and in others, it may come from public health entities, businesses, or community organizations such as the local United Way.

The HealthPartners approach offers one example of how a multisectoral community business model partnership can evolve as each organizational sector begins to commit resources and to take action both within its control and with others where partners are needed. Wherever a population health initiative begins, the partnership process will likely start with sectors whose links to mission and health are relatively straightforward, and it will eventually evolve to include sectors such as agriculture and transportation, where the health impact is less direct.

As demonstrated by HealthPartners, motivated and committed leaders are critical, and they need to recruit appropriate partners with the skills and resources to achieve community priorities. Thus, leaders must have a sophisticated understanding of how health objectives are important not only to the community but also to individual organizations so that individual and community business models work synergistically.

How would such effective partnerships develop? One possibility is by way of the status quo, where each sector makes uncoordinated investments to optimize its own goals, which may or may not include population health improvement. We have ample evidence to show that under this current situation, few—if any—communities are as healthy as they could be.

Another option is to garner adequate accountability by one sector taking lead responsibility for population health improvement, using informal or formal authority to ensure that others play their roles. While this approach may work in some places, in others it may result in conflict or have limited effectiveness. Some concerns related to this approach are that healthcare organizations may overemphasize biomedical approaches, that governmental public health is too underresourced for even its critical traditional functions, and that business time and energy might be challenged by competing goals.

If such concerns manifest themselves, in at least some locations it might be necessary to develop a strong and neutral cross-sectoral coordinating entity or mechanism at the helm. The outside border in Exhibit 4 illustrates this mechanism as a super–health integrator (Kindig 2010).

With appropriate financial resources and authority, such an integrator could align investments and activities across the multiple sectors, which would affect population health

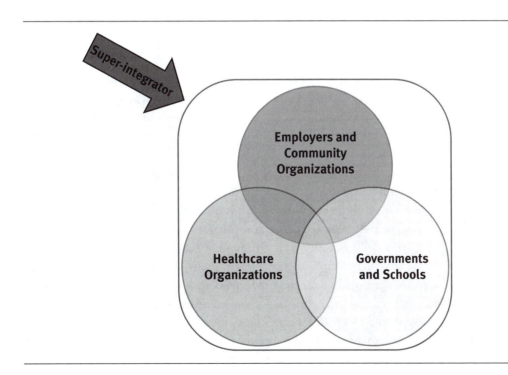

EXHIBIT 4
Super-integrator
Model

factors, such as healthcare, public health, schools, employers, and community organizations (Chang 2012).

To our knowledge, no such mechanism has been fully developed, although pieces exist in many healthy community partnerships. Such an entity likely would not be governmental or corporate, but would certainly need active public- and private-sector involvement. And, as noted, it would need some authority and financial resources to do its work. Such integrators, outcome trusts (Kindig 1997), or accountable health communities (Magnan et al. 2012) might draw on the principles of social entrepreneurship by emphasizing strategic partnerships and leveraging resources to raise levels of performance and accountability. The integrator role in some communities might be played by the local United Way, which has as its three goals health, education, and income and has considerable experience with the corporate community.

We are not naïve about the potential challenges such nontraditional structures pose, but addressing the multiple determinants of population health to optimize our communities' well-being will almost certainly require some form of coordinating authority.

INCENTIVES AND RESOURCES FOR A COMMUNITY PARTNERSHIP BUSINESS MODEL

However such cross-sector business models evolve, new incentives and resources are needed to make the models deliver results.

INCENTIVES

As outlined in another collection of population health essays on incentives featured in a special issue of *Preventing Chronic Disease* (McGinnis 2010), while *moral incentives*, framed as either the right thing to do or corporate social responsibility, can be important motivators to be celebrated, they will not likely alone deliver the performance needed for improving health outcomes.

In some instances, *regulatory incentives,* such as laws requiring seat belt use in vehicles and limiting smoking in public spaces, are appropriate. However, such mandates are often viewed as coercion and can be controversial. It is therefore unlikely that population health objectives will be fully achieved through regulation.

Steady progress will primarily come through stronger *remunerative* or *financial incentives,* whereby material rewards accrue to individuals or organizations in exchange for acting in a particular way. But on the other hand, it is probable that all three types of incentives will be needed to incite broad action and investment to allow a community health business model to develop and thrive. Good intentions will not be adequate—each sector must see how improving population health contributes to its own primary mission, in the form of productive employees for business, and in the form of students equipped to learn for educators. Each sector must also see economic alignment of its business model with the community health business model.

RESOURCES

There is no doubt that new or realigned resources will be required if our population health improvement efforts are to be accelerated. Where can such resources come from in these times when both public and private sectors are facing economic pressure? We suggest five major opportunities for identifying new or reallocating existing resources to bring community health business models alive.

1. Capture Funding from Reduction of Ineffective Healthcare Spending

It is now widely accepted that the United States delivers less health for the dollars invested in healthcare than any other developed nation (IOM 2013). Governmental and business leaders are calling for significant efficiencies to keep public programs healthy and improve corporate competitiveness. Many experts assert that as much as 25 percent of all healthcare expenditures are for services considered to be ineffective. Another recent estimate of such a "health dividend" available from improved effectiveness is $750 billion annually (McCullough et al. 2012).

While challenging, capturing these dollars for reinvestment in more effective programs and policies within and outside of healthcare should be a high priority for both public- and private-sector leaders. Consideration should be given to setting aside a community share from savings anticipated under the implementation of accountable care organizations, which are designed to provide higher-quality care in an efficient manner (Shortell 2013). The Center for Medicare & Medicaid Innovation, part of the Centers for Medicare & Medicaid Services, is devoting resources to population health; its Health Care Innovation Awards program includes promising population health initiatives in asthma and diabetes treatment and in efforts to integrate community-based resources, public health, and clinical services (Center for Medicare & Medicaid Innovation 2012). In addition, the State Innovation Models Initiative includes a major focus on community-based population health initiatives in both its design and testing phases. These demonstrations could lead to policy approaches that result in additional investment from within healthcare into community health.

In addition, as uncompensated care burdens are minimized under healthcare reform, community benefit resources required by the Internal Revenue Service for non-profit hospital tax-exempt status might be redirected from charity care and unreimbursed Medicaid to broad health-promoting investments (Young et al. 2013; CBO 2006; Bakken and Kindig 2012). This amount is considerable; as of 2002, the only year ever examined, the national value of this tax exemption was $12.2 billion, and current estimates project a much higher amount (Bostic et al. 2012).

2. Better Return on Investment from Policies and Programs Outside of Healthcare

Savings from healthcare alone will not be adequate to improve population health outcomes. Increased attention is being paid to "health in all" policies in non–medical care sectors such as housing, agriculture, and education, which are defined as those policies that have a primary impact in a nonhealthcare sector but often have secondary health-promoting features. For example, a new US Department of Housing and Urban Development demonstration project awards rental assistance subsidies to state housing agencies or other nonprofits that partner with state health and human services and Medicaid agencies (Bostic et al. 2012). The federal cabinet–level Public Health and Prevention Council, chaired by the US surgeon general and guided by the Office of the Surgeon General's National Prevention Strategy, also presents a groundbreaking occasion to identify and encourage such opportunities because of the participation of high-profile cabinet-level officials in its work (Office of the Surgeon General 2011).

Current policies can also be evaluated for increased health promotion. For example, Baxter (2010) observes that physical education and nutritional content of food in schools are covered in school wellness policies required by the Child Nutrition Act and by many state laws, but "without local school champions and active parental involvement, good intentions often have been undercut by failed execution or compromised by competition for space in the school day for other subjects."

3. Strengthen Governmental Funding for Population Health Improvement at All Levels

While federal, state, and local budgets are currently stressed, public health and prevention efforts deserve serious attention as the economy recovers. Prevention expenditures are below demonstrated cost-effective levels in classic prevention investments (Trust for America's Health 2008). Also, considerable variation is seen across states and counties for essential services that are taken for granted by many of us, including the accessibility of food, environmental quality, and infectious and chronic disease control. Government funding can play a key role in allowing local public health agencies to carry out their core functions as well as actively contributing to the types of community partnerships envisioned here.

Specifically, a 2012 IOM report recommends setting national targets for cost reduction and improvement in life expectancy, establishing a consistent cost accounting system for public health agencies to provide reliable cost data, doubling the investment in governmental public health from $12 billion to $24 billion, ensuring that all public health departments provide a minimum package of public health services, and raising these resources through a healthcare transaction tax (IOM 2012). It should be noted, however, that these resources are only those needed for governmental public health and do not include investments required in other sectors for other determinants.

4. Focus on Philanthropy

Many private foundations, such as the California Endowment and the Robert Wood Johnson Foundation, are increasingly focused on developing comprehensive neighborhood pilot strategies for health improvement. Similarly, community social service agencies can play—and are playing—increasingly critical organizational and financial roles in catalyzing health business models at the community level. Part of the mission of United Way Worldwide, for example, is to "galvanize and connect . . . individuals, businesses, non-profit organizations and governments [to] create long-term social change that produces healthy, well-educated and financially-stable individuals and families." Some communities have historical patterns of substantial philanthropy that could be emulated elsewhere.

5. Engage Corporate Business Leaders

Employers have a rich history of philanthropy, but they also have a stake in a healthy and productive future workforce. The National Business Coalition on Health, a nonprofit, purchaser-led group, is just one example of business leaders encouraging partnerships between businesses and other local stakeholders (Webber and Mercure 2010). As noted earlier, Porter and Kramer (2011) argue for social responsibility as a business imperative; for businesses to succeed, they must create shared social value.

The involvement of business with healthcare and public health is often focused on reducing healthcare costs and improving employee productivity (Baicker, Cutler, and Song 2010). As important as these factors are, we believe that many other factors contribute to better health, providing a strong rationale for an even wider role for business in making the communities in which they operate healthier. This role can be rooted in core business objectives far beyond corporate social responsibility. According to Andrew Webber, former president and CEO of the National Business Coalition on Health, "Business leaders must understand that an employer can do everything right to influence the health and productivity of its workforce at the worksite, but if that same workforce lives in unhealthy communities, employer investments can be seriously compromised" (Webber and Mercure 2010).

Better community health can contribute to the bottom line in many ways beyond reducing healthcare costs. Catherine Baase, MD, global director of health services at the Dow Chemical Company, has identified the following benefits of business involvement: attracting and retaining talent, engaging employees, supporting human performance, ensuring personal safety, supporting manufacturing and service reliability, ensuring sustainability, and managing brand reputation (Kindig, Isham, and Siemering 2013).

"WHERE WOULD YOU PUT THE MONEY?" INFORMING COST-EFFECTIVE INVESTMENT

Better evidence is needed to inform cost-effective investment. While we argue for the need for a regular, sustainable revenue stream to support population health improvement, we have not directly addressed the question of how these dollars should be allocated. One of the authors of the important Evans-Stoddart population field model notes in his 2003 *American Journal of Public Health* article that "redirecting resources means redirecting someone's income. . . . [M]ost students of population health cannot confidently answer the question . . . well, where would you put the money?" (Evans and Stoddart 2003).

This statement echoes two earlier quotes. The first, by Victor Fuchs in 1974, is as follows:

> How much, then, should go for medical care and how much for other programs affecting health, such as pollution control, fluoridation of water, accident prevention and the like. There is no simple answer, partly because the question has rarely been explicitly asked.

The second is one of our own, from a 1996 Association for Health Services Research presidential address (Kindig 1999):

> Now that we are in a time when attention is turning to fundamental health outcomes, when performance and value purchasing are becoming discussed by business coalitions, when there is serious discussion of a new connection between medicine and public health, we find that our research community has not invested nearly enough in the knowledge and understanding we need to guide policy.

Why don't we know more precisely what to recommend to policymakers to close these gaps? Can't we simply link the huge variation in health outcomes we see across states and communities to financial and nonfinancial policy investments over time? Why have we not simply estimated community level, per capita policy, and programmatic investment in each health factor area (health behaviors, clinical care, social and economic factors, and the physical environment) to derive a base level of investment needed to achieve health benchmarks (Kindig and Mullahy 2010)?

Some limited national- and state-level research and policy analysis has been conducted on this question. The Trust for America's Health estimated in 2008 that investing $10 per person per year in proven community-based programs to increase physical activity, improve nutrition, and prevent smoking could save the United States more than $16 billion annually within five years. In 2009, Kim and Jennings found that at the state level more generous education spending, progressive tax systems, and more lenient welfare program rules help to improve population health. However, the magnitude of the effects was quite small, most likely because using the state as the unit of analysis masks much of the important variation in outcomes and investments at local levels. In cross-national analysis, Bradley and colleagues (2011) argue that an important reason for the poor performance of the US health system is the relative proportion of nonhealthcare social services spending to health services spending; in other developed countries it is 2.00 to 1, whereas in the United States it is 0.91 to 1.

What is wrong here? It is true that going beyond simply describing differences to finding causal pathways is extremely complicated. Methods and data sets to explore these relationships are limited, and so far few studies even show associations of factors producing health disparities—even fewer indicate the relative cost-effectiveness of policies across determinants such as healthcare and behaviors and the social determinants of health.

In addition, little guidance is available because of the lack of comparable investment information across small units of population, such as communities and counties. Tim Casper and I (DAK) examined the availability of such data in a sample of Wisconsin counties for per capita expenditures in select categories of healthcare, public health, human services, income support, job development, and education. We found that even this well-resourced state is challenged by the difficulty in locating usable data, a lack of resources among public agencies to upgrade information technology systems for making data more usable and accessible to the public, and a lack of enterprise-wide coordination and geographic detail in data collection efforts (Casper and Kindig 2012).

While waiting for such improved evidence, an intermediate goal could be to increase investment in public health to make available the minimum package of public health services, as recommended earlier, and to create packages of evidence-based policy options across all determinants that are tailored to individual communities (Kindig 2011a). For example, some communities have good healthcare access and quality while their attention to social and environmental factors is underdeveloped. Enormous variation is seen across the country in such profiles, but it is likely that a reasonable number of representative situations exist for most communities and counties to reference. For each profile, using the best evidence available from sources such as the MATCH What Works (County Health Rankings 2013c) and the Centers for Disease Control and Prevention's "Guide to Community Preventive Services" (Epidemiology Program Office 2002), a set of investment priorities could be developed that covers all the determinants of health. It would be as broad as the global evidence allows but would be tailored to a community's strengths and weaknesses. Options for improving behaviors such as smoking would not be as highly suggested for places already doing well in this factor. The packages would not be prescriptive, but merely a menu of the investments likely to produce the best health outcome improvement. Where possible, options would include the strength of public- and private-sector policies beyond dollar investment in specific programs.

As with most initiatives, the initial set of policy packages would not be the ideal set, for a variety of reasons. We still have incomplete evidence of effectiveness of different programs and policies, particularly regarding cost-effectiveness beyond effectiveness itself. It is not clear which level of investment in a particular determinant or factor is optimal, or where diminishing return sets in and when resources should be moved to other factors. We are limited in evidence for different types of outcomes, particularly disparity reduction.

However, we should not let the perfect be the enemy of the good. A beginning set would be extremely helpful to guide the work in many places where discussions are taking place regarding improving the health of their communities. It would help ensure that local passion and commitment is channeled in an evidence-based direction while preserving autonomy and sensitivity to community preferences.

Next Steps

The approach we outline here is a departure from much current policy and management practice. But new models are needed to drive action—not just thinking—to address the enormous challenge of improving population health. We believe that a community business model that involves all sectors in partnership can function as a road map. We recommend the following next steps to do so.

First, public- and private-sector policymakers should stimulate conversations and efforts to better understand the specific opportunities for improvement within each segment of society. As in the HealthPartners example, care should be taken to identify those improvement opportunities that fall within the sectors' primary control; those not under primary control should move to multisectoral partnerships.

Policymakers should then use these perspectives to make the business case for population health improvement and the resources and policies each type of community actor requires through its national networks and directly to leaders in each sector. For example, healthcare leaders could work with the National Quality Forum and the Institute for Healthcare Improvement to improve outcomes in healthcare, a determinant that they directly control, while reducing total expenditures. They must think beyond healthcare to health and to achieving it through broad community partnerships.

Similarly, business leaders could turn to the Business Roundtable or local chambers of commerce to develop efforts to improve workforce wellness, productivity, and health directly while looking beyond their workforces for ways in which their communities can be healthier. Public health leaders might focus on national public health associations as well as the National Association of Counties (because local public health agencies are often located within the county structure) to find more effective and efficient ways to provide essential public health services while making information available to and engaging partners in the private and public sectors. United Way Worldwide could continue to work toward ensuring that its national vision is increasingly recognized at local levels and highlight examples where local United Way agencies are providing multisectoral leadership.

Finally, foundations and government should collaborate to develop a catalogue of cost-effective health-in-all policies in sectors beyond health, which could be reinforced by financial or regulatory incentives discussed earlier. They should also seek out and disseminate effective examples of work currently being done in communities, as the Robert Wood

Johnson Roadmaps to Health Prize (County Health Rankings 2013b) and the California Endowment (2013) Building Healthy Communities programs are doing. Benchmarks of the minimal and optimal cross-sectoral investments should be developed and promoted.

While we applaud continuing calls to improve health and reduce disparities, progress will require a much more robust incentive and business model strategy than has been the practice to date. Our hope is that the ideas presented here will help to catalyze a collective multisectoral response to this critical social and economic challenge.

ACKNOWLEDGMENTS

We acknowledge the helpful critique of Jo Ivey Boufford, Michael McGinnis, Mary Pittman, Andrew Webber, Lisa Richer, Stephanie Robert, Elizabeth Rigby, and Kirstin Siemering. This article was supported in part by the MATCH grant to the University of Wisconsin Population Health Institute from the Robert Wood Johnson Foundation.

REFERENCES

Baicker, K., D. Cutler, and Z. Song. 2010. "Workplace Wellness Programs Can Generate Savings." *Health Affairs* 29 (2): 304–11.

Bailey, S. B. C. 2010. "Focusing on Solid Partnerships Across Multiple Sectors for Population Health Improvement." *Preventing Chronic Disease* 7 (6): A115.

Bakken, E., and D. Kindig. 2012. "Is Hospital Community Benefit Charity Care?" *WMJ* 111 (5): 215–19.

Baxter, R. J. 2010. "Making Better Use of the Policies and Funding We Already Have." *Preventing Chronic Disease* 7 (5): A97.

Berwick, D., T. Nolan, and J. Whittington. 2008. "The Triple Aim: Care, Health, and Cost." *Health Affairs* 27: 759–69.

Bostic, R., R. Thornton, E. Rudd, and M. Sternhal. 2012. "Health in All Policies: The Role of the US Department of Housing and Urban Development." *Health Affairs* 31 (9): 2130–36.

Bradley, E. H., B. R. Elkins, J. Herrin, and B. Elbel. 2011. "Health and Social Services Expenditures: Associations with Health Outcomes." *BMJ Quality & Safety* 20 (10): 826–31.

Casper, T., and D. A. Kindig. 2012. "Are Community-Level Financial Data Adequate to Assess Population Health Investments?" *Preventing Chronic Disease* 9: E136.

California Endowment. 2013. "The California Endowment: Building Healthy Communities." www.calendow.org/healthycommunities.

Center for Medicare & Medicaid Innovation. 2012. "State Innovation Models Initiative: General Information." http://innovation.cms.gov/initiatives/state-innovations/.

Chang, D. 2012. "What Does a Population Health Integrator Do?" www.improvingpopulationhealth.org/blog/2012/05/what-does-a-population-health-integrator-do.html.

Congressional Budget Office (CBO). 2006. "Nonprofit Hospitals and Tax Arbitrage." www.cbo.gov/sites/default/files/cbofiles/ftpdocs/76xx/doc7696/12-06-hospitaltax.pdf.

County Health Rankings. 2013a. "Our Approach." www.countyhealthrankings.org/our-approach.

———. 2013b. "RWJF Roadmaps to Health Prize." www.countyhealthrankings.org/roadmaps/prize.

———. 2013c. "What Works for Health." www.countyhealthrankings.org/roadmaps/what-works-for-health.

———. 2011. "Find Health Ratings for Your State and County." www.countyhealthrankings.org.

Epidemiology Program Office, Centers for Disease Control and Prevention. 2002. "The Guide to Community Preventive Services Website: www.thecommunityguide.org." www.cdc.gov/epo/communityguide.htm.

Evans, R., and G. Stoddart. 2003. "Consuming Research, Producing Policy?" *American Journal of Public Health* 93 (3): 371–79.

Fuchs, V. 1974. *Who Shall Live? Health, Economics, and Social Choice.* New York: Basic.

Institute of Medicine. 2013. *U.S. Health in International Perspective: Shorter Lives, Poorer Health.* Washington, DC: National Academies Press.

———. 2012. *For the Public's Health: Investing in a Healthier Future.* Washington, DC: National Academies Press.

———. 2011a. "Activity: Roundtable on Population Health Improvement." www.iom.edu/Activities/PublicHealth/PopulationHealthImprovementRT.aspx.

————. 2011b. *For the Public's Health: The Role of Measurement in Action and Account-ability*. Washington, DC: National Academies Press.

Isham, G., D. Zimmerman, D. Kindig, and G. Hornseth. 2013. "HealthPartners Adopts Community Business Model to Deepen Focus on Nonclinical Factors of Health Outcomes." *Health Affairs* 32 (8): 1446–52.

Jacobson, D., and S. Teutsch. 2013. *An Environmental Scan of Integrated Approaches for Defining and Measuring Total Population Health by the Clinical Care System, the Government Public Health System, and Stakeholder Organizations*. Washington, DC: National Quality Forum.

Johnson, M. W., C. M. Christensen, and K. Henning. 2011. *Reinventing Your Business Model*. In *Harvard Business Review on Rebuilding Your Business Model*. Boston: Harvard Business Review Press.

Kania, J., and M. Kramer. 2011. "Collective Impact." *Stanford Social Innovation Review* 64 (Winter): 36–41.

Kim, A., and E. T. Jennings. 2009. "Effects of US States' Social Welfare Systems on Population Health." *Policy Studies Journal* 37 (4): 745–67.

Kindig, D. A. 2011a. "Locally Customized Population Health Policy Packages?" Blog post. www.improvingpopulationhealth.org/blog/2011/08/locally-customized-population-health-policy-packages.html.

————. 2011b. "Unpacking the Triple Aim Model." Blog post. www.improvingpopulation-health.org/blog/2011/01/unpacking_triple_aim.html.

————. 2010. "Do We Need a Super Integrator?" Blog post. www.improvingpopulation-health.org/blog/2010/09/super_integrator.html.

————. 1999 "Beyond Health Services Research." *Health Services Research* 34 (1, Pt. II): 205–14.

————. 1997. *Purchasing Population Health: Paying for Results*. Ann Arbor, MI: University of Michigan Press.

Kindig, D., and E. Cheng. 2013. "Even as Mortality Fell in Most US Counties, Female Mortality Nonetheless Rose in 42.8 Percent of Counties from 1992 to 2006." *Health Affairs* 32 (3): 451–58.

Kindig, D., G. Isham, and K. Q. Siemering. 2013. "The Business Role in Improving Health: Beyond Social Responsibility." Discussion paper, Institute of Medicine. http://iom.edu/Global/Perspectives/2013/TheBusinessRole.

Kindig, D., and J. Mullahy. 2010. "Comparative Effectiveness—of What? Evaluating Strategies to Improve Population Health." *Journal of the American Medical Association* 304 (8): 901–2.

Kindig, D., and G. Stoddart. 2003. "What Is Population Health?" *American Journal of Public Health* 93 (3): 380–83.

Kulkarni, S. C., A. Levin-Rector, M. Ezzati, and C. J. L. Murray. 2011. "Falling Behind: Life Expectancy in US Counties from 2000 to 2007." *Population Health Metrics* 9 (1): 16.

Magnan, S., E. Fisher, D. Kindig, G. Isham, D. Wood, M. Eustis, C. Backstrom, and S. Leitz. 2012. "Achieving Accountability for Health and Health Care." *Minnesota Medicine* (November): 37–39.

McCullough, J. C., F. J. Zimmerman, J. E. Fielding, and S. M. Teutsch. 2012. "A Health Dividend for America: The Opportunity Cost of Excess Medical Expenditures." *American Journal of Preventive Medicine* 43 (6): 650–54.

McGinnis, J. M. 2010. "Observations on Incentives to Improve Population Health." *Preventing Chronic Disease* 7 (5): A92.

Office of the Surgeon General, US Department of Health and Human Services. 2011. *National Prevention Strategy: America's Plan for Better Health and Wellness*. www.surgeongeneral.gov/initiatives/prevention/strategy/.

Pittman, M. A. 2010. "Multisectoral Lessons from Healthy Communities." *Preventing Chronic Disease* 7 (6): A117.

Porter, M. E., and M. R. Kramer. 2011. "Creating Shared Value: How to Reinvent Capitalism—and Unleash a Wave of Innovation and Growth." *Harvard Business Review* 89 (1–2): 1–17.

Shortell, S. 2013. "Bridging the Divide Between Health and Health Care." *New England Journal of Medicine* 309 (11): 1121–22.

———. 2010. "Challenges and Opportunities for Population Health Partnerships." *Preventing Chronic Disease* 7 (6): A114.

Trust for America's Health. 2008. *Prevention for a Healthier America: Investments in Disease Prevention Yield Significant Savings, Stronger Communities*. www.healthyamericans.org/reports/prevention08/Prevention08.pdf.

Webber, A., and S. Mercure. 2010. "Improving Population Health: The Business Community Imperative." *Preventing Chronic Disease* 7 (6): A121.

Young, G., C. Chou, J. Alexander, S. Lee, and E. Raver. 2013. "Provision of Community Benefits by Tax-Exempt U.S. Hospitals." *New England Journal of Medicine* 368 (16): 1519–27.

US Department of Health and Human Services (HHS). 2011. "National Quality Strategy Will Promote Better Health, Quality Care for Americans." News release. www.hhs.gov/news/press/2011pres/03/20110321a.html.

CHRONIC DISEASE MANAGEMENT AND PRIMARY CARE

The Affordable Care Act (ACA) contains a number of policy initiatives that focus on improving care for patients with chronic disease. Chronic disease and disability management are important aspects of population health, as discussed in Chapter 3.

Chronic care comes with a high cost and high variability in treatment. Knowledge on best practices in chronic disease management has accumulated over the past 30 years, and the ACA contains many new policies that promote the application of this knowledge throughout the provider community.

Exhibit 4.1 illustrates the distribution of costs associated with the care of patients with chronic diseases. Note the high cost for people with three or more chronic conditions (89 percent). In addition, the costs of chronic disease care vary greatly throughout the United States (Exhibit 4.2).

THE CHRONIC CARE MODEL

Dr. Edward Wagner of the MacColl Institute for Healthcare Innovation, a leader in the improvement of chronic care, has developed one of the most widely accepted models for chronic disease management. The first important element of Wagner's model is population-based outreach, which ensures that all patients in need of chronic disease management receive it. Next, treatment plans are created that are sensitive to each patient's preferences. The most current evidence-based medicine is employed; this process is aided by clinical information systems with built-in decision support. The patient is encouraged to change risky behaviors and to manage himself better. The actual clinical visit changes in the Wagner model to allow more time for interaction between physicians and patients with complicated clinical issues. Visits for routine or specialized matters are delivered by other healthcare professionals (e.g., nurses, pharmacists, dieticians, lay health workers). Close follow-up supported by clinical information system registries and patient reminders is also characteristic of effective chronic disease management (Improving Chronic Illness Care 2014; Wagner 2000).

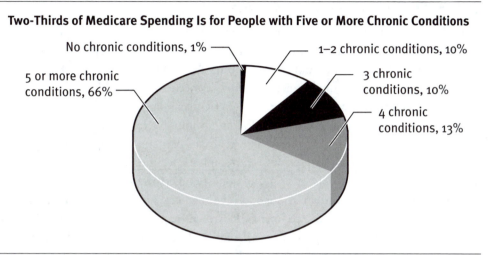

Two-Thirds of Medicare Spending Is for People with Five or More Chronic Conditions

No chronic conditions, 1%

1–2 chronic conditions, 10%

5 or more chronic conditions, 66%

3 chronic conditions, 10%

4 chronic conditions, 13%

Exhibit 4.1
Medicare Spending for Chronic Conditions

SOURCE: The Commonwealth Fund; data from G. Anderson and J. Horvath, *Chronic Conditions: Making the Case for Ongoing Care* (Baltimore, Md.: Partnership for Solutions, Dec. 2002). Used with permission.

Exhibit 4.2
Costs of Care for Medicare Beneficiaries with Multiple Chronic Conditions

		Average	10th Percentile	25th Percentile	75th Percentile	90th Percentile	90th to 10th	75th to 25th
All 3 Conditions	2001	$31,792	$20,960	$23,973	$37,879	$43,973	2.10	1.58
	2005	$38,004	$25,732	$29,936	$44,216	$53,019	2.06	1.48
Diabetes + Heart Failure	2001	$18,461	$12,747	$14,355	$20,592	$27,310	2.14	1.43
	2005	$23,056	$16,144	$18,649	$26,035	$32,199	1.99	1.40
Diabetes + COPD	2001	$13,188	$8,872	$10,304	$15,246	$18,024	2.03	1.48
	2005	$15,367	$11,317	$12,665	$17,180	$20,062	1.77	1.36
Heart Failure + COPD	2001	$22,415	$15,355	$17,312	$25,023	$32,732	2.13	1.45
	2005	$27,498	$19,787	$22,044	$31,709	$37,405	1.89	1.44

COPD = chronic obstructive pulmonary disease.

SOURCE: Commonwealth Fund National Scorecard on U.S. Health System Performance, 2008. Data from G. Anderson and R. Herbert, Johns Hopkins University analysis of Medicare Standard Analytical Files (SAF) 5% Inpatient Data. Used with permission.

THE HITECH ACT AND MEANINGFUL USE

Chronic disease management is information intensive and information dependent. The American Recovery and Reinvestment Act of 2009 (ARRA) includes the Health Information Technology for Economic and Clinical Health Act (HITECH Act), which established programs under Medicare and Medicaid to provide incentive payments for the "meaningful use" of certified electronic health records (EHR) technology.

The goals of the HITECH legislation are to improve healthcare outcomes, facilitate access to care, and simplify care. These goals are particularly important to patients with chronic disease. As regulations were contemplated for the payment of incentives for the installation of health information technology, two perspectives were apparent. Many vendors felt that technical specifications and requirements should be used to certify these new systems for federal incentive payments. However, many clinicians with experience in informatics felt that this new government incentive should only be paid if the EHR systems were used in a meaningful manner to improve patient care. This latter view prevailed. Therefore, the goals of HITECH will be met when the EHR is used in a meaningful way.

Three components of Stage I meaningful use are:

1. Use of a certified EHR in a meaningful manner, such as e-prescribing

2. Use of certified EHR technology for the exchange of health information (exchanging data with other providers of care or business partners, such as labs or pharmacies)

3. Use of certified EHR technology to submit clinical quality and other measures to the HHS

Thus, the first stage of meaningful use is capturing and sharing the data. Meaningful use Stage II involves using the technology in advanced clinical processes, and Stage III involves the meaningful use of an EHR in the context of improved healthcare outcomes. Glandon, Smaltz, and Slovensky (2013) provide a more detailed review of meaningful use and other important government policies related to the use of health information technology in **Reading 4A.** The meaningful use regulations are available at bit.ly/Reform4_1.

POLICIES TO SUPPORT CHRONIC CARE IN THE ACA

The designers of the ACA incorporated a number of tools that can be used to improve the quality of care for patients with chronic disease and for emergency care. These tools include:

- ◆ Comparative effectiveness research
- ◆ Medical homes
- ◆ Shared decision making

Another ACA tool for improved chronic care is the accountable care organization (ACO); because the ACO is more of a financial incentives-based tool, it is addressed in Chapter 6.

EXHIBIT 4.3

Healthcare Systems Map Highlighting Comparative Effectiveness Research and Healthcare Home

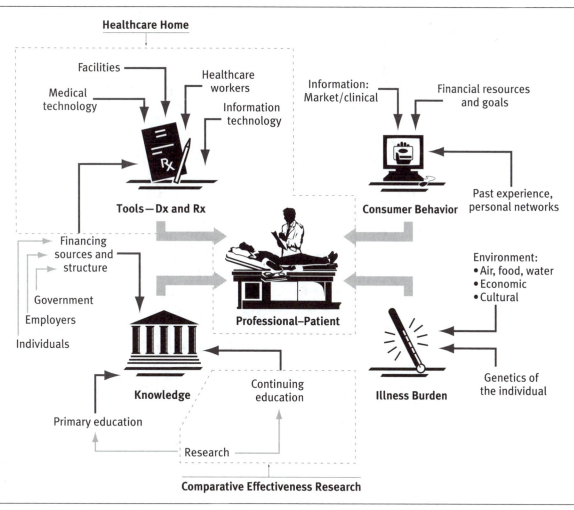

The system elements of comparative effectiveness research and the healthcare home can be located clearly on the healthcare systems map (Exhibit 4.3).

Jorna and Martin in **Reading 4B** provide the results of a recent survey of healthcare systems that are using population health principles and care coordination to improve their chronic disease management.

COMPARATIVE EFFECTIVENESS RESEARCH

The "product line" of American healthcare is immense. The ICD-9[1] contains a multitude of codes—currently more than 13,600 diagnosis codes and 3,700 procedure codes. ICD-10 will increase the number of codes significantly. In this mix of tools for diagnosis and treatment, many common clinical approaches have never been adequately tested as to their efficacy. Most medical researchers are not interested in routine healthcare.

To address this problem, the ACA and the ARRA establish and fund a nonprofit corporation called the Patient-Centered Outcomes Research Institute, or PCORI (ACA §6301, 6302): "The purpose of the Institute is to assist patients, clinicians, purchasers, and policymakers in making informed health decisions by advancing the quality and relevance of evidence concerning the manner in which diseases, disorders, and other health conditions can effectively and appropriately be prevented, diagnosed, treated, monitored, and managed through research and evidence synthesis that considers variations in patient subpopulations, and the dissemination findings with respect to the relative health outcomes, clinical effectiveness, and appropriateness of the medical treatments, and services" (from §6301).

The PCORI complements the work of the National Institutes of Health and the Agency for Healthcare Research and Quality (AHRQ)—both part of the US Department of Health and Human Services. One of AHRQ's responsibilities is to help users to incorporate these research findings into their clinical practice through the use of clinical decision support health information technology.

A major focus for the research topics addressed by the PCORI is chronic disease management. The PCORI can be accessed at bit.ly/Reform4_2.

THE MEDICAL HOME

The medical home (sometimes called the healthcare home) has emerged as an effective tool in the delivery of care to patients with chronic disease. The American Academy of Pediatrics (AAP COPP 1967) introduced the medical home concept in 1967; it then referred to a central location for archiving a child's medical record. In its 2002 policy statement, the AAP expanded the medical home concept to promote care that is accessible, continuous, comprehensive, family centered, coordinated, compassionate, and culturally effective. Because this concept now involves many additional types of health professionals, it has been renamed the healthcare home.

In 2007, the four major primary care associations (American Academy of Family Physicians [AAFP], American Academy of Pediatrics [AAP], American College of Physicians [ACP], and American Osteopathic Association [AOA]) developed a joint statement on the principles for the patient-centered medical home (AAFP 2007) that includes the following:

◆ *Personal physician:* Each patient has an ongoing relationship with a personal physician trained to provide first contact and continuous and comprehensive care.

◆ *Physician-directed medical practice:* The personal physician leads a team of individuals at the practice level who collectively take responsibility for the ongoing care of patients.

◆ *Whole person orientation:* The personal physician is responsible for providing for all the patient's healthcare needs or taking responsibility for appropriately arranging care with other qualified professionals. This includes care for all stages of life and involves acute care, chronic care, preventive services, and end-of-life care.

◆ *Care is coordinated and/or integrated:* Care is coordinated across all elements of the healthcare system (e.g., subspecialty care, hospitals, home health agencies, nursing homes) and the patient's community (e.g., family, public and private community-based services). Care is facilitated by registries, information technology, health information exchange, and other means to ensure that patients get the indicated care when and where they need and want it in a culturally and linguistically appropriate manner.

◆ *Quality and safety:* Quality and safety are hallmarks of the medical home, and evidence-based medicine is emphasized.

◆ *Enhanced access:* Care is facilitated through systems such as open scheduling and expanded hours, and communication between patients, their personal physicians, and practice staff.

◆ *Payment:* Payment appropriately recognizes the added value provided to patients who have a patient-centered medical home.

A recent study on the effectiveness of healthcare homes found three key components needed for success:

◆ individualized and intense caring for patients with chronic illness;

◆ efficient service provision; and

◆ careful selection of specialists (taking into consideration quality and cost).

By carefully implementing these aspects of care, the healthcare homes studied reduced the total cost of care by 15 percent and improved quality, and providers reported a "less frenetic clinical pace" (Milstein and Gilbertson 2009). The healthcare home as both a quality improvement and cost-containment vehicle is detailed in **Reading 4C**.

The ACA builds on this framework of care delivery and expands the concept to include teams of practitioners in addition to physicians. Section 2703 provides states with the authority to make payments for healthcare homes through their Medicaid systems. Each state will develop rules and payment systems to support the healthcare home; the joint principles mentioned in the previous list will likely be the basis for the regulatory framework.

Because primary care is delivered by small or solo practitioners in some regions of the United States, §3502 provides for the establishment of community health teams to support healthcare homes. These interdisciplinary teams will "collaborate with local primary care providers and existing State and community based resources to coordinate disease prevention, chronic disease management, transitioning between health care providers and settings and case management for patients, including children, with priority given to those amenable to prevention and with chronic diseases or conditions" (from §3502). The medical home is being tested by the Centers for Medicare & Medicaid Services under the demonstration authority (§3021), and updates can be found at bit.ly/Reform4_3.

Finally, Title V of the ACA has numerous provisions to increase the supply, quality, and distribution of primary care physicians and other health professionals. In addition, §5501 provides for increased Medicare payments for primary care; in 2013 all states must set their Medicaid rates of payment for primary care services at Medicare rates or higher. In **Reading 4D**, Barton provides overviews of the current definition of primary care and of the current supply and future demand.

SHARED DECISION MAKING

Patient engagement is a key feature of successful primary care and chronic disease management. The ACA provides a new tool for patient engagement: §3506, "Program to Facilitate Shared Decision Making." Shared decision making is a concept that effectively empowers patients and reduces unnecessary costs in the system. This section provides funding to create patient educational and decision-support materials and to disseminate these aids to providers and patients.

The focus of shared decision making is surgical services where no single treatment option is right or wrong; rather, the patient and caregivers consider whether one option or another is right for the patient. For example, among women with early-stage breast cancer, both mastectomy and lumpectomy followed by radiation yield similar mortality benefit. Many women have strong preferences for one or the other, so the quality of care extends beyond the surgeon's technical skills to the decision-making process.

Traditionally, patients have delegated treatment decisions to their physicians: The physician diagnoses the patient's illness, recommends treatment, and then the patient gives informed consent. Policymakers, in turn, have assumed that physicians' decisions reflect medical need and patient demand. However, the remarkable degree of variation in the utilization rates of discretionary surgery raises questions about these assumptions.

For example, Wennberg and colleagues (2007) found that in 2002 and 2003 among the 306 US Hospital Referral Regions (HRRs), the incidence of joint replacement for chronic arthritis of the hip or knee and of surgery for low-back pain varied 5.6-, 4.8-, and 5.9-fold, respectively, from the lowest to the highest region. The authors found that the pattern of variation was remarkably stable over time; for most common procedures, variation among regions was highly correlated with the pattern a decade before the study was completed.

Shared decision making is a tool that can be used to address this problem. Highly sophisticated and evidence-based patient decision aids inform the patient of the benefits and risks of a procedure. Trained health professionals counsel patients on use of the decision tools and support the patient's decision. Performance monitoring is also part of a shared decision making program.

Total system costs can be reduced dramatically through the use of shared decision making. A Cochrane review[2] identified trials of seven conditions commonly treated surgically among the Medicare population: arthritis of the hip and knee; low-back pain from a herniated disc; chest pain (stable angina); enlarged prostate (benign prostatic hypertrophy, or BPH); and early-stage prostate and breast cancers. The review documented that although the decision to have surgery following shared decision making (compared to control groups) varied from study to study, a 21 to 44 percent decline was typical. Patients in shared decision-making arms of the trials were better informed about treatment options and made choices more consistent with their values (Wennberg et al. 2007).

SUMMARY

Chronic disease is an important cost driver in the US healthcare system, and 89 percent of Medicare spending is for people with three or more chronic conditions. Fortunately, a chronic care model has been developed and tested that reduces costs and improves quality for patients with chronic disease.

The ACA (and the ARRA) legislate a number of policies to improve chronic care. The knowledge base for best approaches to the treatment of various chronic diseases increases with comparative effectiveness research. Funding for the acquisition and meaningful use of health information technology to care for chronic patients was included in the HITECH act. An increase in training and payment for primary care providers and the use of the healthcare home is also designed to improve chronic care. Shared decision making is a new tool that improves patient engagement and has been shown to dramatically lower costs in many situations.

NOTES

1. The ICD-9 system is a standardized classification of disease, injuries, and causes of death, by etiology and anatomic localization and codified into a six-digit number.

2. The Cochrane Collaboration, established in 1993, is an international network of people helping healthcare providers, policymakers, patients, and patient advocates, make well-informed decisions about human healthcare by preparing, updating, and promoting the accessibility of Cochrane Reviews: over 4,000 evidence-based medicine studies so far, published online in *The Cochrane Libra*.

APPLICATIONS: DISCUSSION AND RESEARCH

1. What is HIPAA? Why was it passed? What are the potential benefits to healthcare organizations to be gained by compliance with HIPAA standards? What are the potential drawbacks (Glandon, Smaltz, and Slovensky 2013; see **Reading 4A**)?

2. What is the HITECH Act? Why was it passed? What are the potential benefits to healthcare organizations to be gained by responding to the Act's incentives? What are the potential drawbacks (Glandon, Smaltz, and Slovensky 2013; see **Reading 4A**)?

3. Discuss some of the potential conflicts between a patient's right to privacy and information needed for public health and medical research (Glandon, Smaltz, and Slovensky 2013; see **Reading 4A**).

4. What concepts are important to information security policies and procedures? What effect does HIPAA have on healthcare organizations' policies and procedures? Are there any other laws that may affect them (Glandon, Smaltz, and Slovensky 2013; see **Reading 4A**)?

5. Review the PCORI website and examine the research projects they are currently funding. Identify those that have the most likelihood to affect costs in the healthcare system and provide a rationale.

6. What are some of the organizational and management challenges of creating a healthcare home? (Access library resources and search journals such as the *Journal of the American Medical Association*, *New England Journal of Medicine*, *Health Affairs*, *Family Practice Management*, *Annals of Internal Medicine*, or *Pediatrics* and search for "healthcare home.")

7. What other options are available to provide primary care beyond physicians? What are the advantages? Disadvantages? (Assume you have a common complaint [e.g. sore throat, back pain, or cough]. Use the Internet to try to obtain primary care either directly online or at a walk-in clinic. Then determine the advantages and disadvantages.)

8. What ethical issues arise in the use of shared decision making? (Interview doctors and other health professionals to obtain their viewpoints on this question. Be sure to interview both surgeons and their staffs and primary care practitioners.)

REFERENCES

American Academy of Family Physicians (AAFP). 2007. "Joint Principles of a Patient-Centered Medical Home Released by Organizations Representing More Than 300,000 Physicians." Published March 5. www.aafp.org/online/en/home/media/releases/2007/20070305pressrelease0.html.

American Academy of Pediatrics Council on Pediatric Practice (AAP COPP). 1967. *Standards of Child Health Care*. Elk Grove Village, IL: AAP.

Improving Chronic Illness Care. 2014. Accessed July 29. www.improvingchroniccare.org.

Milstein, A., and E. Gilbertson. 2009. "American Medical Home Runs." *Health Affairs* 28 (5): 1317.

Wagner, E. H. 2000. "The Role of Patient Care Teams in Chronic Disease Management." *British Medical Journal* 320 (7234): 569.

Wennberg, J. E., A. M. O'Connor, E. D. Collins, and J. N. Weinstein. 2007. "Extending the P4P Agenda, Part 1: How Medicare Can Improve Patient Decision Making and Reduce Unnecessary Care." *Health Affairs* 26 (6): 1564.

CHAPTER 4

ADDITIONAL READINGS

READING 4A

GOVERNMENT POLICY AND HEALTHCARE REFORM

Gerald L. Glandon, Detlev H. Smaltz, and Donna J. Slovensky

From *Information Systems for Healthcare Management*, 8th ed. (2013), Chapter 3, 51–79. Chicago: Health Administration Press.

LEARNING OBJECTIVES

1. Describe a justification for government intervention in business processes.

2. List five major types of government intervention into the healthcare business, and explain the need for government to invest in healthcare information management and healthcare information technology (HIT).

3. Describe the eight components of the administrative simplification portion of the Health Insurance Portability and Accountability Act.

4. Assess your organization's readiness for transactions and code set development.

5. Analyze why privacy and security are important and why HIT has a key role in protecting privacy and security.

6. Assess four key questions to answer in developing privacy policies.

7. Describe HIT leadership's role in responding to legislation.

OVERVIEW

Much has been written regarding the details of the federal, state, and local government policies that have direct and indirect influences on healthcare information technology (HIT) and its leadership in healthcare organizations (Blumenthal 2006; Feldstein 2001; Goldsmith, Blumenthal, and Rishel 2003; Kleinke 2005; Poon et al. 2006; Taylor et al. 2005). This chapter does not present an exhaustive list of those impacts. Its goal is to provide HIT leadership with the awareness of the potential effects of healthcare legislation on HIT business practices; the tools to identify and respond to current healthcare legislation; and the strategic vision to plan for future challenges that may arise from government interventions. The chapter has three sections:

1. *Government's role in HIT.* This section provides the justification for government intervention in business processes. Understanding why government gets involved will assist you in responding to legislation and anticipating future actions.

2. *Specific healthcare legislations.*

    a. Health Insurance Portability and Accountability Act (HIPAA) of 1996. This major set of legislative and administrative interventions has fundamentally changed HIT for the last decade and will likely change it in the future. It is a complex array of interventions that have been implemented in ways not fully anticipated when the legislation was passed in 1996. This section presents some basic policies and procedures designed to respond to select HIPAA requirements.

    b. American Recovery and Reinvestment Act's Health Information Technology for Economic and Clinical Health Act. This legislation arose from the economic crisis of 2007–2009 but became an enabler, nonetheless, of electronic health record adoption in the United States.

    c. Patient Protection and Affordable Care Act of 2010. This controversial health reform legislation is designed to expand coverage to the uninsured and to improve quality of care and provider accountability.

3. *HIT leadership roles.* The external environment and government have direct, indirect, and substantial roles in healthcare operations. Leaders must understand those roles today and anticipate roles in the future. This section presents an action plan for HIT leadership.

GOVERNMENT'S ROLE IN HIT

Three questions must be asked in assessing the role of government in HIT:

1. Why does the government (at any level) get involved in healthcare or any business practice? Is there justification for government intervention?

2. If yes, how much and what types of intervention are justified?

3. What triggers those interventions?

The easy answer to these questions is that the government recognizes the challenges that the healthcare field faces regarding cost, quality, and access to care (see Gauthier and Serber [2005]). Further, the government has an obligation to intervene to provide access to high-quality, affordable care to all residents.

Justification for Government Intervention

The generic argument for government intervention is that the marketplace does not perform its normal function of optimizing resource-production efficiency and resource-allocation decision making as classical economics theory suggests (Santerre and Neun 2004). As a result of the market's failure, government can—and some say should—intervene to fix the problem. Key reasons for intervention include problems with public goods, externalities, imperfect consumer information, and monopoly. Public goods are those that producers cannot easily exclude people from consuming, and consumption by one person does not reduce the availability for others to consume. A classic example is national defense, but medical research that leads to cures for disease is another. Externalities are costs or benefits related to a market action that parties not related to the transaction incur. For example, cigarette smoking may impose costs on those not involved in the decision to smoke. Imperfect information may give rise to government involvement in markets because people are concerned that profit-seeking businesses may take advantage of people's inability to make informed choices. In each of these cases, the market does not reliably provide the optimal quantity. (See Santerre and Neun [2004] for an extensive discussion of these issues.)

If the market fails to produce a good or service for any of these reasons, government is empowered to intervene in the public interest. Generally, the "fix" is to develop and implement policies that approximate what the market solution would generate, if possible. For healthcare, that intervention is justified because of asymmetric information between purchasers and providers and significant uncertainty about future need for services (Arrow 1963; Poterba 1996). However, some have argued that government interventions are designed to benefit those special interests that influence politicians rather than society as a whole (Blumenthal 2006; Feldstein 2001; Goldsmith, Blumenthal, and Rishel 2003; Kleinke 2005; Taylor et al. 2005).

Examples of the range of government intervention are included in Exhibit 3.1. Correcting externalities has been one of the major reasons for government intervention. HIPAA, described later in this chapter, can be considered an intervention to force a market solution that would not occur without direct government support. Funding for medical research is a more traditional example of this type of intervention and is briefly described as it relates to funding for HIT. The other categories in the exhibit are not directly relevant to this book but are still worthy of note.

Purpose	Government Initiative
Provide public goods	Funding of medical research
Correct for externalities	Tax on alcohol and cigarettes
Impose regulations	Federal Drug Administration
Enforce antitrust laws	Limit hospital mergers
Sponsor redistribution programs	Medicare and Medicaid
Operate public enterprises	Veterans Administration hospitals

EXHIBIT 3.1
Types of Government Market Intervention

SOURCE: Reprinted from Feldstein (2001). Used with permission from Health Administration Press, Chicago.

A significant amount of research in HIT has been funded by the federal government. A primary source of this funding for research and demonstration projects comes from the National Library of Medicine (NLM, www.nlm.nih.gov). The importance of the NLM to current initiatives and emerging features of HIT make it a major change agent. HIT leadership should be familiar with NLM funding priorities. Exhibit 3.2 presents the eight primary functions of the NLM. Assisting healthcare organizations with developing the data systems to support both their clinical operations and health services research is a major portion of NLM's charge. Using the justification for government intervention argument, the government funds these (and other) crucial activities because it believes that private organizations will not spend sufficiently on them. Further, the findings from these efforts will benefit the entire US healthcare system by enabling the development and testing of new technologies and infrastructure support.

GOVERNMENT INTERVENTION IN THE HEALTHCARE FIELD

For most industries, the government largely allows the market to determine costs, efficiency, quality, availability, and firm survival. With the exception of enforcing property rights and legal contracts, the government's role is minor.

Healthcare is different from other industries, however. The government gets involved in healthcare—and, by extension, HIT—because the government has a broad obligation to protect the health and welfare of the population. That obligation extends beyond ensuring that markets function and property rights are enforced (Feldstein 2001). Finding that the health of the population is at risk makes intervention to improve patient safety vital. Evidence that this risk is real comes from a series of prestigious studies, such as the Institute of Medicine's 1999 and 2001 reports. Further, published estimates that nearly 50 million people are uninsured and many more are underinsured (DeNavas-Walt,

Exhibit 3.2
Primary Functions
of the National
Library of Medicine

The National Library of Medicine

1. assists the advancement of medical and related sciences through the collection, dissemination, and exchange of information important to the progress of medicine and health;

2. serves as a national information resource for medical education, research, and service activities of Federal and private agencies, organizations, and institutions;

3. serves as a national information resource for the public, patients, and families by providing electronic access to reliable health information issued by the National Institutes of Health and other trusted sources;

4. publishes in print and electronically guides to health sciences information in the form of catalogs, bibliographies, indexes, and online databases;

5. provides support for medical library development and for training of biomedical librarians and other health information specialists;

6. conducts and supports research in methods for recording, storing, retrieving, preserving, and communicating health information;

7. creates information resources and access tools for molecular biology, biotechnology, toxicology, environmental health, and health services research; and

8. provides technical consultation services and research assistance.

SOURCE: Reprinted from the National Library of Medicine (2004).

Proctor, and Smith 2012; Gauthier and Serber 2005) bring another call for government intervention. Lack of insurance has an effect on the health of the population because lack of insurance may actually lead to preventable morbidity and mortality (a negative health outcome), which in turn cost the US healthcare system more than $65 billion per year (Ayanian et al. 2000; IOM 2003).

As discussed in earlier chapters, healthcare costs have been rising rapidly both in absolute terms and relative to the gross domestic product. These increases in cost are largely paid by governments; thus, budget considerations drive government interest as well. In 2010, 39.2 percent of personal health expenditures were paid by Medicare and Medicaid alone. All levels of government have a major stake in payment rates (CMS 2012b). The conclusion is that quality, access, and cost provide a justification of the government's role in healthcare and thus in HIT. (See Chapter 2 for more details on the expenditures for healthcare services.)

GOVERNMENT AND BUSINESS PRACTICE

Given that government intervention can be justified, how much and what types of intervention are justified? With respect to HIT, patient information privacy and security are the major foci of government intervention. The argument is that social interest in having patient healthcare information protected cannot be left to individual providers. Good business practice dictates that much of what comes under the guise of government intervention should be followed irrespective of the regulations. As addressed in detail in the next section, HIPAA has, among other features, enhanced privacy regulation. Because healthcare delivery organizations are responsible for the health and welfare of their patients, it only makes sense to adopt strict privacy standards even in the absence of government regulation. Therefore, information system managers in healthcare facilities must develop policies and procedures to protect the security of information contained in automated systems throughout the organization.

Government can extend into healthcare business practices in a number of potential ways. Goldsmith, Blumenthal, and Rishel (2003) argue for the need for government-sanctioned and government-supported standardization of at least communication protocols and nomenclature. Without a direct government role, healthcare organizations will adopt technology slowly and in a haphazard fashion. Blumenthal (2006) provides three business arguments justifying government intervention. First, no compelling business case exists for investment in HIT. Better performance is not routinely rewarded in healthcare, and, in fact, poor performance and providing more services generate greater revenue. The savings from implementing HIT do not go to providers but rather benefit insurers and others. Second, for real system benefits to be seen, all components of the fragmented US healthcare delivery system must participate. Without this participation, benefits are incomplete. Interoperability among providers is a necessary step for true sharing to occur, and government needs to impose common communication standards. Third, fraud-and-abuse regulations do not allow physicians to receive subsidies from hospitals. Blumenthal (2006) makes a strong case for the failure of the market to achieve the desired results, and thus government must become more actively involved. HIT leadership must be aware of specific government interventions to effectively manage their organization.

The bottom line is that government has intervened in healthcare markets in significant ways, such as through the Health Insurance Portability and Accountability Act (HIPAA), Health Information Technology for Economic and Clinical Health (HITECH) Act, and the Patient Protection and Affordable Care Act (ACA). The issue with regard to HIT intervention, however, is still somewhat open, but a growing body of evidence suggests that HIT investment will have positive results (Buntin et al. 2011). Economic recovery funding through the HITECH Act implicitly assumes that this investment is good for quality and potentially for cost savings.

Specific Healthcare Legislations

Health Insurance Portability and Accountability Act

As an example of legislation that has had far-reaching effects on HIT, HIPAA has no equal. Begun as a mechanism to ensure that individuals could retain access to health insurance when they changed jobs (portability) (Flores and Dodier 2005; Schmeida 2005), HIPAA also contains a second provision called *administrative simplification* that has far greater impact (CMS 2005a):

> The Administrative Simplification provisions of the Health Insurance Portability and Accountability Act of 1996 (HIPAA, Title II) required the Department of Health and Human Services (HHS) to establish national standards for electronic healthcare transactions and national identifiers for providers, health plans, and employers. It also addressed the security and privacy of health data. As the industry adopts these standards for the efficiency and effectiveness of the nation's healthcare system will improve the use of electronic data interchange.

As this general provision indicates, HIPAA anticipated the development of electronic record keeping in healthcare. The healthcare field was not able internally to develop the standards and rules governing these new technologies for collecting, storing, and transmitting health information (another example of potential market failure mentioned earlier). Many realized that strict government controls would have to be put in place to enable healthcare providers to develop systems that met internal needs and facilitated the transfer of information across institutions (Blumenthal 2006; Goldsmith, Blumenthal, and Rishel 2003; Kleinke 2005). The electronic medium also raised concerns with security and privacy that the government felt it should address. In simple terms, administrative simplification involved setting standards, mandating health plan and provider compliance, and establishing privacy elements (CMS 2005b).

The complete text of HIPAA's Summary of Administrative Simplification Provisions is provided in Exhibit 3.3. Each of the five provisions presented in the exhibit is important because of what it implies. While the translation of these broad provisions to policy details has evolved incrementally since the passage of HIPAA in 1996, the details are now emerging as a result of a series of negotiations among all of the interested parties. Exhibit 3.4 shows the eight components of the administrative simplification provisions that were promulgated to meet the five provisions listed in Exhibit 3.3.

The HIPAA overview reveals specific details of these standards and the timing of their implementation (CMS 2005a). Steps to achieving the goals of improving patient quality and enhancing efficiency through the use of electronic records were developed in stages. The first step was to make employers obtain a national identification number for healthcare transactions. Next, providers were required to have a commonly determined standard identifier—the National Provider Identifier (NPI). These rules set the stage for

Standards for electronic health information transactions. Within 18 months of enactment, the Secretary of HHS is required to adopt standards from among those already approved by private standards developing organizations for certain electronic health transactions, including claims, enrollment, eligibility, payment, and coordination of benefits. These standards also must address the security of electronic health information systems.

Mandate on providers and health plans, and timetable. Providers and health plans are required to use the standards for the specified electronic transactions 24 months after they are adopted. Plans and providers may comply directly, or may use a health care clearinghouse. Certain health plans, in particular workers compensation, are not covered.

Privacy. The Secretary is required to recommend privacy standards for health information to Congress 12 months after enactment. If Congress does not enact privacy legislation within 3 years of enactment, the Secretary shall promulgate privacy regulations for individually identifiable electronic health information.

Pre-emption of state law. The bill supersedes state laws, except where the Secretary determines that the State law is necessary to prevent fraud and abuse, to ensure appropriate state regulation of insurance or health plans, addresses controlled substances, or for other purposes. If the Secretary promulgates privacy regulations, those regulations do not pre-empt state laws that impose more stringent requirements. These provisions do not limit a State's ability to require health plan reporting or audits.

Penalties. The bill imposes civil money penalties and prison for certain violations.

NOTE: Provisions in the original legislation have been modified by subsequent legislation, including the ACA.
SOURCE: Reprinted from CMS (2005b).

EXHIBIT 3.3
HIPAA's Summary of Administrative Simplification Provisions

1. Employer-identifier standard
2. Enforcement
3. National provider-identifier standard
4. Security standard
5. Transaction and code sets standard
6. Place-of-service codes for HIPAA transactions
7. Health insurance reform for consumers (HIPAA Title I)
8. Medicaid HIPAA administrative simplification

SOURCE: Information from CMS (2005a).

EXHIBIT 3.4
Eight Major Components of HIPAA Administrative Simplification Provisions

creating a regional or national data set of electronic information transmission by uniquely identifying the payer source and the provider. This seems insignificant when viewed from within a healthcare organization because they have always used unique numbers to identify patients and to keep patient records distinct. The NPI was novel when applied across organizations, however. The timing of the NPI mandate is current in relation to this discussion in that after May 23, 2007, "healthcare providers may only use their NPIs to identify themselves in standard transactions" (CMS 2005c).

Transactions and *code set standards* warrant additional commentary because they are so vital to the effective implementation and use of the electronic record. The precise definition of these standards is also still in flux. According to the Centers for Medicare & Medicaid Services (CMS 2005d),

> Transactions are activities involving the transfer of healthcare information for specific purposes. Under the Health Insurance Portability & Accountability Act of 1996 (HIPAA), if a healthcare provider engages in one of the identified transactions, they must comply with the standard for that transaction. HIPAA requires every provider who does business electronically to use the same healthcare transactions, code sets, and identifiers. HIPAA has identified ten standard transactions for Electronic Data Interchange (EDI) for the transmission of healthcare data. Claims and encounter information, payment and remittance advice, and claims status and inquiry are several of the standard transactions. Code sets are the codes used to identify specific diagnosis and clinical procedures on claims and encounter forms. The HCPCS, CPT-4 and ICD-9 codes with which providers are familiar, are examples of code sets for procedures and diagnose.

This generic statement gives rise to an array of specific rules designed to enable organizations to collect data in a consistent manner. Unless everyone uses a common nomenclature for defining all clinical and administrative terms, there will be no capacity to communicate. *Interoperability* is the term that describes the goal to its fullest extent. To assist providers and others in this pursuit, CMS has provided information on the web that can be easily accessed and applied. The posted information is a series of checklists to be used by healthcare organizations to determine their readiness; download the information from www.cms.gov/Regulations-and-Guidance/HIPAA-Administrative-Simplification/EducationMaterials/Educational-Materials.html. In addition, CMS makes available a series of ten documents, listed in Exhibit 3.5, to assist organizations in dealing with issues appropriate to their particular need. (Discussing these documents is beyond the scope of this book; however, HIT leadership must be aware of their existence and importance.)

The Need for Information Privacy and Security

HIT "systems contain sensitive information. Clinical systems process medical information about individual patients; human resources information systems contain personal

EXHIBIT 3.5
Checklist Aids
for Transactions
and Code Set
Development

The HIPAA Information Series for Providers consists of ten papers that can aid healthcare organizations in transactions and code-sets development as well as other HIPAA issues:

- HIPAA 101
- Are You a Covered Entity?
- Key HIPAA Dates and Tips
- What Electronic Transactions and Code Sets Are Standardized Under HIPAA?
- Is Your Software Vendor or Billing Service Ready for HIPAA?
- What to Expect from Your Health Plans
- What You Need to Know About Testing
- Trading Partner
- Final Steps for Compliance with Electronic Transactions and Code Sets
- Enforcement

These documents can be downloaded from www.cms.gov/Regulations-and-Guidance/ HIPAA-Administrative-Simplification/EducationMaterials/Educational-Materials.html.

---

information about employees; and financial and decision-support systems include proprietary data used for planning, marketing, and management of the enterprise" (Stahl 2003). HIPAA has placed special emphasis on privacy, and the implications of safeguarding privacy to HIT leadership are expansive.

To give some idea of the nature and extent of privacy and security issues even after HIPAA's enactment, the Health Privacy Project (www.healthprivacy.org) has compiled anecdotes reported in the national press. The sheer number of events suggests their importance. In 2012 *Healthcare Finance News* reported the top ten security breaches for that year (McNickle 2012). These breaches affected many institutions, including the Utah Department of Health, Emory Healthcare, and the University of Arkansas for Medical Sciences. Following are examples from the Health Privacy Project's (2007) web publication, *Health Privacy Stories*:

◆ "The California state Department of Health Services inadvertently revealed the names and addresses of up to 53 people enrolled in an AIDS drug assistance program to other enrollees by putting benefit notification letters in the wrong envelopes. . . . The department learned about the mix-up after 12 people in the drug assistance program phoned to say they had received letters addressed to someone else. . . . The department is looking into ways to make the system more foolproof, such as using envelopes with window addresses, said health services Director Sandra Shewry. HIV/AIDS services and advocacy groups said this was the first known breach of that database. 'I would hope this is an anomaly,' said Jeff Bailey, director of client services for AIDS Project Los Angeles" (Engel 2007).

◆ "A desktop computer containing personal information for up to 38,000 patients treated at Veterans Affairs Department medical centers in Pittsburgh and Philadelphia over the past four years was reported missing from the Reston, VA offices of VA contractor Unisys Corp. The VA and Unisys [say] the computer contained names, addresses, Social Security numbers and dates of birth. It may also have included insurance carrier and billing information, claims data and medical information" (Robeznieks 2006a).

Needless to say, ensuring the security of clinical information systems must be a top priority for healthcare leaders and HIT managers alike. Clinical information systems refer to the following types of health and healthcare records:

1. *Patient care systems* include information technology used in the course of providing care, services, or treatments, such as order entry and results reporting; electronic medical records; and lab, pharmacy, and radiology systems. Data contained in these systems—including medical histories, medication lists, physician orders, diagnoses, treatment plans, and test results—are extremely private and thus should be accessible only to those involved in care delivery. Breach of security in this instance has legal and ethical ramifications for the healthcare delivery organization.

2. *Public health information systems,* according to Stahl (2003), "support disease prevention and surveillance programs. Protecting public health requires the acquisition and storage of health-related information about individuals. Public health benefits sometimes conflict with threats to individual privacy. Individuals concerned about privacy who avoid clinical tests and treatments may endanger the health of others in the community." For example, a person with a sexually transmitted infection may opt to not test and/or report the presence of the infection, which could then lead to the spread of the disease (Gostin, Hodge, and Valdiserri 2001). A security breach of public health information systems could lead to a person or groups facing discrimination in employment or insurance eligibility.

3. *Medical research information systems* are repositories of medical diagnoses, health conditions, disease data, risk factors, and other health-related details culled from patient records. The purpose of such a system is to enable clinical researchers and other investigators to understand disease risks, patterns, and contributing factors observed in a patient population. Lau and Catchpole (2001) emphasized the importance of respecting the patients' privacy rights as well as protecting the information contained in these systems by restricting access and use to authorized personnel.

Following are some of the ways healthcare delivery organizations have addressed privacy concerns to comply with HIPAA standards:

◆ Form HIPAA task forces.

◆ Install a new compliance office or function dedicated to managing HIPAA-related challenges, or designate an existing office or function (e.g., chief information officer, medical records, risk management) to address or prevent issues (Marietti 2002).

◆ Use information system software designed by a vendor to meet the specific purpose, needs, and concerns identified by the organization. In this way, HIPAA patches to existing programs, and some in-house work is required to ensure the applications interface with one another (Wilson and McPherson 2002).

◆ Implement changes to some business processes and procedures. Marietti (2002, 55) projected that "80 percent to 85 percent of HIPAA compliance issues will depend on adjusting human behavior."

Findings from studies of the HIPAA regulations have emerged. First, the immediate impact has been on the research community. Evidence suggests that HIPAA compliance makes recruitment and retention of subjects into research projects more difficult (Wipke-Tevis and Pickett 2008). Second, some specific examples now exist regarding how process improvements (automated access verification) can assist organizations to demonstrate compliance (Hill 2006). Third, the change process is still incomplete because privacy and security rules are being revised/updated frequently, such as a new rule announced in January 2013 (HHS 2013). Checklists are still being published to help organizations meet HIPAA requirements (HIPAA Survival Guide 2013).

A number of studies have examined the impact of privacy rules on healthcare organizations, giving rise to a set of inappropriate responses (as observed by consultants) related to privacy (Upham and Dorsey 2007). Some concerns center on the application of privacy rules to other activities or innovations in healthcare. For example, in 2007 Paul Tang, then the chair of the board of the American Medical Informatics Association, indicated that electronic health record vendors often included contract provisions that may require providers to violate patient privacy standards (Conn 2007). Similarly, in the wake of mass tragedies, access to the perpetrator's health record often is cited as a reason to relax privacy constraints. Peel (2007) discussed this issue in the context of the Virginia Tech massacre in April 2007, in which a student killed 32 people on that campus. Peel concluded that privacy constraints would not likely prevent these events. More recently, there is the case of James Holmes—the gunman who opened fire at an Aurora, Colorado, movie theater, killing 12 and injuring about 50 people. Prior to the shooting, Holmes was reportedly being seen by a mental health specialist at the University of Colorado, where Holmes was a student (Meyer and Ingold 2012). The specialist contacted a university threat-assessment team but did not invoke a "72-hour psychiatric hold" because Holmes was leaving the university. Under pressure from news sources that are trying to piece together the events that led up to the tragedy, the University of Colorado released thousands of e-mails related to Holmes. However, the university did not make available any records or documents related to the crime or Holmes's mental health status (Meyer and Ingold 2012). As consumers continue to provide information over the Internet, the collection, availability, and security of their data will remain a major concern (Nelson 2006).

At the level of information sharing across organizations was a study commissioned by the California Healthcare Foundation to look at privacy from the perspective of developing regional health information organizations (RHIOs). The study was trying to determine what needed to be done at the systems level to facilitate RHIO development. It resulted in a number of findings and substantial recommendations on developing and implementing security policies for RHIOs. The analyses identified the following four key questions that must be addressed to develop privacy policies (Rosenfeld, Koss, and Siler 2007):

1. Who will have access to patient information?

2. Which information will be accessible?

3. What are acceptable purposes of patient information exchange?

4. What circumstances justify patient information exchange?

In addition, the study reported a number of common elements that are important to consider in developing privacy policies across organizational entities, including the following:

◆ Privacy policies are local.

◆ Organizations participating in the RHIO influence the privacy policies.

◆ Privacy policies need to be developed early and revisited often.

◆ Work on privacy policies is ongoing.

◆ Privacy policies are unique to the environment; thus, best practices have yet to follow.

◆ Building consensus on privacy policies takes time.

◆ The consumer role in privacy policy development is limited.

HIPAA was not the first effort by government to assure the public that the privacy of an individual's medical information would be secure. The Privacy Act of 1974 established key provisions to protect the privacy of patients (CMS 2005e). Enacted before the conception of electronic health records prevalent today, the legislation protected all patient records with "personal identifiers" (social security number or other). Under the Privacy Act, every patient can access and, if necessary, correct his or her individual records, and it generally prohibits disclosure of these records—but that applied only to federal agencies.

The individual's right to genetic privacy was also addressed in Oregon's Genetic Privacy Act of 1995, which provides legal protection for medical information, tissue samples, and DNA samples. Harris and Keywood (2001, 415) pointed out that individuals "have a powerful interest in genetic privacy and its associated claim to ignorance"; however, "any claims to be shielded from information about the self must compete on equal terms with claims based in the rights and interests of others." Further, Cummings and Magnusson (2001, 1089) stated that "As genetic privacy legislation is developed and enacted at state and federal levels, the needs of individuals must be balanced with the needs of institutions and of research in the larger context of societal needs."

Now, the Patient Protection and Affordable Care Act of 2010 has increased the rigor of the HIPAA rules further by requiring a unique Health Plan Identifier and both standards and rules for financial transactions.

HEALTH INFORMATION TECHNOLOGY FOR ECONOMIC AND CLINICAL HEALTH ACT

President Obama signed the American Recovery and Reinvestment Act (ARRA) in February 2009. This comprehensive stimulus package is designed to address the 2007–2009 economic crisis. ARRA contains many provisions, including tax relief (federal); unemployment benefit expansion; social welfare spending; and spending for specific sectors such as energy, education, and healthcare. The healthcare spending is diverse, allocating funds or subsidies for Medicaid, health research and construction, benefits for the newly uninsured, prevention and wellness, and research on the effectiveness of healthcare treatments, among many other provisions.

A major part of ARRA is called the Health Information Technology for Economic and Clinical Health (HITECH) Act. It is designed to promote the expansion of the electronic health record (EHR) because of its perceived social benefits. A total of about $22 billion was allocated to the HITECH Act, with the bulk ($19.2 billion) devoted directly to EHR adoption. An additional $2 billion went to the Office of the National Coordinator for Health Information Technology (ONCHIT 2011) to support the agency's varied activities for promoting information exchange, training health professionals for information technology, and enhancing interoperability. ONCHIT is the body responsible for implementing the incentives for EHR use and establishing an HIT Policy Committee and an HIT Standards Committee. These committees are charged with developing recommendations for adopting health information infrastructure and standards for information exchange, respectively (Recovery.gov n.d.).

Adoption of EHR

From a broad social perspective and consistent with our earlier justification for government intervention, the benefits of the meaningful use of EHRs include the following, as identified by HealthIT.gov (n.d.):

◆ Complete and accurate information

◆ Better access to information

◆ Patient empowerment

One can argue whether the government or private sector is better at realizing these goals, but some opine that the benefits of sharable electronic information accrue to society at large and thus cannot be fully captured by any private provider or organization. Consequently, investing in this public good can be justified.

Meaningful Use

The HITECH Act provides the authority to make changes that can improve healthcare quality, safety, and efficiency through the use of EHR and the exchange of electronic health information. ONCHIT has released regulations to define appropriate standards for the certification of EHR technologies and the means by which providers can receive financial incentives to adopt and use those systems (see www.healthit.gov/policy-researchers-implementers /about-certification). An example of one of the many features of the HITECH Act is the meaningful use provision, which offers incentives to organizations that adopt and implement EHRs. The underlying assumption is that EHRs can provide benefits to providers and patients. The benefits may not be realized, however, without sufficient intensity of use. Consequently, CMS developed a set of standards called *meaningful use*. These standards allow hospitals and individual providers deemed eligible to obtain incentive payments by meeting specific criteria; the incentives for adoption by clinical professionals are substantial, as seen in Exhibit 3.6.

For professionals applying in 2011, the maximum payment was $44,000 over the period. Notice the built-in incentives to begin the process early: The initial payment was lower for eligible professionals who delayed EHR. Eligible professionals for Medicare's incentive program include doctors of medicine, osteopathy, dentistry, podiatry, optometry, and chiropractic medicine. For Medicaid, the professionals who may participate include nurse practitioners, certified nurse midwifes, and select physician assistants. Hospitals eligible for participation in Medicare incentives include those receiving inpatient prospective

Exhibit 3.6

CMS Meaningful Use Incentive Payment Schedule for Medicare-Eligible Professionals

Payment Amounts	If a Medicare-Eligible Professional Qualifies to Receive First Payment in 2011	If a Medicare-Eligible Professional Qualifies to Receive First Payment in 2012	If a Medicare-Eligible Professional Qualifies to Receive First Payment in 2013	If a Medicare-Eligible Professional Qualifies to Receive First Payment in 2014	If a Medicare-Eligible Professional Qualifies to Receive First Payment in 2015
Payment amount for 2011	$18,000				
Payment amount for 2012	$12,000	$18,000			
Payment amount for 2013	$8,000	$12,000	$15,000		
Payment amount for 2014	$4,000	$8,000	$12,000	$12,000	
Payment amount for 2015	$2,000	$4,000	$8,000	$8,000	
Payment amount for 2016		$2,000	$4,000	$4,000	
Total Payment Amount	$44,000	$44,000	$39,000	$24,000	

SOURCE: CMS (n.d.[a], 2010b).

payment, critical access hospitals, and Medicare Advantage hospitals. Medicaid qualifications include inpatient hospitals with 10 percent Medicaid patient volume or any children's hospital.

The catch in EHR incentive participation is that the level of use must be deemed "meaningful." Incentive payments come in three stages. Stage 1 (implemented in the 2011–2012 period) involves installing certified information systems that capture structured patient data and give the ability to share that data with the patient or other healthcare professionals. Stage 2 (scheduled for 2014) requires more collection and reporting to advance clinical processes. Stage 3 (scheduled for 2016) requires actual improved outcomes. The HIT requirement for meaningful use is clearly detailed in Stage 1. Eligible providers must report providing all 15 Core Measures, a choice of 5 out of 10 menu objectives, and 6 clinical quality measures. The 15 Core Measures are listed in Exhibit 3.7. Each of the core measures has detailed definitions and reporting requirements. Consult this government

EXHIBIT 3.7

15 Core
Measures for
CMS Meaningful
Use Standards
for Eligible
Professionals

1. Implement computerized physician order entry
2. Perform drug–drug and drug–allergy checks
3. Maintain up-to-date problem list of current and active diagnoses
4. Use e-prescribing (eRx)
5. Maintain active medication list
6. Maintain active medication allergy list
7. Record demographics
8. Record and chart changes in vital signs
9. Record smoking status for patients aged 13 or older
10. Report ambulatory clinical quality measures to CMS/states
11. Implement clinical decision support
12. Provide patients with an electronic copy of their health information, upon request
13. Provide clinical summaries for patients for each office visit
14. Establish capability to exchange key clinical information
15. Protect electronic health information

SOURCE: CMS (2010a).

publication for the specifications: www.cms.gov/EHRIncentivePrograms/Downloads
/EP-MU-TOC.pdf. As an example, the following is the specification for the measure
computerized physician order entry (CPOE):

> Requirement: More than 30 percent of unique patients with at least one medication in
> the medication list and seen by the eligible professional must have at least one medi-
> cation entered using CPOE. You can be excluded from this core measure if you write
> fewer than 100 prescriptions during the reporting period.

The ten menu objectives (see Exhibit 3.8) are also required, and their specifications
are found on the website mentioned earlier. While this list of objectives gives you some
choice, the first two are public health–oriented and thus one of the two must be selected.
Basically, meaningful use demands that providers demonstrate that they can effectively
communicate population-based information from their practice.

Eligible professionals also must report six clinical quality measures. Three of the
six are core, and the three others can be selected from a large list of measures (see Exhibit
3.9). The three primary and three alternate core measures (which are available should the
primary measures not apply to the provider's patient population) include the following:

◆ Primary measures

 – Hypertension: Blood pressure measurement

EXHIBIT 3.8
10 Menu
Objectives for
CMS Meaningful
Use Standards

1. Submit electronic data to immunization registries
2. Submit electronic syndromic surveillance data to public health agencies
3. Perform drug formulary checks
4. Incorporate clinical lab-test results
5. Generate lists of patients by specific conditions
6. Send reminders to patients for preventive/follow-up care
7. Provide patient-specific education resources
8. Provide electronic access to health information for patients
9. Perform medication reconciliation
10. Maintain summary-of-care record for transitions of care

SOURCE: CMS (2010a).

-    Preventive care and screening: Tobacco use assessment and tobacco cessation intervention

-    Adult weight screening and follow-up

◆ Alternate measures

-    Weight assessment and counseling for children and adolescents

-    Preventive care and screening: Influenza immunization for patients aged 50 or older

-    Childhood immunization status

The remaining three quality measures must be selected from the 38 measures listed in Exhibit 3.9.

EXHIBIT 3.9
Clinical Quality
Measures for CMS
Meaningful Use
Standards

1. Diabetes: Hemoglobin A1c poor control
2. Diabetes: Low-density lipoprotein (LDL) management and control
3. Diabetes: Blood pressure management
4. Heart failure (HF): Angiotensin-converting enzyme (ACE) inhibitor or angiotensin receptor blocker (ARB) therapy for left ventricular systolic dysfunction (LVSD)
5. Coronary artery disease (CAD): Beta-blocker therapy for CAD patients with prior myocardial infarction (MI)
6. Pneumonia vaccination status for older adults
7. Breast cancer screening
8. Colorectal cancer screening

(continued)

EXHIBIT 3.9
Clinical Quality
Measures for CMS
Meaningful Use
Standards
(Continued)

9. Coronary artery disease (CAD): Oral antiplatelet therapy prescribed for patients with CAD
10. Heart failure (HF): Beta-blocker therapy for LVSD
11. Antidepressant medication management: (a) effective acute phase treatment, (b) effective continuation phase treatment
12. Primary open angle glaucoma (POAG): Optic nerve evaluation
13. Diabetic retinopathy: Documentation of presence or absence of macular edema and level of severity of retinopathy
14. Diabetic retinopathy: Communication with the physician managing ongoing diabetes care
15. Asthma pharmacologic therapy
16. Asthma assessment
17. Appropriate testing for children with pharyngitis
18. Oncology breast cancer: Hormonal therapy for stage IC-IIIC estrogen receptor/ progesterone receptor (ER/PR) positive breast cancer
19. Oncology colon cancer: Chemotherapy for stage III colon cancer patients
20. Prostate cancer: Avoidance of overuse of bone scan for staging low-risk prostate cancer patients
21. Smoking and tobacco use cessation, medical assistance:
    a. Advising smokers and tobacco users to quit
    b. Discussing smoking and tobacco use cessation medications
    c. Discussing smoking and tobacco use cessation strategies
22. Diabetes: Eye exam
23. Diabetes: Urine screening
24. Diabetes: Foot exam
25. Coronary artery disease (CAD): Drug therapy for lowering LDL cholesterol
26. Heart failure (HF): Warfarin therapy patients with atrial fibrillation
27. Ischemic vascular disease (IVD): Blood pressure management
28. Ischemic vascular disease (IVD): Use of aspirin or another antithrombotic
29. Initiation and engagement of alcohol and other drug-dependence treatment: (a) initiation, (b) engagement
30. Prenatal care: Screening for human immunodeficiency virus (HIV)
31. Prenatal care: Anti-D immune globulin
32. Controlling high blood pressure
33. Cervical cancer screening
34. Chlamydia screening for women
35. Use of appropriate medications for asthma
36. Low back pain: Use of imaging studies
37. Ischemic vascular disease (IVD): Complete lipid panel and LDL control
38. Diabetes: Hemoglobin A1c control (<8.0%)

SOURCE: CMS (2010a).

The set of reporting requirements that apply to eligible hospitals includes 14 core measures, 5 of 10 menu objectives, and 15 quality measures. Details on these items are found in the following documents posted on the CMS website (www.cms.gov/Regulations-and-Guidance/Legislation/EHRIncentivePrograms/Meaningful_Use.html):

◆ ALL Stage 1 EHR Meaningful Use Specification Sheets for Eligible Hospitals

◆ Hospital Attestation Worksheet

◆ Critical Access Hospital Payment Tip Sheet

◆ EHR Incentive Program for Medicare Hospitals

◆ EHR Incentive Program for Critical Access Hospitals—Spanish Version

◆ Medicaid Hospital Incentive Payments Calculations

We have only discussed Stage 1 of meaningful use. Stages 2 and 3 are on the books but are not yet fully developed, and Stage 2 meaningful use core and menu measures were not released until October 2012 and are not scheduled to be implemented until fiscal year 2014. Those working with HIT *must* know where to go for the latest information, as these requirements are updated and revised occasionally. This website offers relevant information: www.cms.gov/Regulations-and-Guidance/Legislation/EHRIncentivePrograms/Stage_2.html.

The evidence of the impact of EHR adoption for hospitals and physicians is disappointing, despite the financial incentives and emphasis. Davis (2009) reports, using detailed HIMSS Analytics databases, that by 2008 few hospitals had attained any of the top four levels of adoption. Only 5.8 percent of respondents reported implementing CPOE and clinical decision support systems, which are level 4 or higher. Nearly 16 percent of respondents had not yet installed laboratory information systems, pharmacy information systems, or radiology information systems, which are the minimum necessary to advance from the bottom level of EHR adoption. Davis concluded that for hospitals to meet meaningful use criteria by 2013, they had to have reached at least level 4. The numbers for physicians were equally discouraging. EHR adoption in US hospitals and physician practices lags in comparison with adoption rates in other industrialized countries (Jha et al. 2008).

PATIENT PROTECTION AND AFFORDABLE CARE ACT

No single legislation in the past several years represents the government's attempt to address a host of social problems in healthcare more than the Patient Protection and Affordable Care Act. Signed on March 23, 2010, HR 3590 and the accompanying HR 4872 (Health

Care and Education Reconciliation Act of 2010) proposed historic changes to the US healthcare delivery and financing system. Designed to expand coverage, the ACA contains a host of provisions with short-term and far-reaching implications. Due to its size, however, most individuals tend to focus on issues of importance to them only. For example, the American Hospital Association (2010) released a summary highlighting eight key features of the legislation important to AHA's constituents:

1. Coverage: expansion of insurance to more than 30 million Americans

2. Delivery system reforms: changes in incentives facing providers to enhance quality, reduce costs, and improve care coordination; this section has the accountable care organization authorization

3. Medicare and Medicaid payment: efforts to reduce the rate of increased spending on these programs, with hospitals being the major target; provisions for a drug discount program, payments to rural hospitals, and enhancements to primary care physicians are also included here

4. Workforce and graduate medical education: expansion and alteration of workforce training to alleviate the shortages in select portions of the healthcare workforce

5. Wellness and prevention: allocation of resources to the Prevention and Public Health Fund and insurer requirement to cover immunizations and screenings with zero cost sharing

6. Quality, disparities, and comparative effectiveness: begins the movement to pay for quality and penalties for hospital-acquired conditions

7. Regulatory oversight: provisions to identify and reduce fraud and abuse, including the continuation of the RAC audits

8. Revenue: to pay for much of these features, the law taxes high cost health insurance plans and imposes fees on select industries

Many of the ACA features cause stress for HIT, but the following deserve special mention. First, accountable care organizations (ACOs) assign responsibility (accountability) to the organization for patients who may not obtain all or even most of their care from the host organization (Kaiser 2012; Miller 2009). Finding the patient, effectively exchanging information with other providers, and ensuring the privacy and confidentiality of that information outside of organizational boundaries are a challenge. That information is exchanged both ways, so even if the institution is not sponsoring an ACO, it may be asked to provide clinical information on select patients.

Second, pay-for-performance initiatives demand greater linkages between provider cost and clinical performance than is customary (Rosenthal and Dudley 2007; Rosenthal and Camillus 2007). The discussion in Chapter 4, regarding management across organizational boundaries, is put to the test as clinical (chief medical officers and chief nursing officers) and financial (chief financial officers) leaders demand accurate and timely data for evaluation, improvement, and contracting purposes.

Third, expansion of covered lives is taxing to HIT in a number of ways. Having more patients can be a minor stressor, but (depending on current capacity) sufficient volume growth might require added facilities. In addition, at least some new patients are likely to be unfamiliar with the delivery system and thus less compliant with completing forms and documentations necessary to manage the care process. Further, some added patients may be "sicker" and may present new problems to the clinicians, testing the provider's documentation, coding quality, and select systems in unforeseen ways.

Fourth, as Gawande (2010) pointed out, there is a host of pushback efforts to the ACA as there was to Medicare and Medicaid decades before, which emphasizes Gawande's argument that "the battle for health-care reform has only begun." More than any individual ACA feature causing concern for HIT leadership is that the timing of implementation is highly uncertain. Planning for an unknown future makes life difficult for HIT management, but that may justify the salary that HIT leadership receives.

HIT LEADERSHIP ROLES

While government involvement through HIPAA, the HITECH Act, and the ACA may seem difficult for information technology specialists to fully understand, it is particularly baffling for those outside of HIT. The consequence of this difficulty is that it requires HIT leadership (chief information officer [CIO] and others) to understand, anticipate, and explain the impact of these legislations. They must be prepared for new and/or changes in government regulations and policies by developing and then implementing a number of activities and programs, including comprehensive environmental scanning and organizational education, information security policies and procedures, disaster preparedness and recovery planning, and information privacy and confidentiality protection.

ENVIRONMENTAL SCANNING AND ORGANIZATIONAL EDUCATION

The first responsibility of HIT leadership is to fully understand the operational and resource implications of all legislations. Internally, the team must understand what it has to do differently as a result and determine what extra staffing, expertise (consultants), hardware and software, and time are needed. The steps for this activity are as follows:

1. Determine breadth and scope of impending or current legislation.

2. Assess current organizational readiness for the impact.

3. Perform a gap analysis within the organization.

4. Recommend strategies to meet legal/regulatory changes.

    a. Develop staffing and critical expertise needed to address changes.

    b. Specify hardware and software needs.

    c. Estimate total financial implications of the recommendations.

5. Identify clinical and other resources within the organization that are necessary in meeting the standards.

6. Outline a timeline for implementation with key dates and milestones.

Naturally, difficulty may be encountered in effectively accomplishing these tasks once the legislation is in place and the deadlines are looming. Consequently, HIT leadership should be constantly monitoring the horizon for proposed legislation to get a head start on planning for its passage. To do this, HIT leadership should be engaged with those responsible for legislative affairs within the organization (if such a role exists). Getting a "heads up" from this source is vital. State and national associations—such as the Healthcare Information and Management Systems Society, American College of Healthcare Executives, Healthcare Financial Management Association, and American Hospital Association, among many others—are good sources of this "pre" data. A body of literature is available as well that documents the many and varied impacts of HIPAA, the HITECH Act, and the ACA. It is important for HIT leadership, either directly or through surrogates, to monitor and stay up-to-date on this literature. For example, Houser, Houser, and Shewchuk (2007) use the nominal group technique (NGT) for gathering information regarding the impact of HIPAA privacy rules on the release of patient information. "The NGT approach is a consumer-oriented formal brainstorming or idea-generating technique that is assumed to foster creativity and to be particularly effective in helping group members articulate meaningful disclosures in response to specific questions" (Houser, Houser, and Shewchuk 2007, 2).

Because the nature of government legislation, such as HIPAA, can be highly complex, HIT leadership should be prepared to educate senior leadership on the implications of these regulatory interventions. Senior leadership includes the chief executive officer as well as the chief operating officer (if the organization has that position), chief medical officer, chief nursing officer, and chief financial officer. Generally, the person responsible for strategic planning, the head of the legal department, the head of human resources, and the head of development should be educated also in HIT-related legislative matters.

INFORMATION SECURITY POLICIES AND PROCEDURES

Healthcare organizations must establish enterprisewide standards to maintain data security and protect the privacy and confidentiality of information, particularly patient records. Data security involves two essential elements: (1) protecting against system failures or external catastrophic events, such as fires, storms, deliberate sabotage, and other destructive acts of man and nature that could result in critical information being lost, and (2) controlling access to computer files by unauthorized personnel.

DISASTER PREPAREDNESS AND RECOVERY PLANNING

The HIT steering committee must ensure that effective data backup and recovery procedures are implemented at all processing sites throughout the organization. Critical data files should be copied to removable disk packs or tapes and stored in a secure location away from the processing sites, preferably in a different building. The CIO should develop a data backup plan for approval by the steering committee. The plan should specify which files require duplication and how often backup procedures should be conducted. Recovery procedures to be used if catastrophic events occur should also be included.

The need for disaster planning was underscored by the terrorist attacks in New York City on September 11, 2001. If that event was not convincing, Hurricane Katrina and the resulting challenges surely were. Disaster plans must be implemented, tested periodically, and refined. Testing of the plan provides training for employees and helps identify shortcomings in technology and procedures before they need to be used. A disaster-plan notebook should be developed and stored at the healthcare facility, at an off-site storage location, and at the homes of key employees who are involved in recovery procedures (Vecchio 2000).

Consultants can be used to assist in disaster planning and recovery. For example, IRM International offers a disaster recovery program that includes four phases: assessment, documentation consolidation, disaster plan development, and testing and refinement. See www.irminternational.com/rptcard.html for a disaster recovery report card that rates disaster-planning readiness.

In addition, data can be lost through computer viruses, which are increasingly prevalent and destructive. Each computer program should be inspected by virus-protection software every time the program is run. Acquisition of software should be subject to central review and approval, and particular care must be exercised to ensure that software downloaded from the Internet or obtained over networks is scanned and proven to be virus free. All incoming e-mail messages should be scanned for viruses, and employees should be trained not to open suspicious files attached to an e-mail, text, or any other electronic communication.

INFORMATION PRIVACY AND CONFIDENTIALITY PROTECTION

As suggested in the earlier discussion related to HIPAA, the HITECH Act, and the ACA, protecting information privacy and confidentiality should be a major concern of the HIT leadership. A comprehensive information security policy should include three elements:

Physical Security	Technical Safeguards	Management Policies
Hardware	Passwords	Written security policy
Data files	Encryption	Employee training
	Audit logs	Disciplinary actions for violations

(1) physical security, (2) technical controls over access, and (3) management policies that are well known and enforced in all organizational units (Stahl 2003) (see Exhibit 3.10).

Understanding the processes of information privacy and confidentiality is not a necessary step to successful implementation at the systems level. While the past decade offers many examples of how individual systems have accomplished these goals, evidence indicates that many organizations are still not compliant with basic security standards (Davis and Having 2006). Some in the healthcare field have called for systematic incentives from industry or insurers to induce organizations to adopt privacy and security technology (e.g., Lang 2006). Despite substantial improvements, however, violations of basic privacy rights by hospitals and other providers are still a challenge (Hiltzik 2012). For an up-to-date list of privacy rule violations and settlements, see www.hhs.gov/ocr/office/news/index.html.

Prior to implementation of HIPAA standards, the Mayo Clinic, based in Rochester, Minnesota, developed a comprehensive set of plans to keep electronic medical records secure. A multidisciplinary team formulated the policy and provided management oversight of the security program. Leaders of the Mayo Clinic effort suggested that a confidentiality policy should include the following elements (Olson, Peters, and Stewart 1998, 29):

◆ Access rights—who has access and for what reasons

◆ Release of information to the patient, other healthcare providers, and third parties

◆ Special handling, if any, for specific information (e.g., HIV results, psychiatric notes)

◆ Special handling, if any, for particular patients (e.g., employees or VIPs)

◆ Availability of medical information, including retention policies

◆ Integrity of medical information, including authentication, completeness, and handling of revisions or addenda

◆ Approved methods for communication of medical information

SUMMARY

This chapter presents three major ideas. First, it presents and explores government's role in HIT. Government intervention in business processes can be justified if markets fail in their role of allocating scarce resources. Understanding why government gets involved assists healthcare and HIT leaders in responding to legislation and anticipating future actions. In healthcare, there are compelling reasons for government intervention, including a weak business case for information technology investment by providers, system fragmentation and lack of interoperability, and regulatory restrictions from fraud-and-abuse standards.

Second, the chapter explores specific legislations—HIPAA, the HITECH Act, and the ACA. These major government legislative and administrative interventions have fundamentally changed HIT. Passed by the US Congress in 1996, HIPAA—particularly two of its components—has a direct impact on healthcare information systems. The administrative simplification provisions of the law are designed to improve efficiency in the healthcare system by establishing uniform, national standards to be used for the electronic transmission of certain financial and administrative transactions. The privacy protection components of HIPAA restrict disclosure of health information to the minimum needed for patient care and administrative support. Patients have gained new rights to access their medical records and to know who has accessed them. HIPAA compliance requires that most healthcare organizations and their software vendors make modifications to computer software to meet the data standards and privacy protection provisions of the law. Changes to business processes and procedures are needed as well. Education and training of employees is particularly important.

The HITECH Act, which is part of the American Recovery and Reinvestment Act of 2009, is designed to facilitate the transition of physicians, hospitals, and other healthcare providers to full users of EHR. Through Medicare and Medicaid reimbursement, the HITECH Act offers financial incentives for adoption and meaningful use of EHR. The HITECH Act established the Office of the National Coordinator for Health Information Technology to foster the electronic exchange and use of health information as well as to enforce health information privacy and security. The ACA is intended to decrease the number of uninsured by introducing incentives and insurance-coverage regulations for both employers and the general population. It also seeks to improve health outcomes and insurance eligibility by eliminating exclusions for preexisting conditions.

Healthcare information systems contain sensitive information. Policies and procedures are needed to protect the confidentiality of information about patients, employees, finances, and organizational strategies. This information is contained in patient care systems, public health systems, and medical research systems. While benefits of public health and medical research systems sometimes conflict with threats to individual privacy, federal and state governments have asserted that providers have a legal and moral obligation to protect patients' rights to privacy. Consequently, all of the laws passed at the federal, state, and local levels of government are aimed at protecting medical information privacy while improving the delivery and outcomes of care.

Finally, the chapter explores HIT leadership roles. The external environment and the government have direct, indirect, and substantial roles in healthcare operations. HIT leaders must understand those roles today and anticipate roles in the future. This section presents an action plan for HIT leadership. In response to HIPAA and other HIT-related legislations—and for ethical reasons as well—healthcare organizations and HIT leadership need enterprisewide standards and policies to maintain data security and protect the confidentiality of certain information. A comprehensive information security program requires disaster protection and recovery procedures as well as procedures for limiting access to certain information stored in computer databases.

WEB RESOURCES

A number of organizations (through their websites) provide more information on the topics discussed in this chapter:

- ◆ American National Standards Institute (www.ansi.org)

- ◆ Center for Democracy & Technology, Health Privacy (www.healthprivacy.org)

- ◆ Data Interchange Standards Association (www.disa.org)

- ◆ IRM International (www.irminternational.com/rptcard.html), a checklist for disaster recovery

- ◆ National Committee on Vital and Health Statistics (http://ncvhs.hhs.gov/index.htm)

- ◆ National Uniform Claim Committee (www.nucc.org)

- ◆ US Department of Health & Human Services:

  - – Office of Civil Rights (www.hhs.gov/ocr/office/news/index.html) offers news releases announcing all of the major settlements of privacy and security breaches.

  - – HealthCare.gov (www.healthcare.gov) provides information on evolving health insurance options available.

  - – Centers for Medicare & Medicaid Services (www.cms.gov) points to detailed information about CMS's core programs and to research and data of value to HIT professionals. General HIPAA information can be found here: www.cms.gov/Regulations-and-Guidance / HIPAA-Administrative-Simplification/HIPAAGenInfo/index. html. Details of the EHR Incentive Programs are on www.cms.gov/

Regulations-and-Guidance/Legislation/EHRIncentivePrograms
/index.html.

◆   Workgroup for Electronic Data Interchange (www.wedi.org)

REFERENCES

American Hospital Association (AHA). 2010. "Detailed Summary of 2010 Health Care Reform
Legislation." Legislative Advisory, April 19. Chicago: AHA.

Arrow, K. 1963. "Uncertainty and the Welfare Economics of Medical Care." *American Economic* Review 52: 941–73.

Ayanian, J. Z., J. S. Weissman, E. C. Schneider, J. A. Ginsburg, and A. M. Zaslavsky. 2000.
"Unmet Health Needs of Uninsured Adults in the United States." *Journal of the American
Medical Association* 284 (16): 2061–69.

Blumenthal, D. 2006. *Health Information Technology: What Is the Federal Government's
Role?* The Commonwealth Fund Commission on a High Performance Health System #907.
New York: Commonwealth Fund.

Buntin, M., M. Burke, M. Hoaglin, and D. Blumenthal. 2011. "The Benefits of Information
Technology: A Review of the Recent Literature Shows Predominantly Positive Results."
Health Affairs 30 (3): 464–71.

Centers for Medicare & Medicaid Services (CMS). 2012b. "National Health Expenditure
Tables: Historical." Accessed January 9, 2013. www.cms.gov/Research-Statistics-Data-
and-Systems/Statistics-Trends-and-Reports/NationalHealthExpendData/National
HealthAccountsHistorical.html.

———. 2010a. Medicare and Medicaid EHR Incentive Program: Meaningful Use Stage 1
Requirements Overview. Accessed May 15. www.cms.gov/Regulations-and-Guidance/
Legislation/EHRIncentivePrograms/Downloads/MU_Stage1_ReqOverview.pdf.

———. 2010b. "Flow Chart: Determine Eligibility for Medicare and Medicaid Electronic
Health Record (EHR) Incentive Programs." Published September. www.cms.gov/MLN
Products/Downloads/Eligibility_Flow_Chart-ICN905343.pdf.

———. 2005a. "HIPAA: Overview." Accessed January 2, 2008. www.cms.hhs.gov/HIPAA
GenInfo/01_Overview.asp.

————. 2005b. "Health Insurance Portability and Accountability Act of 1996: Summary of Administrative Simplification Provisions." Accessed January 2, 2008. www.cms.hhs.gov/ HIPAAGenInfo/Downloads/SummaryofAdministrativeSimplificationProvisions.pdf.

————. 2005c. "National Provider Identifier Activities Begin in 2005." Accessed January 2, 2008. www.cms.hhs.gov/NationalProvIdentStand/Downloads/NPIdearprovider.pdf.

————. 2005d. "Transactions and Code Sets Regulations." Accessed January 2, 2008. www. cms.hhs.gov/TransactionCodeSetsStands/.

————. 2005e. "Privacy Act of 1974: Overview." Accessed January 2, 2008. www.cms.hhs. gov/PrivacyActof1974/.

Conn, J. 2007. "IT Guru Says Some E-vendor Contracts Violate Privacy." *Modern Healthcare*. Accessed January 10, 2008. www.modernhealthcare.com/apps/pbcs.dll/ article?AID=/20070719/FREE/70719007/0/FRONTPAGE.

Cummings, L. A., and R. Magnusson. 2001. "Genetic Privacy and Academic Medicine: The Oregon Experience." *Academic Medicine* 76 (11): 1089–93.

Davis, D., and K. Having. 2006. "Compliance with HIPAA Security Standards in U.S. Hospitals." *Journal of Healthcare Information Management* 20 (2): 108–15.

Davis, M. 2009. *The State of U.S. Hospitals Relative to Achieving Meaningful Use Measurements.* Chicago: HIMSS Analytics.

DeNavas-Walt, C., B. Proctor, and J. Smith. 2012. *Income, Poverty, and Health Insurance Coverage in the United States: 2011.* Washington, DC: US Census Bureau. Also available at www.census.gov/prod/2012pubs/p60-243.pdf.

Engel, M. 2007. "Mix-Up Breaches Confidentiality of Dozens in State AIDS Program." *Los Angeles Times*, March 3.

Feldstein, P. J. 2001. *The Politics of Health Legislation: An Economic Perspective.* Chicago: Health Administration Press.

Flores, J. A., and A. Dodier. 2005. "HIPAA: Past, Present, and Future Implications for Nurses." *Online Journal of Issues in Nursing* 10 (2): 5.

Gauthier, A., and M. Serber. 2005. *A Need to Transform the U.S. Healthcare System: Improving Access, Quality, and Efficiency.* New York: Commonwealth Fund.

Gawande, A. 2010. "Now What?" Talk of the Town column. *New Yorker.* Accessed April 21, 2011. www.newyorker.com/talk/comment/2010/04/05/100405taco_talk_gawande.

Goldsmith, J., D. Blumenthal, and W. Rishel. 2003. "Federal Health Information Policy: A Case of Arrested Development." *Health Affairs (Millwood)* 22 (4): 44–55.

Gostin, L. O., J. G. Hodge, and R. O. Valdiserri. 2001. "Informational Privacy and the Public's Health: The Model State Public Health Privacy Act." *American Journal of Public Health* 91 (9): 1388–92.

Harris, J., and K. Keywood. 2001. "Ignorance, Information, and Autonomy." *Theory of Medical Bioethics* 22 (5): 415–36.

HealthIT.gov. n.d. "What Is Meaningful Use?" Accessed May 22, 2012. www.healthit.gov/policy-researchers-implementers/meaningful-use.

Health Privacy Project. 2007. "Health Privacy Stories." Accessed July 1. www.healthprivacy.org/usr_doc/Privacystories.pdf.

Hill, L. 2006. "How Automated Access Verification Can Help Health Organizations Demonstrate HIPAA Compliance: A Case Study." *Journal of Healthcare Information Management* 20 (2): 116–22.

Hiltzik, M. 2012. "Her Case Shows Why Healthcare Privacy Laws Exist." *Los Angeles Times.* Accessed March 15, 2013. http://articles.latimes.com/2012/jan/04/business/la-fi-hiltzik-20120104.

HIPAA Survival Guide. 2013. "HIPAA Privacy Rule Checklist Under HITECH." Accessed March 14. http://store.hipaasurvivalguide.com/checklists.html.

Houser, S., H. Houser, and R. Shewchuk. 2007. "Assessing the Effects of the HIPAA Privacy Rule on Release of Patient Information by Healthcare Facilities." *Perspectives in Health Information Management* 4 (1): 1–11.

Institute of Medicine (IOM). 2003. *Hidden Costs, Value Lost: Uninsurance in America.* Washington, DC: National Academies Press.

Jha, A., D. Doolan, D. Grandt, T. Scott, and D. Bates. 2008. "The Use of Health Information Technology in Seven Nations." *International Journal of Medical Informatics* 77: 848–54.

Kaiser. 2012. *Building ACO Foundations: Lessons from Kaiser Permanente's Integrated Delivery Model: Case Study.* Danvers, MA: HealthLeaders Media Rounds.

Kleinke, J. D. 2005. "Dot-Gov: Market Failure and the Creation of a National Health Information Technology System." *Health Affairs (Millwood)* 24 (5): 1246–62.

Lang, R. D. 2006. "Patient Safety and IT: A Need for Incentives." *Journal of Healthcare Information Management* 20 (4): 2–4.

Lau, R. K., and M. Catchpole. 2001. "Improving Data Collection and Information Retrieval for Monitoring Sexual Health." *International Journal of STD and AIDS* 12 (1): 8–13.

Marietti, C. 2002. "HIPAA: Blueprint for Privacy and Security." *Healthcare Informatics* 19 (1): 55–60.

McNickle, M. 2012. "Top 10 Data Security Breaches in 2012." *Healthcare Finance News.* Accessed August 13. www.healthcarefinancenews.com/news/top-10-data-security-breaches-2012.

Meyer, J., and J. Ingold. 2012. "Source: Psychiatrist Rejected Offer to Put James Holmes on Psych Hold." *The Denver Post.* Accessed March 15, 2013. www.denverpost.com/breakingnews/ci_22129860/cu-expected-release-nearly-3-800-emails-referencing.

Miller, H. 2009. *How to Create Accountable Care Organizations.* Pittsburgh: Center for Healthcare Quality and Payment Reform.

National Library of Medicine (NLM). 2004. "National Library of Medicine Functional Statement." Accessed June 5, 2012. www.nlm.nih.gov/about/functstatement.html.

Nelson, S. 2006. "Privacy and Medical Information on the Internet." *Respiratory Care* 51 (2): 183–87.

Office of National Coordinator for Health Information Technology (ONCHIT). 2011. *Federal Health Information Technology Strategic Plan, 2011–2015.* Washington, DC: US Government Printing Office.

Olson, L. A., S. G. Peters, and J. B. Stewart. 1998. "Security and Confidentiality in an Electronic Medical Record." *Healthcare Information Management* 12 (1): 27–37.

Peel, D. 2007. "Will Violating Privacy Preserve Mass Murder?" *Modern Healthcare.* Accessed January 4, 2008. http://modernhealthcare.com/apps/pbcs.dll/article?AID=/20070427/FREE/70426007.

Poon, E. G., A. K. Jha, M. Christino, M. M. Honour, R. Fernandopulle, B. Middleton, J. New-house, L. Leape, D. W. Bates, D. Blumenthal, and R. Kaushal. 2006. "Assessing the Level of Healthcare Information Technology Adoption in the United States: A Snapshot." *BMC Medical Informatics and Decision Making* 6: 1.

Poterba, J. 1996. "Government Intervention in the Markets for Education and Health Care: How and Why?" In *Individual and Social Responsibility: Child Care, Education, Medical Care, and Long-Term Care in America,* edited by V. Fuchs. Chicago: University of Chicago Press.

Recovery.gov. n.d. "The Recovery Act." Recovery.gov. Accessed May 24, 2012. www.recovery.gov/About/Pages/The_Act.aspx.

Robeznieks, A. 2006a. "Another Computer with VA Data Goes Missing." *HIT Strategist,* August 8.

Rosenfeld, S., S. Koss, and S. Siler. 2007. "Privacy, Security and the Regional Health Information Organization." California Healthcare Foundation. Accessed August 1. www.chcf.org/documents/chronicdisease/RHIOPrivacy Security.pdf.

Rosenthal, M., and J. Camillus. 2007. *How Four Purchasers Designed and Implemented Quality-Based Purchasing Activities: Lessons from the Field.* Agency for Healthcare Research and Quality Pub. No. 07-RG008. Washington, DC: AHRQ.

Rosenthal, M., and A. Dudley. 2007. "Pay for Performance: Will the Latest Payment Trend Improve Care?" *Journal of the American Medical Association* 297 (7): 740–44.

Santerre, R. E., and S. P. Neun. 2004. *Health Economics: Theories, Insights, and Industry Studies.* Mason, OH: Thompson South-Western.

Schmeida, M. 2005. "Health Insurance Portability and Accountability Act of 1996: Just an Incremental Step in Reshaping Government." *Online Journal of Issues in Nursing* 11 (1): 7.

Stahl, M. J. (ed.). 2003. *Encyclopedia of Health Care Management.* Thousand Oaks, CA: Sage Publications.

Taylor, R., A. Bower, F. Girosi, J. Bigelow, K. Fonkych, and R. Hillestad. 2005. "Promoting Health Information Technology: Is There a Case for More-Aggressive Government Action?" *Health Affairs (Millwood)* 24 (5): 1234–45.

Upham, R., and A. Dorsey. 2007. "Living Day-to-Day with HIPAA Privacy: The Top 10 Most Inappropriate Responses Overheard in the Healthcare Workplace." HIPAAdvisory. Accessed January 4, 2008. www.hipaadvisory.com/action/privacy/daytoday.htm.

US Department of Health & Human Services (HHS). 2013. "New Rule Protects Patient Privacy, Secures Health Information." News Release. Published January 17. www.hhs.gov/news/press/2013pres/01/20130117b.html.

Vecchio, A. 2000. "Plan for the Worst Before Disaster Strikes." *Health Management Technology* 21 (6): 28–30.

Wilson, K. J., and C. E. McPherson. 2002. "It's 2002: How HIPAA-Ready Are You?" *Health Management Technology* 23 (1): 14–15, 20.

Wipke-Tevis, D. D., and M. A. Pickett. 2008. "Impact of the Health Insurance Portability and Accountability Act on Participant Recruitment and Retention." *Western Journal of Nursing Research* 30 (1): 39–53.

READING 4B

POPULATION HEALTH: COORDINATING CARE TO PROVIDE EFFECTIVE POPULATION HEALTH MANAGEMENT

Heather Jorna and Stephen A. Martin, Jr.

From *Futurescan 2014: Healthcare Trends and Implications 2014–2019* (2014), Chapter 1, 5–10. Chicago: Society for Healthcare Strategy & Market Development of the American Hospital Association and Health Administration Press, a division of the Foundation of the American College of Healthcare Executives.

Hospitals and healthcare systems are focusing more attention on population health management as a tool to improve the health of their communities and patient bases.

Provisions in the Patient Protection and Affordable Care Act explicitly promote a population health approach by accelerating the transition to value-based payment models and by expanding access to healthcare services among newly insured populations. As hospitals increasingly are being held accountable for health outcomes, leaders need to proactively manage the health of populations beyond the acute care setting.

Population health management integrates public health principles into the health-care delivery system. By focusing on upstream factors, such as health promotion and care coordination, population health management aims to deliver holistic healthcare that addresses a broad array of determinants of health to prevent chronic and acute disease. This approach to care significantly expands the traditional role of hospitals beyond their walls and into the community (HRET 2012; Stoto 2013).

The 2012 Annual Survey of Hospitals, conducted by the American Hospital Association, found that 98 percent of CEOs believe that hospitals need to investigate and implement population health management strategies. This task will require leaders to improve quality and patient safety, increase care coordination across the healthcare continuum, improve communication and information-sharing mechanisms, and expand preventive services and chronic disease management initiatives. To achieve these goals, hospital leaders are looking beyond traditional partnerships, such as those with physicians and other clinicians, and are exploring relationships with community organizations, payors, and other health providers.

This year's *Futurescan* survey assessed the foundational elements necessary for population health management. The results reveal that within the next five years, a majority of hospitals will likely focus on (1) improving care coordination for their own patient base, while forming partnerships with community organizations, payors, and other health providers; (2) improving communication and care coordination mechanisms; and (3) sharing electronic health information to improve the health of populations.

DEGREE OF CONTROL ACROSS THE CARE CONTINUUM

Hospitals plan to work with other stakeholders to improve the patient experience across the care continuum, exercising various degrees of control by partnering with the community (AHA 2013; HRET 2012), affiliating with medical groups, and engaging and educating patients. Human capital and financial resources will factor into the decision whether a hospital will control the complete continuum of care or be a noncontrolling participant in the complete continuum of care.

Large hospitals and healthcare systems have increasingly aligned themselves with primary care and specialty practices; through these relationships, hospitals gain control of the continuum of care and use integrated electronic medical records to consolidate primary, specialty, and acute care encounters (Gamble 2012). Smaller and rural hospitals are more likely to collaborate with larger organizations than lead their own integration efforts (HRET 2013). Integrated delivery systems that already own facilities spanning a variety of health services (preventive, acute, post-acute, ancillary) have the resources and facilities to assume a greater degree of control and leadership in coordinating care across populations.

The *Futurescan* survey results support this trend: A majority of hospital leaders recognize the importance of population health strategies to achieve value-based care, expect some type of participation within the next five years, and are in the process of evaluating their role and degree of control in coordinating care.

Futurescan Survey Results: Population Health

How likely is it that the following will be seen in your hospital's area by 2019?

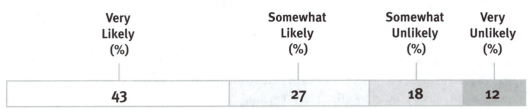

Very Likely (%)	Somewhat Likely (%)	Somewhat Unlikely (%)	Very Unlikely (%)
43	27	18	12

Your hospital or health system **will control** a complete continuum of care in your service area through a variety of relationships.

21	32	29	19

Your hospital or health system will be a **noncontrolling** participant in a complete continuum of care in your service area through a variety of relationships.

51	42	7	1

Formal mechanisms will be in place in your service area to ensure seamless coordination across the care continuum (e.g., documented handoff processes for transition management, integrated health information portal).

55	37	8	1

A formal communication structure will be established between your hospital or system and community partners to promote population health (e.g., regular meetings, representation of community partners on board or planning committees).

NOTE: Percentages may not total to exactly 100% due to rounding.

What Practitioners Predict

Hospitals or health systems will participate in a continuum of care in their service area. A majority (70 percent) of survey respondents report that by 2019 it is likely that their hospital or health system will be in control of a complete continuum of care in their service area. Approximately half of the CEOs in the survey believe that their hospital or health system will be a noncontrolling partner in a care continuum by that time.

Formal mechanisms will ensure coordination across the continuum of care. Of CEOs surveyed, nearly 93 percent predict that mechanisms such as documented handoff processes and an integrated health information portal will be in place to ensure seamless coordination across the care continuum in their area by 2019.

Hospitals or health systems will work with community partners to promote population health. Almost all (92 percent) of the CEOs surveyed report it is likely that by 2019 a formal structure of communications, including regular meetings, will be

(continued)

Futurescan Survey Results: Population Health

How likely is it that the following will be seen in <u>your hospital</u> by 2019?

Very Likely (%)	Somewhat Likely (%)	Somewhat Unlikely (%)	Very Unlikely (%)
76		22	2 ◊

Your hospital will be partnering with community organizations to support population health management initiatives (e.g., community needs assessments, chronic disease management).

80		17	3 1

Your hospital will be participating in a health information exchange (HIE), which allows electronic sharing of health information among provider organizations.

12	42	31	15

Your hospital will require that its governing board have at least one member with population health expertise.

43	49	7 1	

Your hospital will have effective measures of "population health" to support the community health improvement mandate.

Note: Percentages may not total to exactly 100% due to rounding.

◊ Less than 0.5%

(continued from previous page)

established between their hospital or health system and community partners to promote population health. Ninety-eight percent believe their organizations will work with community partners to promote population health management initiatives, such as community needs assessments or chronic disease management, by that time.

Hospitals or health systems will participate in a health information exchange (HIE). Almost all (97 percent) of the survey respondents predict that their organization will participate in an HIE that allows sharing of health information among providers by 2019.

Practitioners are divided about population health expertise on boards. Just over half of CEOs in the survey report it is likely that their hospital or health system will require that its governing board include at least one population health expert.

Population health measures will be established. Almost all CEOs surveyed (92 percent) predict that their hospitals or health systems will have effective measures of "population health" in place to support the community health mandate by 2019.

Formal Mechanisms to Coordinate Across the Continuum of Care

Hospitals and healthcare systems are confident that formal care coordination structures that ensure seamless coordination across the care continuum, such as documented handoff processes and integrated health portals, will be in place by 2019. The formal mechanisms should optimize the use of health information across the continuum of care, resulting in fewer non-value-added treatments and better use of health resources to improve patient health and quality of care.

To become active participants in their own healthcare, patients must be engaged and given tools to manage their own health. Whether these tools include an integrated health portal, patient navigator, social worker, case manager, or community health worker, hospitals can adopt various mechanisms to drive patient involvement and accountability (AHA 2013).

Degree of Community Partnership

More and more hospitals are recognizing the value of addressing the health of populations beyond the traditional acute care setting. To successfully engage populations outside of their four walls, hospitals have to form community-based partnerships. These partnerships have the ability to (1) engage communities outside the hospital setting (HRET 2013), (2) expand the scope of the population served by the hospital, (3) align community needs with hospital offerings, and (4) address upstream disease prevention in the community. Formal collaboration structures indicate a commitment to sustaining strong relationships with outside organizations. Post-acute care providers; government and commercial payors; employers; social and community services providers; public health agencies; local, state, and federal policy makers; physicians and other clinicians; and hospitals all play various roles in effectively engaging the patient in population health initiatives (AHA 2013). The specific groups with which a hospital collaborates are determined by the community's needs and the hospital's goals.

Participation in Health Information Exchanges

The *Futurescan* survey reveals important trends in electronic exchange of health data. The findings suggest that hospitals view information sharing as an important step toward better understanding and addressing the health status of populations. Participation in health information exchanges (HIEs) across the health system will be essential for monitoring and identifying population health trends, identifying opportunities for population health interventions, and predicting the impact of those interventions. Developing robust health information technology is essential for population health management because it will (1) allow providers to target at-risk populations in greatest need of services, (2) make the data actionable, and (3) generate alerts to providers about patient needs (Institute for Health Technology Transformation 2012). Although implementing an HIE presents myriad challenges, these systems will be crucial for managing population health.

IMPLICATIONS FOR HOSPITAL LEADERS

The aggregate *Futurescan* survey results indicate a strong commitment to population health advancement within the next five years. The degree and type of involvement a hospital will pursue will depend on the hospital's type, institutional culture, and competing priorities. Exhibit 1.1 lists key considerations for different hospital categories.

CONCLUSION

The *Futurescan* survey results support a paradigm shift toward population health management across the entire continuum of care within the next five years. Forward-looking hospitals are engaging in challenging but necessary changes that promote population health. Whether improving the overall health of their population through better care coordination or working with community partners to improve the health of the broader community, hospitals are

EXHIBIT 1.1
Key Considerations by Hospital Type

Small/Rural Hospitals	• Take a more noncontrolling, network- or affiliation-type approach to population health initiatives because of their limited size and resources. • Can leverage their influence and relationships within communities to ensure successful programs.
Integrated Delivery Systems	• Have more opportunities to assume a coordinating role in population health initiatives with several community partners (e.g., a population health "integrator" role) because of their size and geographic reach. • Possess resources to engage in advocacy and policy efforts that promote better health and well-being.
Academic Medical Centers	• Face the challenge of aligning population health across their threefold mission—patient care, research, and medical education. • Often have high standing in their communities and can leverage their influence and prestige to engage partners.
Other	• Specialty hospitals can leverage their expertise to implement targeted population health programs in their communities (e.g., childhood obesity, heart health programs). • Faith-based hospitals can garner the support of religious organizations to supply volunteers for and financially support population health initiatives. • Stand-alone hospitals have fewer established affiliations and may therefore take a noncontrolling or networking-type approach to population health initiatives.

committing resources to promote population health. Participating in an HIE and sharing health data with other providers will allow hospitals to effectively address population health trends.

Hospital and healthcare system leaders recognize that advancing population health will enable them to thrive in a value-based landscape. With strong collaborations, formal structures that enable care coordination, and the ability to leverage health data, hospitals can create population health initiatives that will lead to success in the evolving care environment.

REFERENCES

American Hospital Association (AHA). 2013. *Engaging Health Care Users: A Framework for Healthy Individuals and Communities.* Published January. Chicago: American Hospital Association. www.aha.org/research/cor/content/engaging_health_care_users.pdf.

————. 2012. "Annual Survey of Hospitals." Unpublished survey conducted November 2011 to January 2012. Data accessed July 2013.

Gamble, M. 2012. "Primary Care Strategy: The Most Important Decisions Hospitals Can Make." *Becker's Hospital Review.* Posted March 27. www.beckershospitalreview.com/ hospital-physician-relationships/primary-care-strategy-the-most-important-decisions-hospitals-can-make.html.

Health Research & Educational Trust (HRET). 2013. *The Role of Small and Rural Hospitals and Care Systems in Effective Population Health Partnerships.* Published June. Chicago: Health Research & Educational Trust. www.hpoe.org/Reports-HPOE/The_Role_Small_Rural_Hospital_Effective_Population_Health_Partnership.pdf.

————. 2012. *Managing Population Health: The Role of the Hospital.* Published April. Chicago: Health Research & Educational Trust. www.hpoe.org/Reports-HPOE/managing_population_health.pdf.

Institute for Health Technology Transformation. 2012. *Population Health Management: A Roadmap for Provider-Based Automation in a New Era of Healthcare.* New York: Institute for Health Technology Transformation. http://ihealthtran.com/pdf/PHMReport.pdf.

Stoto, M.A. 2013. *Population Health in the Affordable Care Act Era.* Published February 21. Washington, DC: AcademyHealth. www.academyhealth.org/files/AH2013pophealth.pdf.

READING 4C
THE PATIENT-CENTERED MEDICAL HOME SOLUTION TO THE COST–QUALITY CONUNDRUM

Michael Ewing

From *Journal of Healthcare Management* 58 (4): 258–66.

EXECUTIVE SUMMARY

The U.S. healthcare system has been plagued by rising costs while achieving relatively poor-quality outcomes, and the situation continues to worsen. One solution is the patient-centered medical home (PCMH) model of primary care. This model focuses on care coordination and development of long-term physician–patient relationships that are expected to lead to better quality care and higher rates of patient satisfaction than have previously been achieved. Although the PCMH features a number of core principles, significant differences are seen across models.

Three of the most prevalent models are those offered by the American Academy of Family Physicians, National Demonstration Project, and National Committee for Quality Assurance (NCQA). After analysis, the NCQA approach emerged as the recommended model due to its specificity and comprehensiveness. Research suggests that the PCMH, and specifically the NCQA model, can achieve both increases in quality and reductions in cost. However, this finding is tempered by the challenges inherent in implementation.

INTRODUCTION

The problem of increasing costs accompanied by merely average quality care in the U.S. healthcare system is well documented. As of 2012, according to the Kaiser Family Foundation (KFF, 2012), healthcare expenditures in the United States comprised 17.9% of gross domestic product, equating to $8,402 spent on healthcare per person. The same report projects that by 2020, healthcare expenditures will be nearly one fifth of the economy, at 19.8%. Furthermore, not only is the U.S. healthcare system the most expensive in the world but it is 48% more costly per capita than the system ranked second in healthcare expenditures, that of Switzerland (KFF, 2012).

However, the extensive spending on the U.S. healthcare system does not yield outstanding quality. Instead, by most measures, healthcare in the United States is at best average compared to other countries. The World Health Organization (WHO, 2011) ranks the U.S. system 37th in the world, behind some countries considered to be less developed, such as Cyprus and Costa Rica. Moreover, while the United States is the world leader in medical research, it lags the other Organisation for Economic Co-operation and Development (OECD, 2011) nations in terms of life expectancy and infant mortality.

These findings have given rise over the past 40 years to many solutions to improve quality of care in the United States while lowering costs. The remainder of this essay analyzes a key element emerging from health reform—the patient-centered medical home (PCMH)—as a potential solution to this conundrum.

BACKGROUND

The concept of the medical home was first introduced into the practice of pediatrics by the American Academy of Pediatrics in the 1960s. At that time, the term referred to a primary care practice that partnered with families in caring for children. As the model grew, it began to take on many of the principles now associated with the PCMH, such as coordinated and comprehensive care. In 1978, WHO met to discuss the medical home, specifically endorsing primary care's role in carrying the medical home forward. WHO believed that primary care was integral to maintaining an individual's health and identified specific functions that primary care providers should perform toward that end. These included the following (Robert Graham Center, 2007):

◆ Address the prevailing health needs of the community

◆ Educate the public about health issues

◆ Provide preventive services

The broad scope of primary care makes pediatrics ideal for accomplishing these tasks and participating in the medical home. But while WHO detailed the benefits of primary care in the late 1970s, it was not until the 1990s that the principles of primary care and the PCMH were linked (Robert Graham Center, 2007).

At that time, the Institute of Medicine (IOM, 1996) mentioned the medical home in conjunction with supporting the tenets of primary care, and in its 2001 report *Crossing the Quality Chasm*, IOM declared patient-centered care to be a main goal of the healthcare system. This report had a major impact on family medicine (Steiger and Balog, 2010). In response, in an effort to better understand how to transform primary care practices into medical homes, several family medicine organizations, including the American Academy of Family Physicians (AAFP), American Academy of Family Physicians Foundation, American Board of Family Medicine, Association of Departments of Family Medicine, Association of Family Medicine Residency Directors, North American Primary Care Research Group, and Society of Teachers of Family Medicine, formed the Future of Family Medicine Project. The group declared that every individual should have a medical home to receive needed services, and organizations such as those involved in the Project, as well as quality organizations such as NCQA, began to develop models to implement their versions of the PCMH (Robert Graham Center, 2007).

The chronic care model also influenced the development of the PCMH concept. This model was developed by the MacColl Center for Health Care Innovation in the early 1990s and was published in 1998 (ICIC, n.d.). The case management principles of this approach to chronic care have been demonstrated to lower costs and provide higher quality healthcare to patients with chronic diseases (RWJF, 2012). For example, TEAMcare, a chronic care model intervention, was shown to result in better outcomes for patients who suffered from depression and other chronic diseases (Katon et al., 2010). Given that 50% of U.S. residents have at least one chronic disease, care coordination and other principles championed by the chronic care model are important applications to incorporate into PCMH models (Robert Graham Center, 2007).

Another profound influence on the PCMH was the overall movement toward patient safety. As physicians and hospitals were hit with decreased Medicare reimbursements in the 1990s, they were forced to adapt to remain profitable and maintain their income. Much of this adaptation occurred through decreased nurse staffing, and many hospitals began to see patients only in terms of their diagnosis and the corresponding payment for treating it through diagnosis-related groups (Simpson, 2003). More recently, this approach has been rejected by many practitioners in favor of patient-centered care (Porter, 2009), which was largely brought about by IOM's groundbreaking reports *To Err Is Human* (1999) and *Crossing the Quality Chasm* (2001).

In *To Err Is Human,* IOM paints a grim picture of patient safety in the United States. The study found that between 44,000 and 98,000 individuals die each year from hospital errors (IOM, 1999). This statistic sparked a strong movement toward better patient safety practices and improved quality.

IOM followed *To Err Is Human* with *Crossing the Quality Chasm* (IOM, 2001), which sets out specific steps for healthcare organizations to follow toward delivering improved patient care. It recommends six goals for improvement, among them the practice of patient-centered care. IOM defines patient-centered care as "providing care that is respectful of and responsive to individual patient preferences, needs, and values, and ensuring that patient values guide all clinical decisions." To achieve this goal, organizations are encouraged to ensure that patients have autonomy in deciding their care and that physicians partner with their patients in making decisions. Physicians were thus charged with providing patients with adequate knowledge and transparency to make their own informed decisions (IOM, 2001).

SOLUTIONS

As solutions to the conundrum of high cost and below-average quality in healthcare, a number of PCMH models have emerged. This section focuses on three of the most prevalent models of the PCMH: those promulgated by AAFP, the National Demonstration Project (NDP), and the National Committee for Quality Assurance (NCQA).

AMERICAN ACADEMY OF FAMILY PHYSICIANS

AAFP, in conjunction with the American Academy of Pediatrics, the American Osteo-pathic Association, and the American College of Physicians, released its model of the PCMH in 2007. The model features the following seven components of a patient's medical home (Robert Graham Center, 2007), each of which is described in more detail below:

◆ Personal physician

◆ Physician-directed medical practice

◆ Whole-person orientation

◆ Coordinated care

◆ Quality and safety

◆ Enhanced access

◆ Payment reform

Having a personal physician implies a strong personal relationship between physi-cian and patient. This relationship must be continually developed over time as the physi-cian provides acute and chronic care. An important precursor to fulfilling this expectation is that the patient has chosen a usual source of care, providing the basis for developing what IOM refers to as a "continuous healing relationship." Establishing this relationship is integral to the PCMH, as it allows primary care physicians to provide high-quality, coordinated care over an extended period.

A physician-directed medical practice adheres to a team-based approach to primary care headed by the physician or another clinician. A key characteristic of this concept is that the team places the patient first, meaning care should be coordinated between primary care and specialty physicians as well as that between physicians and their care teams. It also stresses the importance of feedback from the patient in promoting continuous improve-ment (Porter, 2009).

The whole-person orientation of the PCMH entails treating the patient through a comprehensive approach as a complex being in the context of illness. That is, the patient's physical, mental, and social health needs must be considered in the course of diagnosis and treatment. Thus, the physician must oversee all of these aspects of the patient or be able to refer the patient to an appropriate specialist.

Coordinated care is a highly organized care delivery approach. For this component, the primary care physician manages a patient's care by coordinating with other health profession-als, usually subspecialists. One important aspect of this feature is the use of health information technology to seamlessly integrate care (Porter, 2009) to ensure that accurate information is shared between care teams and that the patient receives the right care at the right time.

Quality and safety are fundamental to the PCMH approach. Quality improvements are inherent within the other principles of the PCMH, but the pursuit of quality brings voluntary participation in scientific quality measurements. It also implies that care is provided on the basis of widely accepted national practice guidelines established by scientific research.

Improved access in the PCMH refers to an environment that features open scheduling and the provision of nontraditional care by care teams through Internet or telephone conferencing. It is important that the patient have access to his or her medical home in some fashion 24 hours a day, every day.

In the PCMH, payment must be tied to the delivery of higher-quality care; specifically, it should be connected to value-adding steps of the healthcare process. Important steps to creating a better payment system include adding incentives for coordinating care and providing care in nontraditional ways, such as through e-mail or phone consultations. It is also important to motivate physicians to enter primary care practice to alleviate the shortage of those physicians. As primary care is the foundation of the PCMH, it is important to create incentives to entice new doctors to the primary care arena and to make sure reimbursement is adequate to keep them there.

In creating its PCMH model, AAFP and its partner organizations sought to enumerate the basic medical home principles so that other models may be similarly built.

NATIONAL DEMONSTRATION PROJECT

The NDP was a two-year pilot program initiated in 2006 by TransforMED, a division of AAFP. The project was designed to determine the impact of TransforMED intervention on a physician practice's ability to adopt the PCMH model of care. A total of 337 practices applied to participate; of those, 36 were chosen for the project. The practices were randomly split into an intervention group and a self-directed group. TransforMED provided guidance to the intervention group on implementing PCMH over two years, and the self-directed group was largely left to implement the model without assistance (Nutting et al., 2009).

Over the course of the study, TransforMED used the intervention group to implement its model of the PCMH. This model was similar to the AAFP model but featured some fundamental differences, especially as implemented at the beginning of the project. The most fundamental aspect that differentiates the NDP model from the AAFP model is the NDP's greater emphasis on information technology to assist in patient access and open scheduling. Whereas AAFP built its model on the pillars of primary care, the NDP model was built on technology. The NDP model is also physician centered; it does not use other clinicians for PCMH activities. It lacks provisions for mental healthcare (Stewart et al., 2010) and does not call for payment reform, one of the seven components of the AAFP model (Stange et al., 2010b).

By the end of the study, the NDP model grew to be more similar to the AAFP model and the nationally accepted guidelines for the PCMH. Its current version is based on three pillars: patient-centered care, a wholeperson orientation, and a continuous patient–physician relationship. It seeks to provide the patient with greater access and coordination through information technology, suggesting that a PCMH's website should enhance patients' access to lab results and other necessary information pertinent to the PCMH's patients. Patients in practices that adopt the NDP model should be able to receive an appointment the same day they request it. In addition, the PCMH should optimize its space for efficient workflow and patient visit spaces. The practice should employ coordinated, multidisciplinary care to improve quality by developing relationships between the practice and other health professionals, such as pharmacists and therapists. Finally, the PCMH should be a comprehensive practice, providing or coordinating all of a patient's needs, including acute and chronic care management, promotion of wellness, and preventive services (Stewart et al., 2010).

The NDP model advanced the application of the AAFP model by carrying it into implementation at primary care practices.

NATIONAL COMMITTEE FOR QUALITY ASSURANCE

The final model considered is that developed by NCQA. The organization proposed this model, based on its Physician Practice Connections (PPC) evaluation system, to give ambulatory practices a guidebook for instituting the PCMH (NCQA, 2011).

In 2008, NCQA created the PPC-PCMH Recognition Program, which evaluates practices on the PPC criteria as they relate to medical homes. These criteria were updated in 2011 to include additional requirements related to healthcare IT meaningful use (NCQA, 2011).

The NCQA model for PCMHs is reflected in the evaluation's requirements. Each practice is graded on aspects of care delivery in six recognition categories:

- Enhancing access

- Identifying and managing populations

- Planning and managing care

- Providing self-care support and community resources

- Tracking and coordinating care

- Measuring and improving performance

Enhanced access and continuity are defined as the extent to which the practice accommodates patients during and after office hours using team-based care. Identification and management of patient populations refers to collecting data on each patient. Planning and managing care includes using evidence-based practices to improve the treatment of patients' maladies. Tracking and coordinating care involves detailing referrals and coordinating treatment for patients and sets the practice up to achieve high marks in the final category, measuring and improving performance (NCQA, 2011).

An environment of continuous improvement is integral to PCMH (NCQA, 2011). The NCQA model focuses on enhancing organization and data collection to inform how higher-quality care is delivered. Allowing for more seamless administration of care and better tracking of patient outcomes provides for an atmosphere of quality. Care is focused on the patient, and better information infrastructure promotes the monitoring of chronic diseases and preventive care (NCQA, 2012).

RECOMMENDATION

Of the three models examined, this analysis finds that the NCQA model is preferred for practices, mostly because of the significant amount of research into it (much of it supportive) and the paucity of research into other models. A study involving Community Care of North Carolina saw a 23% decrease in emergency department utilization and costs over 7 years. A different study involving Oklahoma Medicaid demonstrated a $29 reduction in per capita member costs over the course of 2 years. A study of NCQA model–based PCMHs involving the Intermountain Healthcare Medical Group demonstrated a marked decrease in emergency room utilization and better chronic disease management (PCPCC, 2009). The NCQA model provides for not only healthier patients but more satisfied patients compared to those in a typical primary care practice structure. In a study involving a Humana PCMH program, patient satisfaction improved or stayed the same, compared to patients' experience before the PCMH intervention, in 45 out of 61 cases (categories used to measure patient satisfaction) (Grumbach & Grundy, 2010). Taken together, the findings from these studies suggest that practices operating under an NCQA-model PCMH achieve better patient outcomes at a lower cost than can be achieved using other PCMH models.

Studies have also revealed that physician practice staff members are happier in the PCMH. One group health study found that only 10% of staff in PCMH pilot programs felt high levels of exhaustion compared to 30% in control practices. The same study also found better retention and satisfaction among primary care physicians compared to non-PCMH practices (Grumbach & Grundy, 2010). This is an important outcome, as the primary care physician shortage is a notable problem—this model helps ensure in a competitive market that practices can recruit and retain the physicians they need by affording them a satisfying work experience.

One main reason for the success of the NCQA approach to PCMHs is that a practice's designation as an NCQA-recognized home can lead to opportunities to new bonuses and payments. As a national committee, NCQA can determine a practice's eligibility for new incentives for achieving quality care outcomes (NCQA, 2011). Another benefit of the NCQA model is that it incorporates information technology, which aligns with the framework of meaningful use. By adopting NCQA's model for PCMHs, practices can take advantage of the incentives offered by the U.S. Department of Health and Human Services for adopting electronic medical records (EMRs) as outlined in the Health Information Technology for Economic and Clinical Health Act.

Even though the PCMH has demonstrated better outcomes and lower costs, operating under this care delivery model is a big commitment for a practice to undertake. The PCMH is more of a transformation than a simple project. Evidence from the NDP details the time and effort it takes to implement the PCMH model. As shown by that project, after 2 years, several of the practices that were seeking to implement the PCMH were still trying to do so, and many were fatigued with the process. Even highly motivated practices were susceptible to burnout from the arduous process of incorporating new technology into the practice (Stewart et al., 2010). These findings serve as a caution that only highly motivated physicians and practices should attempt to implement a PCMH, with the understanding that implementation should not be undertaken step-by-step. Instead, evidence suggests that practices have greater success when they completely revamp at one time (Stange et al., 2010b). The often impractical nature of a complete overhaul is one reason explaining the difficulty practices experience in installing the PCMH model.

Another reason is the direct costs involved. EMRs are notoriously expensive and difficult to implement. They can cost $100,000 or more, not including the cost of training. Furthermore, many practices have difficulty transferring data to an EMR, and practices can experience slowdowns in production due to this process. Another economic cost of implementation is the uncertainty of payment reform. Billing remains tied to traditional care structures, even though reimbursement is slowly changing. The fact that reimbursement schedules are lagging advancements in new forms of care leads to uncertainties about how new forms of care, such as group consultation and telemedicine, will be reimbursed (Stange et al., 2010a). Overall, a number of costs and uncertainties accompany the PCMH, but once applied, its principles are sound, as demonstrated by numerous studies.

CONCLUSION

The NCQA model of the patient medical home has proven its effectiveness, a factor that separates it from the other two models analyzed in this essay. All PCMH models have been shown to provide improved patient quality at a decreased cost compared to traditional primary care practice; however, implementing the PCMH is complicated by a number of factors. The cost and effort involved and the need to choose among a number of different models can make executing this primary care model difficult. Even with this difficulty, however, the PCMH model represents an exciting movement for primary care. Its incorporation of technology and its dedication to coordination of care provide the basis for an improved system. This option emerges at a time that change is crucial to keep the U.S. healthcare system solvent.

Healthcare expenditures in the United States now account for a greater percentage of the economy than ever before, and if no measures are taken to stem those expenditures, the current system will continue to provide below-average care at an extraordinary cost.

REFERENCES

Grumbach, K., & Grundy, P. (2010). Outcomes of implementing patient centered medical home interventions. Retrieved from http:// www.pcpcc.net/files/evidnece_outcomes_in_pcmh.pdf

Improving Chronic Illness Care (ICIC). (n.d.). The MacColl Center for Health Care Innovation. Retrieved from http:// www.improvingchroniccare.org/index.php?p=The_MacColl_Center&s=93

Institute of Medicine (IOM). (1996). *Primary care: America's health in a new era. Washington, DC: National Academies Press.*

Institute of Medicine (IOM). (1999, November). *To err is human: Building a safer health system.* Washington, DC: National Academies Press.

Institute of Medicine (IOM). (2001, March). *Crossing the quality chasm: A new health system for the 21st century.* Washington, DC: National Academies Press.

Kaiser Family Foundation (KFF) (2012, May). *Health care costs: A primer.* Retrieved from http://www.kff.org/insurance/upload/7670-03.pdf

Katon, W. J., Lin, E. H., Von Korff, M., Ciechanowski, P., Ludman, E. J., Young, B., . . . McCulloch, D. (2010). Collaborative care for patients with depression and chronic illnesses. *New England Journal of Medicine,* 363 (27), 2611–2620.

Nutting, P., Miller, W., Crabtree, B., Jaén, C., Stewart, E., & Stange, K. (2009). Initial lessons from the first National Demonstration Project on practice transformation to a patient-centered medical home. *Annals of Family Medicine,* 7(3), 254–260.

National Committee for Quality Assurance (NCQA). (2011). NCQA patient centered medical home. Retrieved from http:// www.ncqa.org/Programs/Recognition/PatientCenteredMedicalHome

National Committee for Quality Assurance (NCQA). (2012). Requirements for NCQA recognition as a patient-centered medical home. Retrieved from http:// www.ncqa.org/Programs/Recognition/PatientCenteredMedicalHome

Organisation for Economic Co-operation and Development (OECD) (2011). *OECD Factbook 2011–2012: Economic, environmental and social statistics*. Retrieved from http://www. oecd-ilibrary.org/economics /oecd-factbook-2011-2012_factbook-2011-en

Patient-Centered Primary Care Collaborative (PCPCC). (2009). Proof in practice. Retrieved from http://www.pcpcc.net/sites/default/files/media/PilotGuidePip.pdf

Porter, S. (2009). Academy launches comprehensive patient centered medical home resources. *Annals of Family Medicine, 7*(4), 378–379

Robert Graham Center. (2007). The patient centered medical home. Retrieved from http:// graham-center.org

Robert Wood Johnson Foundation (RWJF). (2012). Model elements. Retrieved from http:// www.improvingchroniccare.org/index.php?p=Model_Elements&s=18

Simpson, R. (2003). Back to basics with IT and patient-centered care. *Nursing Management, 34*(4), 14.

Stange, K. C., Miller, W. L., Nutting, P. A., Crabtree, B. F., Stewart, E. E., & Jaén, C. R. (2010a). Context for understanding the National Demonstration Project and the patient-centered medical home. *Annals of Family Medicine, 8*(Suppl. 1), S2–S8, S92.

Stange, K., Miller, W., Nutting, P., Crabtree, B., Stewart, E., & Jaén, C. R. (2010b). Summary of the National Demonstration Project and recommendations for the patient-centered medical home. *Annals of Family Medicine, 8*(Suppl. 1), S80–S92.

Steiger, N., & Balog, A. (2010). Realizing patient-centered care: Putting patients in the center, not the middle. *Frontiers of Health Services Management, 26*(4), 15–24.

Stewart, E. E., Nutting, P. A., Crabtree, B. F., Stange, K. C., Miller, W. L., & Jaén, C. R. (2010). Implementing the patient-centered medical home: Observation and description of the National Demonstration Project. *Annals of Family Medicine, 8*(Suppl. 1), S21–S32, S92.

World Health Organization (WHO). (2011). *World health statistics*. Retrieved from http:// www.who.int/en/

READING 4D

PRIMARY CARE

Phoebe Lindsey Barton
From *Understanding the U.S. Health Services System*, 4th ed. (2010), Chapter 13, 331–38. Chicago: Health Administration Press.

INTRODUCTION

Even the most effective system of health promotion, health protection, and disease prevention will not forestall the need for treatment of illness, injury, and disease. A primary care system provides appropriate treatment for common diseases and injuries, essential drugs, and basic dental care, and it identifies potentially serious physical or mental health conditions that require prompt referral for more intensive levels of care.

This chapter defines primary care, discusses who provides it, and addresses how patients access and use it. The chapter concludes with a discussion of policy issues related to primary care.

DEFINING PRIMARY CARE

Primary care is usually the patient's first contact with the treatment system. Roemer's model of a health services system defines primary care as the entry point into the health services system, wherein:

- illness or disease is diagnosed and initial treatment is provided;

- episodic care for common, nonchronic illnesses and injuries is rendered;

- prescription drugs to treat common illnesses or injuries are provided;

- routine dental care—examinations, cleaning, repair of dental cavities—occurs; and

- potentially serious physical or mental health conditions that require prompt referral for secondary or tertiary care are diagnosed.

The Institute of Medicine (IOM), which established its first conference on primary care in 1978, convened a Committee on the Future of Primary Care in the early 1990s to reexamine its initial definition of primary care. The IOM committee issued the following revised definition of primary care in 1994:

> Primary care is the provision of integrated, accessible health care services by clinicians who are accountable for addressing a large majority of personal health care needs, developing a sustained partnership with patients, and practicing in the context of family and community (IOM 1995).

Central to this definition are concepts of integrated services, accessibility, provider accountability, provider–patient partnerships, and care oriented to family and community needs. In 1995, the IOM released its comprehensive study on primary care, *Primary Care, America's Health in a New Era.*

Although most primary care is provided on an ambulatory basis, some types of secondary care may also be provided on an ambulatory basis. The terms *primary care* and *ambulatory care* therefore overlap but are not synonymous. The data presented in the sections that follow, although inclusive of primary care, are compiled as ambulatory care visits and may include contacts or visits for secondary care. Despite these limitations, the data provide insight into categories of primary care providers and utilization of primary care services.

PRIMARY CARE PROVIDERS

The IOM definition of primary care emphasizes the provision of care by clinicians. The first category of clinicians that comes to mind is generally physicians. Exhibit 13.1 shows the distribution of ambulatory care visits to physicians' offices, by type of physician specialty, for 2006. The use of specialty physicians increases as a person ages.

Physician assistants, nurse practitioners, nurse midwives, nurses, and other categories of providers are also considered clinicians. The definition of primary care provider may be expanded to also include physical and speech therapists, mental health providers, diagnostic and therapeutic laboratory staff, podiatrists, optometrists, home health aides, respiratory therapists, and social workers (Nichols 1996).

ACCESS TO AND UTILIZATION OF PRIMARY CARE

Because primary care is the entry level to diagnosis and treatment of illness, injury, and disease in a comprehensive health services system, it would seem logical that all members of society would have unobstructed access to the system. However, financial and other barriers may limit access to primary and other health services. People with public or private health insurance are more likely to have a connection to one or more primary care providers. People with limited or no health insurance obtain episodic primary and other care from a variety of sources. The Community and Migrant Health Center Program, for example, provides comprehensive primary health services to migrant workers and their families and to persons with low incomes who pay on a sliding-scale basis.

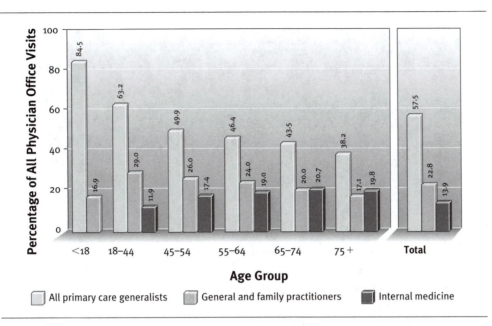

EXHIBIT 13.1
Visits to Primary
Care Generalist
and Specialist
Physicians, by Age
Group, 2006

SOURCE: This exhibit was created using data from *Health, United States, 2008*, published by the National Center for Health Statistics in 2009.

One measure of access to primary care is the average number of visits to physicians and other primary care providers, including hospital outpatient and emergency departments, per person per year.[1] Exhibit 13.2 shows that the average number of physician visits per person per year dropped from a high of 6 visits in 1993 to 3.3 in 1995 and then increased to 3.8 in 2006. The increase is likely attributable to several factors, including increased Medicaid coverage of children and increased utilization of physician services for chronic health problems, some associated with an aging population. Although perhaps most of these contacts are for primary care, some are for more intensive care. Of physician contacts, 80 percent take place in the physician's office, 11 percent in hospital emergency departments, and 9 percent in hospital outpatient departments (USDHHS 1995a; NCHS 2008).

Contacts with a primary care provider are associated with perceived and/or diagnosed health status, age, gender, race/ethnicity, and income. Exhibit 13.3 shows the number of physician contacts by age and by gender. After reaching age 18 years, women typically have more physician contacts per year than do men. Some of this difference is related to reproductive health and childbearing.

Exhibit 13.4 shows the proportion of the population that had a dental visit in 2006. More females than males typically visit a dentist in a year. What these data do not reflect are the visits for restorative and cosmetic dental care that may be occurring among people with higher incomes.

EXHIBIT 13.2
Number of Annual
per Person Visits
to Primary Care
Providers, Select
Years, 1987–2006

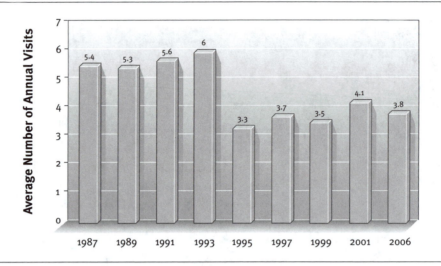

SOURCE: This exhibit was created using data from Health, United States, 2008, published by the National Center for Health Statistics in 2009.

NOTE: Sites of contact include physician's offices, hospital outpatient facilities, and emergency departments.

EXHIBIT 13.3
Number of Annual
Visits to Physicians,
by Age and
Gender, 2006

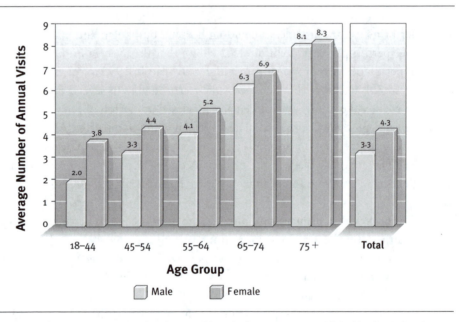

SOURCE: This exhibit was created using data from Health, United States, 2008, published by the National Center for Health Statistics in 2009.

NOTE: Sites of contact include physician offices, hospital outpatient facilities, and emergency departments.

EXHIBIT 13.4
Dental Visits in
the Past Year, by
Gender, 2006

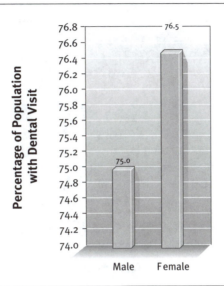

SOURCE: This exhibit was created using data from *Health, United States, 2008*, published by the National
Center for Health Statistics in 2009.

Exhibit 13.5 shows the number of physician visits per year by race and by age. The
proportion of whites, blacks, Hispanics, and other racial and ethnic groups who saw a
dentist in 2006 is shown in Exhibit 13.6; a higher proportion of whites and Asians had a
dental visit than did other racial and ethnic groups.

PRIMARY CARE ISSUES IN THE U.S. HEALTH SERVICES SYSTEM

The U.S. health services system faces several major policy issues related to primary care:
access to care, the availability of primary care providers, and reimbursement for primary
care providers.

ACCESS TO PRIMARY CARE

Primary care, as the entry into the treatment system, is important for dealing with routine
illnesses and injuries but also for diagnosing and initiating therapy for more severe illnesses
and diseases. Unrestricted access to primary care, if appropriately pursued, should result
in improved health status for individuals and for a population. When access to primary
care is limited or impeded, however, an individual's health status may deteriorate and in
turn negatively affect the health of a population. Based on the IOM definition, a comprehensive health services system should ensure that primary care and other health services
are accessible.

EXHIBIT 13.5

Annual Number
of Physician Visits,
by Age and Race/
Ethnicity, 2006

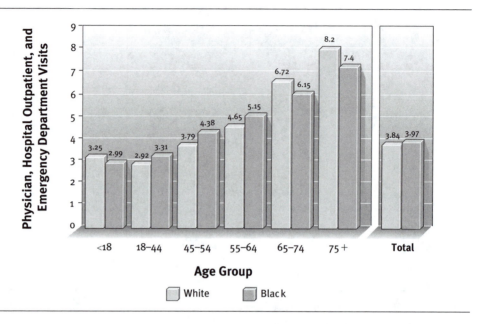

SOURCE: This exhibit was created using data from *Health, United States, 2008*, published by the National
Center for Health Statistics in 2009.

EXHIBIT 13.6

Dental Visits in the
Past Year, by Race/
Ethnicity and Age,
2006

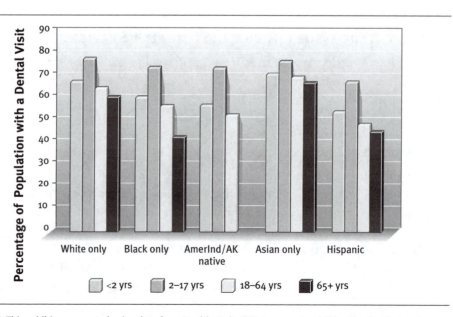

SOURCE: This exhibit was created using data from *Health, United States, 2008*, published by the National
Center for Health Statistics in 2009.

AVAILABILITY OF PRIMARY CARE PROVIDERS

Access to primary care depends, in part, on the type and number of primary care providers available to serve a population. Primary care and other generalist physicians constitute only about one-third of U.S. physicians, an inverse ratio to that of health services systems in other industrialized countries. Efforts have been made (e.g., revising basic medical school training and limiting the number of available slots for specialist training) to increase the number of primary care physicians in the U.S. system. The lengthy pipeline for physician training, however, suggests that the supply and the ratio will not dramatically change in the short term.

REIMBURSEMENT FOR PRIMARY CARE PHYSICIANS

The provision of primary care services has traditionally been reimbursed at lower rates than more intensive levels of services, and primary care and generalist physicians have generally had lower incomes than their specialist counterparts. One effect of this differential is an implicit devaluing of primary care providers and a tendency for people to self-refer to a range of specialists rather than to access care through a primary provider.

The U.S. health services system's move toward managed care signaled a change in the valuation of primary care providers. Many forms of managed care focus on the primary care provider as the point of entry for other levels of care and services. Primary care physicians and other providers found themselves in demand, and the market forces of supply and demand resulted in increased incomes for primary care providers. How all the managed care forces will play out over time is not yet clear. Some reports indicate that some managed care entities are reducing or eliminating their gatekeeping functions, which were often filled by primary care physicians (Ferris et al. 2001; Lawrence 2001).

THE FUTURE OF PRIMARY CARE

Primary care is the backbone of our health services system, but alarms have been clanging about the potential erosion of primary care. Thomas Bodenheimer (2006), a practicing primary care physician, reports that

> Primary care is facing a confluence of factors that could spell disaster. Patients are increasingly dissatisfied with their care and with the difficulty of gaining timely access to a primary care physician; many primary care physicians, in turn, are unhappy with their jobs, as they face a seemingly insurmountable task; the quality of care is uneven; reimbursement is inadequate; and fewer and fewer medical students are choosing to enter the field.

At the same time alarms are being raised about primary care, others are calling for greater expansion of the field. A recent report from the Pan American Health Organization (2008) discusses the global interest in integrating mental health care into primary care.

None of these concerns is trivial. The fate of primary care as a discipline rests in some part on proposed reforms for the U.S. health services system. Few would anticipate that such reforms will occur quickly or smoothly.

SUMMARY

Primary care—the first level of diagnosis and treatment of illness, injury, and disease—has transitioned from the edges of the delivery system toward its center. This transition is changing the ways primary care providers are trained, the demand for their services, and the reimbursement for primary care.

NOTE

1. Physician and other health care visits generally indicate a face-to-face visit between provider and patient. The term *contacts* is often used to include telephone and face-to-face communication.

KEY WORDS

access to care
ambulatory care
Community and Migrant Health Center Program
gatekeeping
Institute of Medicine (IOM)
nurse practitioner
physician assistant
primary care
utilization of services

BIBLIOGRAPHY

Bodenheimer, T. 2006. "Primary Care—Will It Survive?" *New England Journal of Medicine* 355 (9): 861–64.

Ferris, T. G., Y. Chang, D. Blumenthal, and S. D. Pearson. 2001. "Leaving Gatekeeping Behind—Effects of Opening Access to Specialists for Adults in a Health Maintenance Organization." *New England Journal of Medicine* 345 (18): 1312–17.

Institute of Medicine (IOM). 1995. *Primary Care: America's Health in a New Era.* Washington, DC: National Academies Press.

Lawrence, D. 2001. "Gatekeeping Reconsidered." *New England Journal of Medicine* 345 (18): 1342–43.

National Center for Health Statistics (NCHS). 2009. *Health, United States, 2008.* Hyattsville, MD: NCHS. [Online information; retrieved 5/24/09.] www.cdc.gov/nchs/hus.htm.

————. 2008. *National Nursing Home Survey, 2004.* Washington, DC: NCHS.

Nichols, L. 1996. *Nonphysician Health Care Providers: Uses of Ambulatory Services, Expenditures, and Sources of Payment.* AHCPR Pub. No. 96-0013. National Medical Expenditure Survey Research Findings, 27. Rockville, MD: Public Health Service/Agency for Health Care Policy and Research.

Pan American Health Organization. 2008. "Integrating Mental Health into Primary Care." [Online information; retrieved 12/12/08.] www.who.int/mental_health/policy/services/mentalhealthintoprimarycare/en/index.html.

U.S. Department of Health and Human Services (USDHHS). 1995a. *Health, United States, 1995.* Pub. No. (PHS) 96-1232. Hyattsville, MD: USDHHS.

CHAPTER 5

PRODUCTIVITY AND QUALITY

Title III of the Affordable Care Act (ACA), "Improving the Quality and Efficiency of Health Care," contains numerous major policy changes to improve healthcare delivery in the United States. A frequent criticism of the US healthcare system has been the uneven quality and safety in care delivery and the significant differences in the cost of care throughout the country (Wennberg, Berkson, and Rider 2008). The sections in Title III are based on a systems approach to solving these problems.

Exhibit 5.1 shows which portions of the systems view are addressed by these policy changes. These sections in the ACA are intended to connect the knowledge of best clinical practices (evidence-based medicine) and best operational practices (e.g., Lean Six Sigma process improvements) with the tools of clinical care delivery. A healthcare organization that can effectively acquire this knowledge and implement new systems of care will succeed in meeting the policy goals of the ACA.[1]

PRODUCTIVITY

VALUE-BASED PURCHASING

The first section of Title III (3001) is the hospital value-based purchasing program; its position is an important message to the healthcare provider community. Medicare is making one of the most significant policy shifts since its inception: changing from paying for the volume of services delivered to paying for quality. This program began in October 2012, and many detailed regulations have been developed for its full implementation. The regulations regarding this program are at bit.ly/Reform5_1.

The principles of this program are based the concept of reducing Medicare hospital diagnosis-related group (DRG) payments and then redirecting these funds to hospitals that meet clinical quality targets as defined by the Centers for Medicare & Medicaid Services (CMS) in a number of clinical areas, including:

EXHIBIT 5.1
Total Health System Model: Productivity and Quality Portion

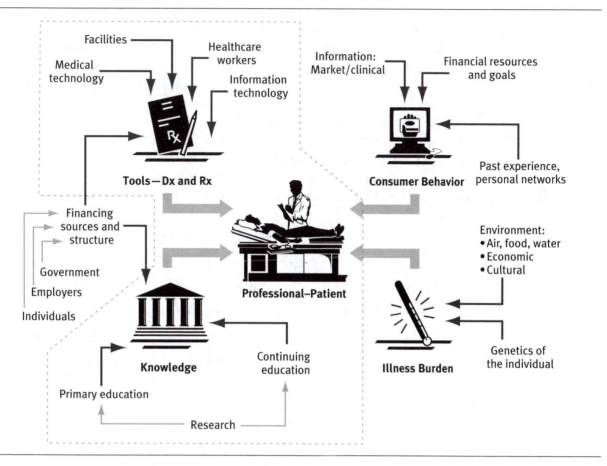

- ◆ acute myocardial infarction (AMI);

- ◆ heart failure;

- ◆ pneumonia;

- ◆ surgeries, as measured by the Surgical Care Improvement Project (Joint Commission 2014); and

- ◆ healthcare-associated infections.

Medicare will likely expand this list, and the amount of DRG payment linked to quality will rise.

Physicians are also included in the value-based purchasing approach of Title III. The ACA builds on the existing Physician Quality Reporting System (PQRS), which uses a combination of incentive payments and payment adjustments to promote reporting of quality information by eligible professionals (EPs). EPs include Medicare physicians, practitioners, and therapists. A detailed list of EPs is at bit.ly/Reform5_2.

The program provides an incentive payment to practices with EPs that satisfactorily report data on quality measures for covered services furnished to Medicare beneficiaries. Beginning in 2015, the program also applies a downward payment adjustment to EPs who do not satisfactorily report data on quality measures for covered professional services.

This program is improved in the ACA by an expansion of its scope and integration with the "meaningful use" policies of the HITECH Act (see Chapter 4). Medicare now posts on a public website information on physician participation in PQRS, electronic prescribing (eRx) and the electronic health record incentive program. Beginning in 2014, the Physician Compare website will also include quality of care ratings for group practices. Ratings for individual physicians and other healthcare professionals will be added in the future.

All of the Medicare quality comparison websites can be found here:

Physician Compare	www.medicare.gov/physiciancompare
Hospital Compare	www.medicare.gov/hospitalcompare
Home Health Compare	www.medicare.gov/homehealthcompare
Nursing Home Compare	www.medicare.gov/nursinghomecompare

In addition to public reporting, a value-based payment system is outlined in §3007 that is built on the PQRS framework. The Value-Based Payment Modifier (VM) program will provide comparative performance information to physicians as part of Medicare's efforts to improve the quality and efficiency of medical care and the move toward physician reimbursement that rewards value rather than volume.

In 2016, groups with ten or more EPs who submit claims to Medicare under a single tax identification number will be subject to the VM, based on their performance in 2014. These groups will need to register and choose one of the PQRS group practice quality reporting methods. If a group does not choose to report quality measures as a group, and at least 50 percent of the EPs within the group report PQRS measures individually, CMS will calculate a group quality score based on their reporting. Failing to report will result in a negative 2 percent VM adjustment to 2016 payment under the physician fee schedule. The VM adjustment is in addition to the PQRS payment adjustment (see bit.ly/Reform5_3).

The VM program provides an incentive for physicians to report as groups. Health policy experts have long argued that a solo physician practice may be too small to effectively measure quality. In addition, system improvements in the delivery of care are much easier to measure at the group level. Therefore, these value purchasing methods have been developed. In fact, §3007 states, "The Secretary shall, as appropriate, apply the payment modifier established under this subsection in a manner that promotes systems-based care."

The movement to value purchasing throughout the United States is detailed in **Reading 5A**.

PRODUCTIVITY IMPROVEMENTS

Section 3401, with its lack of details except for the payment reduction formulas, provides a stark contrast to the detailed treatment of quality improvement in the ACA. This section may be one of the most important aspects of healthcare reform to providers, as it reduces the normal market basket update of Medicare prices by the average business productivity improvement in the United States and specific percentages detailed in the ACA (which range from 0.25 to 0.75 percent). Trade associations that represent these providers will likely press Congress to change these formulas over the years, but the policy direction is clear in the ACA. The healthcare system must implement changes to improve its productivity to match the other industries in the United States.

The calculation of these adjustments is complex and can found each year in the CMS proposed rules for the inpatient prospective payment system, which are released in the spring. Comments are received in the summer, and the final rule for the upcoming year published in the early fall. An example is here: bit.ly/Reform5_4.

QUALITY

QUALITY REPORTING

The ACA is a health reform bill (not just health insurance reform) and contains significant policies to report on and support the improvement of the quality of healthcare delivery in the United States. Sections 3011 and 3012 call for the development of a national strategy for quality improvement and the coordination of this strategy among the many federal and state agencies involved in the healthcare system. The federal agencies are listed in Exhibit 5.2.

Reading 5B provides an overview of the national strategy and many related private sector initiatives.

Section 3013 advances the progress toward quality improvement by providing funding and authority for the continued refinement and construction of quality measures. Section 3014 provides for multi-stakeholder input into the quality improvement process, and §3015 expands the use of these measures for public reporting of quality—much of which is now available on www.healthcare.gov. Because the first sections of Title III outline

- Department of Health and Human Services
- Centers for Medicare & Medicaid Services
- National Institutes of Health
- Centers for Disease Control and Prevention
- Food and Drug Administration
- Health Resources and Services Administration
- Agency for Healthcare Research and Quality
- Office of the National Coordinator for Health Information Technology
- Substance Abuse and Mental Health Services Administration
- Administration for Children and Families

- Department of Commerce Office of Management and Budget
- United States Coast Guard
- Federal Bureau of Prisons
- National Highway Traffic Safety Administration
- Federal Trade Commission
- Social Security Administration
- Department of Labor
- United States Office of Personnel Management
- Department of Defense
- Department of Education
- Department of Veterans Affairs
- Veterans Health Administration
- Any other federal agencies and departments with activities relating to improving healthcare quality and safety, as determined by the president

a value-based purchasing strategy, these quality measures will likely be used as the basis for payment. Quality measures will be developed in the areas of:

◆ health outcomes and functional status of patients;

◆ the management and coordination of healthcare across episodes of care and care transitions for patients across the continuum of providers, healthcare settings, and health plans;

◆ the experience, quality, and use of information provided to and used by patients, caregivers, and authorized representatives to inform decision making about treatment options, including the use of shared decision making (see Chapter 4);

◆ tools and preference-sensitive care (Dartmouth Atlas 2007);

◆ the meaningful use of health information technology (see Chapter 4);

◆ the safety, effectiveness, patient-centeredness, appropriateness, and timeliness of care (IOM 2001);

◆ the efficiency of care;

- the equity of health services and health disparities across health disparity populations and geographic areas;

- patient experience and satisfaction;

- the use of innovative strategies and methodologies; and

- other areas determined appropriate by the secretary of the Department of Health and Human Services (HHS).

HEALTH PLANS AND MEDICAID

Because quality reporting for Medicare is currently robust, the ACA extends these policies to health plans and Medicaid. Section 1001/2717 mandates the development and public reporting requirements to:

- improve health outcomes through the implementation of activities such as quality reporting, effective case management, care coordination, chronic disease management, and medication and care compliance initiatives;

- implement activities to prevent hospital readmissions through a comprehensive program for hospital discharge that includes patient-centered education and counseling, comprehensive discharge planning, and postdischarge reinforcement by healthcare professionals;

- implement activities to improve patient safety and reduce medical errors through the appropriate use of best clinical practices, evidence-based medicine, and health information technology; and

- implement wellness and health promotion activities.

Section 2701 mandates the creation and reporting of Medicaid quality measures. Because this activity must be done with the states, the process will be slow and complex.

HEALTH PLAN QUALITY RATING SYSTEM

An important aspect of the ACA is the availability of health plans to individuals and small employers through health insurance exchanges (see Chapter 8). Section 1311(c)(3) directs the secretary to develop a system that rates qualified health plans (QHPs) based on relative quality and price. It also requires marketplaces to display QHP quality ratings on their websites to help consumers select QHPs. This feature was not available on the initial operation of the exchange but will be implemented in 2015. In addition, §1311 also requires public display of information by each marketplace to allow individuals to assess enrollee experience among comparable plans. HHS is developing a QHP enrollee survey that evaluates consumer experience.

Additional information on the Quality Reporting System can be found at bit.ly/Reform5_5.

SUPPORT FOR QUALITY AND PRODUCTIVITY IMPROVEMENT

The Agency for Healthcare Research and Quality (AHRQ) has emerged as one of the key federal agencies to support healthcare reform. Section 3501 gives the agency additional mandates and funding to continue research to:

- identify best practices in the delivery of healthcare services;

- find changes in processes of care and systems used by providers that will reliably result in intended health outcomes, improve patient safety and reduce medical errors (such as skill development for healthcare providers in team-based healthcare delivery and rapid-cycle process improvement), and facilitate adoption of improved workflow;

- identify healthcare providers—including healthcare systems, single institutions, and individual providers—that

  - deliver consistently high-quality, efficient healthcare services and

  - employ best practices that are adaptable and scalable to diverse healthcare settings or effective in improving care across diverse settings;

- assess research, evidence, and knowledge about what strategies and methodologies are most effective in improving healthcare delivery; and

- determine methods to translate such information rapidly and effectively into practice and to document the sustainability of those improvements.

AHRQ has an excellent website (www.ahrq.gov) that contains the results of studies already undertaken in these areas, and it updates this site frequently. Healthcare organizations that wish to make significant improvements in their operations should fully utilize this exceptional resource.

SUMMARY

Although much of the controversy and press coverage surrounding the enactment of the ACA focused on its health insurance provisions, the ACA also makes significant strides toward improving the quality and efficiency of the US healthcare system.

A value-based purchasing system is being implemented for Medicare, and Medicare fee-for-service payments will be reduced. Quality reporting will be improved and expanded for physicians, health plans, and Medicaid. A national strategy for quality improvement will be developed and the dissemination of advances in quality and productivity will be increased through the AHRQ.

APPLICATIONS: DISCUSSION AND RESEARCH

1. What are the advantages and disadvantages of moving from fee-for-service to value-based purchasing for hospitals? For doctors? (Interview a hospital CFO or clinic business office manager and obtain their opinions on this question. Also ask them how they plan to move from fee-for-service to value-based revenue.)

2. How can a hospital meet the productivity targets set by CMS? (Access library resources to review journals such as *Healthcare Executive*, *Journal of Healthcare Management*, *Quality Progress*, *Journal of Quality and Participation*, and *Quality Management Journal*. Use the search terms *productivity*, *process improvement*, *Lean*, and *Six Sigma* with *healthcare*.)

3. What are the principal efforts led by employers since 2000 to usher in a new era in value-based purchasing (de Brantes 2014; see **Reading 5A**)?

4. Value-based payments are one side of a two-sided value-based purchasing coin. What is the other side, and why is it so essential to the long-term sustainability of the movement (de Brantes 2014; see **Reading 5A**)?

5. What forms of provider organizations are likely to develop in response to the different types of value-based payments being piloted (de Brantes 2014; see **Reading 5A**)?

6. Discuss how passage of the ACA has changed or will change the quality of services delivered to the consumer, the ultimate stakeholder in healthcare services (Acquaviva and Johnson 2014; see **Reading 5B**).

7. Construct an evidence-based timeline of future quality improvement activities and legislative initiatives. Include levers such as value-based purchasing, the role of

QIOs, consumer demographics, business groups, accreditors, and the HITECH Act (Acquaviva and Johnson 2014; see **Reading 5B**).

8. Discuss the impact that trends in federal quality improvement initiatives will have on healthcare delivery in the state in which you reside. What federal legislative initiatives are controversial in your state or have a high degree of support? Why (Acquaviva and Johnson 2014; see **Reading 5B**)?

9. Compare and contrast the mandated quality improvement reporting activities and nonmandated, judgment-driven reporting activities in the health sectors discussed in this chapter. In your opinion, what are the pros and cons of each approach (Acquaviva and Johnson 2014; see **Reading 5B**)?

NOTE

1. *Make It Happen: Effective Execution in Healthcare Leadership* (Health Administration Press, 2011), by the author, outlines an integrated system to quickly and efficiently implement strategy.

REFERENCES

Dartmouth Atlas. 2007. "Preference-Sensitive Care." Accessed July 22, 2014. www.dartmouthatlas.org/keyissues/issue.aspx?con=2938.

Institute of Medicine (IOM). 2001. *Crossing the Quality Chasm: A New Health System for the 21st Century.* Washington, DC: National Academies Press.

Joint Commission. 2014. "Surgical Care Improvement Project." Published June 23. www.jointcommission.org/surgical_care_improvement_project/.

Wennberg, D., D. Berkson, and B. Rider. 2008. "Addressing Overuse, Underuse and Misuse of Care." *Healthcare Executive* 23 (4): 8.

ADDITIONAL READINGS

READING 5A

HOW PURCHASERS SELECT AND PAY FOR VALUE: THE MOVEMENT TO VALUE-BASED PURCHASING

François de Brantes

From *The Healthcare Quality Book*, 3rd ed. (2014), Chapter 20, 525–40. Edited by M. S. Joshi, E. R. Ransom, D. B. Nash, and S. B. Ransom. Chicago: Health Administration Press.

In early 2012, the Congressional Budget Office (CBO) issued a report on several decades' worth of pilots and demonstrations by the Centers for Medicare & Medicaid Services (CMS), all aimed at improving the quality and affordability of healthcare in the United States (Nelson 2012b). The news was sobering and highly informative and can be summarized simply: Quality improves when physicians, nurses, and other clinicians take a high-touch approach; affordability improves when payment models are designed with built-in savings.

The simplicity of these findings underscores the complexity of reforming the US healthcare system. If reform were simple, the findings would suggest that successful strategies could have been implemented long ago to the great benefit of all. And yet they have not. Why?

Most US workers receive healthcare coverage through their employer. The employer, in turn, contracts with an administrator, either to purchase healthcare coverage on behalf of the employees or to administer the benefits that the employer pays for directly. Employees are therefore removed from many of the purchasing decisions. Employers themselves are removed from the actual function of healthcare delivery and from the payment for services because the third-party administrator organizes and manages those functions. Attempts to control the rise of healthcare costs, reflected in premiums paid to the third-party administrator or in medical claims paid by the employer, led to a succession of strategies that have, for the most part, failed to produce widespread effective results. They have, however, led to the introduction of value-based Medicare payment efforts, which should yield significant benefits. The evolution to today's value-based purchasing movement has gone through several prior phases.

EVOLUTION OF VALUE-BASED PURCHASING

The concept of value-based purchasing was imported into healthcare from industry and applied on the premise that plans would compete for employers' and employees' premium dollars by demonstrating greater effectiveness in caring for covered members and greater efficiency in paying for care services. The primary strategy to achieve efficiency was to consolidate the purchasing power of payers and health plan sponsors and obtain discounts from physicians, hospitals, and ancillary care providers. The primary strategy to achieve effectiveness was to standardize measures of quality across plans and create a common way of assessing plan quality. Efforts by the National Committee for Quality Assurance (NCQA), described in the previous chapter, helped create the methodology for assessing plan performance on effectiveness of care in a standard way.

Even before value-based purchasing at the plan level lost its ability to improve quality and control costs for the majority of Americans covered by health insurance, purchasers had started to understand that providers did not change their behaviors for one plan alone. They changed their behaviors for all plans. In fact, researchers observed little difference in the quality of care between managed care networks and non–managed care networks (McGlynn et al. 2003; Schuster, McGlynn, and Brook 1998; Wennberg 1999), especially as purchasers demanded that plans increase the size of their networks. With the expansion of networks came the reduction in relative purchasing power. Purchaser focus has, as a result, shifted from individual plan performance to individual provider performance, evidenced by the creation of the Leapfrog Group in 2000, Bridges to Excellence in 2003, and the Patient-Centered Primary Care Collaborative in 2006. With the release of the Institute of Medicine's report *Crossing the Quality Chasm* (IOM 2001), purchasers realized that serious gaps remained in the quality of care in the United States and that variations in quality at the individual provider level were significant. Reducing the variation and increasing the overall level of quality have become purchasing imperatives, especially in light of continued cost increases.

However, the movement from plan selection to provider selection was not a direct one. While many large employers worked together to form the organizations mentioned previously, many others focused almost exclusively on managing the demand for healthcare through employee-based interventions such as disease management and shared decision making. Many of these interventions, when tried by Medicare on a larger scale, have proven ineffective (Nelson 2012a).

The value-based purchasing movement has thus evolved from trying to get managed care organizations to compete for patients by delivering better value, to getting plan members to improve their personal healthcare consumption habits, to trying to affect provider behavior. Therein lies the reason that change has been so long in coming. Employers assumed that health plans that contract with providers would have an incentive to test payment models that would motivate the contracted providers to deliver higher-quality, more affordable care. However, health plans have barely innovated in the way they pay providers. Instead, the large employers in the United States have pushed for and piloted innovative payment models.

That activity, described in this chapter, has reached a new level thanks to the significant payment reform activities introduced by the Affordable Care Act (ACA). The ACA not only creates a burning platform for fee-for-service (FFS) payments but empowers the Center for Medicare & Medicaid Innovation (CMMI 2013), housed within CMS, to pilot new payment and delivery system models and to propagate those models throughout Medicare if they prove successful. The final pages of this chapter briefly touch on these innovations.

BACKGROUND AND TERMINOLOGY

The payment systems that range between the two poles of FFS and capitation assign varying levels of financial risk to providers. The pole with the least risk is FFS, while the pole with the most risk is capitation. In FFS, physicians are neither responsible for the probability that a patient will require services nor at risk for the value of the service delivered. They bill a service to the payer, and if the service conforms to the payer's administrative requirements, the payer will pay the agreed-upon fee. The physician's only financial risk is that the cost of providing the service may be greater than the fee received. In capitation, the opposite is true. Providers are at risk both for the probability that a patient will require a service and for the cost (not necessarily the value) of delivering all the care the patient needs. These two forms of risk are called probability risk and technical risk.

Employers and, more recently, Medicare have experimented with programs that fit within the spectrum bounded by these poles (Exhibit 20.1):

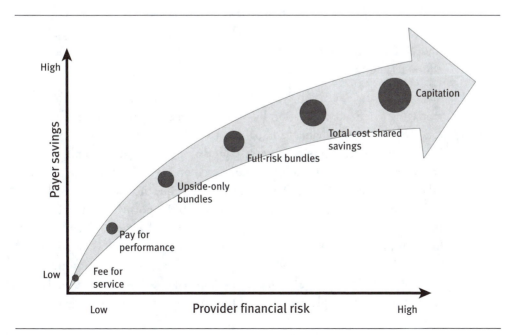

EXHIBIT 20.1
Provider Payment Models in Value-Based Purchasing

◆ *FFS* entails a minimal amount of risk for the provider. FFS encourages physicians to provide more services, which can be useful when payers want to encourage use of services—for example, immunizations and screenings for certain diseases or conditions. Medicare, which is the largest payer in the United States, primarily pays physicians according to the FFS model.

◆ *Pay for performance* is the most prevalent method that attempts to counter the FFS model's tendency to reward the volume rather than the value of care by tying a portion of the payment to certain performance criteria. This chapter describes the work done by employers in this domain and lessons learned to date.

◆ *Upside-only bundles* group the services that center on a specific procedure, an acute medical event, or even a chronic condition. According to the CBO report, the most successful payment experiment undertaken by CMS as of early 2012 was the bundled payment demonstration of the early 1990s (Nelson 2012b). This form of payment does not lay probability risk on the provider, but it does entail technical risk because the provider is at risk for the frequency, mix, and costs of services produced within the defined bundle. Upside-only bundled payments are designed to insulate the providers against any downside risk but create the potential for financial gain if the actual costs of care are lower than the predefined budget for the bundle. This chapter describes the private-sector efforts to launch bundled payments in the United States.

◆ *Full-risk bundles*, in contrast to upside-only bundles, put the provider at full risk for any costs in excess of (or eligible for the full reward of any costs under) the defined price negotiated with the payer. This chapter also describes efforts related to this model.

◆ *Total cost of care shared-savings models* contain the costs associated with managing a defined population by picking a target rate of increase of the total costs of care; providers and payers share the savings realized through a lower-than-expected rate of increase. Many of these programs do not include penalties for going over budget and are based on a Medicare demonstration called the Physician Group Practice Demonstration, the results of which are summarized in the previously referenced CBO report (Nelson 2012b). In 2008–2009, several academic researchers launched a coordinated call for what they termed the *accountable care organization*, which is designed around the same principles as the Physician Group Practice Demonstration (Rittenhouse, Shortell, and Fisher 2009; Shortell and Casalino 2008). The ACA includes the implementation of this model in a formal pilot that launched in 2012.

◆ *Capitation* defines a specific budget for an entire patient population, and the providers are at full risk for all costs incurred above that budget. Even in its heyday in the mid-1990s, capitation was never widely adopted, principally because of the inherent financial risks assumed by the provider organizations. Further, many states require providers to file as insurance companies with state insurance regulators if they take on capitated payments for a patient population, thus increasing the administrative burden of such an approach.

CASE STUDY: BRIDGES TO EXCELLENCE: A PAY-FOR-PERFORMANCE MODEL

In 2003 several large employers, including General Electric, Ford, Procter & Gamble, and UPS, launched Bridges to Excellence (BTE) to tie physician payments to the achievement of certain quality criteria. The concept was simple and continues to be implemented by employers and health plans throughout the United States (Health Care Incentives Improvement Institute 2013a). It asks physicians to demonstrate the quality of care delivered by submitting clinical data to an independent third-party evaluator. Physicians receive a financial reward per patient managed if their quality score exceeds a certain threshold. Like most pay-for-performance programs, BTE is an upside-only program. Physicians are never penalized; they are only rewarded on the basis of the premise that better quality care will lead to better financial outcomes. Since the program began, many variations have been launched, and much research has been published on the topic. The seminal work on designing a pay-for-performance program was done by Meredith Rosenthal and Adams Dudley (2007). In addition, several papers have been published on BTE and the lessons learned from its implementation. These lessons may be summarized as follows:

◆ *Avoid "tournament-style" programs* that retroactively rank providers in deciles or quartiles and distribute rewards based on that ranking. The primary drawback of this design is its uncertainty. A physician or a hospital could work hard to improve all year and never get a reward.

◆ *Measure what matters.* Outcome measures should be selected in careful consideration of the desired goal of the pay-for-performance program (de Brantes, Wickland, and Williams 2008). If the goal is to increase immunization rates, the measure should be immunization rates. If the goal is to achieve better outcomes for patients with chronic conditions, then blood pressure, cholesterol, and blood sugar levels may be appropriate measures.

◆ *Create meaningful incentives.* The research is clear. To pierce through the noise of FFS payment, a strong signal is needed. The greater the signal, the higher the response. De Brantes and D'Andrea (2009) studied the response of physician practices in several communities to the size of an offered bonus and found that response rises with the size of the bonus. Many pay-for-performance programs expect high response rates with paltry incentives, only to be disappointed.

◆   *Know that better-quality care can cost less.* This fundamental premise that led the BTE founders to launch the program was proven true (Rosenthal et al. 2008).

The lessons learned from BTE, as well as its seminal work in creating tools to measure systems in physician offices and the quality of care delivered to patients with certain chronic conditions, led to the design and implementation of incentive programs to reward patient-centered medical homes (PCMHs).

PATIENT-CENTERED MEDICAL HOMES

The PCMH concept is close to 50 years old. First introduced by the American Academy of Pediatrics, it was subsequently revised and adopted by a number of primary care specialty associations (e.g., the American Association of Family Physicians) as part of an overall effort in the early 2000s to address the future of family medicine (Robert Graham Center 2007). The observations were simple: The Medicare resource-based relative value scale (RBRVS) system had started to create significant distortions in the value of services, significantly favoring interventions to the detriment of evaluation and management. Medical school graduates were quick to respond to this shift, moving into specialties that provided far greater FFS billing opportunities, and the ranks of family practitioners started to significantly shrink.

The response to the report on the future of family medicine (Robert Graham Center 2007), in conjunction with the Institute of Medicine report *Crossing the Quality Chasm* (IOM 2001) and the rising costs of healthcare, pointed policymakers, payers, and providers in the direction of shoring up primary care. IBM took a central role in launching the Patient-Centered Primary Care Collaborative (2013), which continues to serve as a general resource on the implementation of PCMH pilots across the United States.

The initial approach was to look at the design of primary care and its functions and figure out incentive or payment models that would suit the design and functions. This approach was evident in the proposal by Goroll and colleagues (2007) that soon became the rallying point for many field experiments. Goroll and colleagues calculated the cost of running a physician practice and then divided the needed revenue across a patient panel to arrive at a fixed payment per patient.

The path chosen was simple: First, design the form of the practice and its functions, and that design will lead to a financial incentive model. The challenge of such a path is that it does not provide incentives for the value of care delivered in these medical homes. Such incentives, if provided, would lead to innovation in primary care delivery regardless of the specific setting. In fact, a divide exists between researchers who propose specific forms of the delivery system—accountable care organizations and PCMHs—and those who propose specific incentives to drive care improvement, such as pay for performance, bundled payments, and shared savings. Interestingly, the ones focusing on the former are mostly from academia, whereas the ones focusing on the latter are mostly from the business community.

Some important early lessons have been learned about PCMHs:

◆ *It is very difficult to transform a traditional physician practice into the type of PCMH described and defined in the report on the future of family medicine.* Crabtree and colleagues (2010) describe the challenges encountered in a large national PCMH demonstration effort.

◆ *Evidence of financial impact is mixed.* Analyses suggest that pilot participants (those that were selected to participate in a PCMH pilot and are receiving an incentive for doing so) have better results than a random sample of physicians in the same community. Exhibit 20.2 shows that patients managed by PCMH pilot practices had fewer hospitalizations and shorter lengths of stay (resulting in fewer bed days) than patients managed by non-PCMH pilot practices. However, Exhibit 20.3 shows that practices designated as PCMHs by the NCQA that were not participating in a pilot did not obtain better

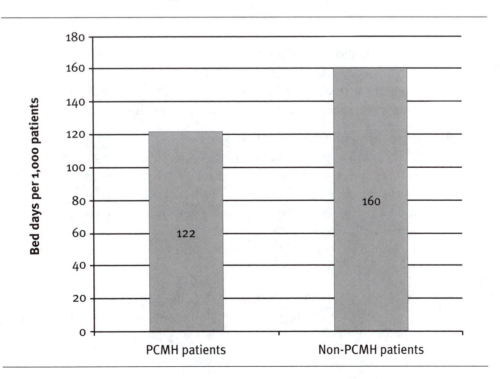

EXHIBIT 20.2
Bed Days per Thousand Patients

Exhibit 20.3

Potentially
Avoidable
Complications
(PACs) per
Thousand Patients
with Chronic
Conditions by Type
of Practice

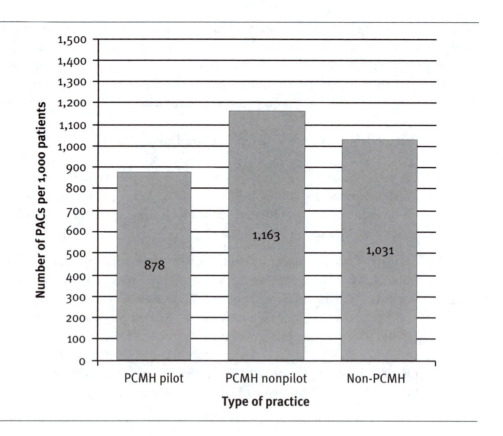

results than other physicians in their community, whereas pilot participants did. The measures used in Exhibit 20.3 are the rates of potentially avoidable complications (PACs), which were approved in 2011 by the National Quality Forum as measures of comprehensive outcomes of care.

◆ *The search for a sustainable funding model for PCMH practices continues.* PCMH practices must fit into the larger context of a delivery system that associates a financial risk with its members' decisions on the type and frequency of services rendered. Therefore, health plans and physicians continue to explore incentives that would cause practices to transform in a manner consistent with the report on the future of family medicine while reducing the total medical spending associated with a population of patients. Options include

– creating prospective budgets, especially for patients with chronic conditions, and assigning the financial risk to the practice for costs in excess of that budget;

– defining a global cost per member per month for all patients based on historical trends and creating a mechanism to share gains with the practice on the basis of actual costs; and

– establishing bonuses linked to a scorecard of cost and quality that are to be paid in addition to the routine FFS payments.

Pay for performance has natural limits because these programs simply attempt to counter the basic incentive of FFS, not to replace it. The following case study looks at the next rung on the ladder of value-based purchasing.

CASE STUDY: PROMETHEUS PAYMENT: A NEW FRONTIER IN VALUE-BASED PURCHASING

In the mid-1990s, Medicare launched a demonstration project to pay hospitals and physicians a single fee for a bundle of services related to a cardiac bypass procedure. The CBO reported that this project was one of the more successful payment reform initiatives undertaken by CMS. Approximately ten years later, CMS launched a new demonstration called the Acute Care Episode Demonstration, which expanded on the first project but was still limited to bundling all inpatient-stay services for specific procedures.

After the launch of BTE, large employers realized that more fundamental payment reform would be needed to respond to the Institute of Medicine's reports on the quality of care in the United States and launched the Provider Payment Reform for Outcomes, Margins, Evidence, Transparency, Hassle-reduction, Excellence, Understandability, and Sustainability (PROMETHEUS) Payment effort. Following the same process used to create BTE, a design team composed of experts in healthcare economics, law, and delivery set about to create a new payment model that would appropriately and fairly shift financial risk to providers, making them responsible for the cost and quality of care delivered to patients for specific procedures, acute medical events, and chronic conditions.

The concepts and design were summarized in several papers (e.g., de Brantes, D'Andrea, and Rosenthal 2009) and served as a launchpad for actual implementations to pilot the model and evaluate it. The model has since been implemented in several communities across the United States, some of which have been and continue to be supported by charitable foundations; others are supported by private-sector payers (Health Care Incentives Improvement Institute 2013b).

One of the more important concepts was that providers, not the employer or payer, would be responsible for the cost of defects and waste. The main challenge in designing the PROMETHEUS Payment model was to impute the financial risk associated with care failures to providers, while limiting their probability risk as much as possible. Splitting these risks—performance and probability—would create more focus on providers to understand how to manage financial risk by reducing defects as opposed to managing financial risk by limiting the probability that a health event occurs, which providers are not particularly adept at doing. The PROMETHEUS Payment model was the first to quantify the cost of defects in episodes of chronic, procedural, and acute medical care. It named these defects PACs, which were subsequently endorsed by the National Quality Forum as measures of comprehensive outcomes of care. PACs became the foundation for the incentives in the PROMETHEUS Payment model because employers immediately grasped what they meant and understood the importance of reducing them to increase value in the delivery of medical care. When analyzed, PACs are converted into a dollar-denominated rate that represents the percentage of costs in any episode that can be attributed to PACs.

Exhibit 20.4 illustrates the variation in rates of PACs for patients with certain chronic conditions, from a large national database of commercially insured plan members. These data demonstrate the significant opportunity to reduce costs in the United States while improving the quality of care. Exhibit 20.5 illustrates the total costs in dollars consumed by PACs and the typical care for 21 patient conditions and procedures as measured

EXHIBIT 20.4

Rates of PACs Among Commercially Insured Patients with Certain Chronic Conditions

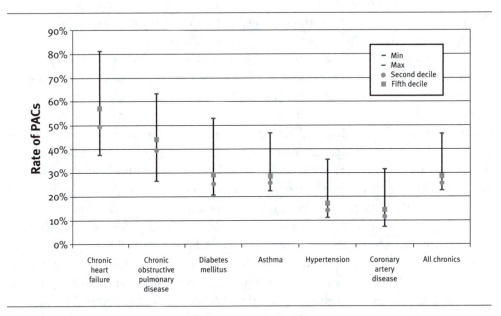

SOURCE: Adapted from de Brantes, Rastogi, and Painter (2010).

NOTE: Each line represents the range, from minimum to maximum, of average PAC rates in different US states. The dot represents the PAC rate for the 20th percentile, and the square represents the PAC rate for the 50th percentile.

EXHIBIT 20.5

Regional Health Plan's Total Episode Costs, by Patient Condition or Procedure, Split Between Typical Costs and PAC Costs

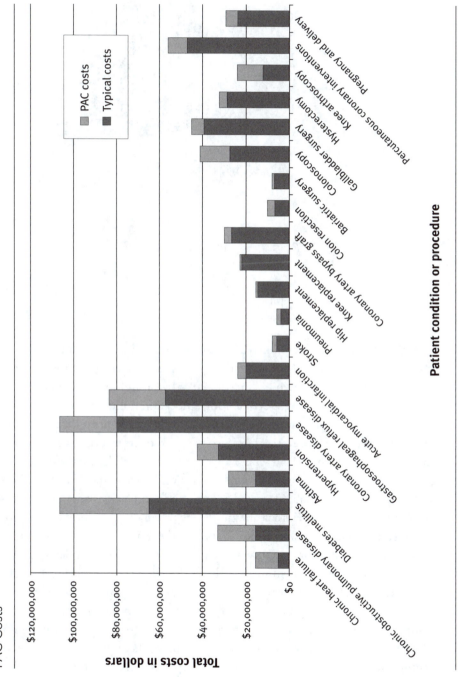

EXHIBIT 20.6
Regional Health
Plan's Total
Episode Costs
Split Between PAC
Costs and Typical
Costs, Expressed
as Percentage of
Total

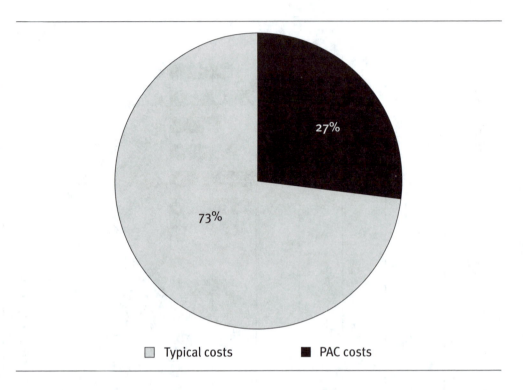

27%

73%

☐ Typical costs   ■ PAC costs

in a regional health plan's commercial claims data set. Exhibit 20.6 represents the same data, aggregated across the episodes and expressed as a percentage of total costs.

For any employer, Exhibit 20.6 paints a clear and unambiguous picture: $1 of every $4 spent on certain episodes of chronic, procedural, and acute care is spent on PACs or defects in the care process. In a global economy in which firms that produce products compete for value and are severely punished when products fail, the contrast between what happens within those firms and what happens in healthcare delivery could not be starker. In response to these data, mainstream publications such as the *New York Times* (Chen 2009) and *Time* (Pickert 2009) started asking a simple question: Shouldn't healthcare services come with a warranty? That question is the driving force behind bundled payments. A bundled payment is a global fee for a specific medical event, condition, or procedure, and it includes an implicit warranty. If a patient is readmitted after being discharged following a total knee replacement surgery, the readmission costs are absorbed by the providers and not charged to the payer as an additional expense. If a patient with diabetes receives poor management and ends up repeatedly in the emergency department, those costs are absorbed by the providers and not charged separately to the payer. Bundled payments replicate, in effect, the dynamics that exist with most other purchases made by consumers or companies—the consumer negotiates or accepts the price up front, and if the product has a defect, the responsibility lies with the manufacturer, not the buyer. Furthermore, employers who had increasingly started to shift the cost of healthcare services to employees could use bundled prices as a mechanism to move market share from one provider to another on the basis of the price of the bundle. Several new consumer-directed tools such as Castlight (Castlight Health 2013) and Healthcare Blue Book (2013) are designed to provide consumable information to plan members, helping them understand the trade-offs in selecting different providers for a specific procedure.

In 2008, the Robert Wood Johnson Foundation awarded a three-year grant to pilot the PROMETHEUS Payment model, to test the operational processes and determine how this type of bundled payment could be implemented on a larger scale in the United States. Three sites, each with a unique set of challenges, were selected and evaluated by a third party. That evaluation was published in late 2011 (Hussey, Ridgely, and Rosenthal 2011). Between 2008 and 2012, the model was launched at several other sites, some funded by other charitable foundations and some supported by regional health plans. In addition, the enactment of the ACA in 2010 changed the landscape, in particular by creating the CMMI and its push to launch payment reform initiatives.

Significant challenges to implementation remain, despite the promise to control costs, increase quality, and engage plan members in value-based purchasing. The combination of antiquated claims processing and member benefits systems, coupled with provider resistance to revenue contraction, creates a significant weight of inertia. Hussey, Ridgely, and Rosenthal (2011) summarized some of these challenges in their evaluation of the PROMETHEUS Payment model pilot sites. Despite those challenges, hundreds of provider organizations filed letters of intent with the CMMI as an initial step in applying to participate in that organization's bundled payment pilot. Furthermore, private-sector bundled payment initiatives have sprung up, including a statewide effort in California led by the Integrated Healthcare Association; an effort in Wisconsin led by an alliance of multiple stakeholders; and efforts in New Jersey, North Carolina, and South Carolina led by those states' Blue Cross and Blue Shield plans.

CONCLUSIONS AND KEY LESSONS

Despite the challenges inherent in designing and implementing value-based payment models, the private sector—and in particular the leading employers in the United States—have paved the way for federal efforts to move away from basic FFS payments. Keys to success have stemmed from careful consideration of stakeholder needs and the desire to maintain a balanced and fair approach in shifting financial risk to providers.

Key principles of a successful design ensure that

- ◆ incentives meet provider needs (in particular, incentives have to be measurable, attainable, and meaningful);

- ◆ performance measures meet provider and purchaser needs, create a return on investment for purchasers, are achievable yet not easy, and are standard as opposed to custom; and

◆ operational structures to implement new payment models meet purchaser and plan needs, are relatively simple and easy for purchasers to implement, and keep the administrative burden on plans to a minimum.

REFERENCES

Castlight Health. 2013. Accessed December 18. www.castlighthealth.com.

Center for Medicare & Medicaid Innovation (CMMI). 2013. Accessed December 18. www. innovations.cms.gov.

Chen, P. W. 2009. "Can Health Care Come with a Warranty?" *New York Times* June 25. www. nytimes.com/2009/06/25/health/25chen.html.

Crabtree, B. F., P. A. Nutting, W. L. Miller, K. C. Stange, E. E. Stewart, and C. R. Jaén. 2010. "Summary of the National Demonstration Project and Recommendations for the Patient-Centered Medical Home." *Annals of Family Medicine* 8 (Suppl. 1): S80–S90.

de Brantes, F. S., and G. D'Andrea. 2009. "Physicians Respond to Pay-for-Performance Incentives: Larger Incentives Yield Greater Participation." *American Journal of Managed Care* 15 (5): 305–10.

de Brantes, F. S., G. D'Andrea, and M. B. Rosenthal. 2009. "Should Health Care Come with a Warranty?" *Health Affairs* 28 (4): w678–w687.

de Brantes, F. S., A. Rastogi, and M. Painter. 2010. "Reducing Potentially Avoidable Complications in Patients with Chronic Diseases: The Prometheus Payment Approach." *Health Services Research* 45 (6): 1854–71.

de Brantes, F., P. Wickland, and J. Williams. 2008. "The Value of Ambulatory Care Measures: A Review of Clinical and Financial Impact from an Employer/Payer Perspective." *American Journal of Managed Care* 14 (6): 360–68.

Goroll, A. H., R. A. Berenson, S. C. Schoenbaum, and L. B. Gardner. 2007. "Fundamental Reform of Payment for Adult Primary Care: Comprehensive Payment for Comprehensive Care." *Journal of General Internal Medicine* 22 (3): 410–15.

Health Care Incentives Improvement Institute. 2013a. "Bridges to Excellence: Premise." Accessed December 18. www.hci3.org/what_is_bte/premise.

———. 2013b. "PROMETHEUS Implementations." Accessed December 18. www.hci3.org/implementations.

Healthcare Blue Book. 2013. Accessed December 18. http://healthcarebluebook.com.

Hussey, P. S., M. S. Ridgely, and M. B. Rosenthal. 2011. "The PROMETHEUS Bundled Payment Experiment: Slow Start Shows Problems in Implementing New Payment Models." *Health Affairs* 30 (11): 2116–24.

Institute of Medicine (IOM). 2001. *Crossing the Quality Chasm: A New Health System for the 21st Century.* Washington, DC: National Academies Press.

McGlynn, E. A., S. M. Asch, J. Adams, J. Keesey, J. Hicks, A. DeCristofaro, and E. A. Kerr. 2003. "The Quality of Health Care Delivered to Adults in the United States." *New England Journal of Medicine* 348 (26): 2635–45.

Nelson, L. 2012a. "Lessons from Medicare's Demonstration Projects on Disease Management and Care Coordination." Working paper 2012-01. Issued January 18. Washington, DC: Congressional Budget Office. www.cbo.gov/doc.cfm?index=12664.

———. 2012b. "Lessons from Medicare's Demonstration Projects on Value-Based Payment." Report. Issued January 18. Washington, DC: Congressional Budget Office. www.cbo.gov/publication/42925.

Patient-Centered Primary Care Collaborative. 2013. Accessed December 18. www.pcpcc.net.

Pickert, K. 2009. "Cutting Health-Care Costs by Putting Doctors on a Budget." *Time* (US) July 6. www.time.com/time/nation/article/0,8599,1908477,00.html.

Rittenhouse, D. R., S. M. Shortell, and E. S. Fisher. 2009. "Primary Care and Accountable Care—Two Essential Elements of Delivery-System Reform." *New England Journal of Medicine* 361 (24): 2301–3.

Robert Graham Center. 2007. *The Patient Centered Medical Home: History, Seven Core Features, Evidence and Transformational Change.* Washington, DC: Robert Graham Center. www.graham-center.org/online/graham/home/publications/monographs-books/2007/rgcmo-medical-home.html.

Rosenthal, M. B., F. de Brantes, A. Sinaiko, M. Frankel, R. D. Robbins, and S. Young. 2008. "Bridges to Excellence—Recognizing High-Quality Care: Analysis of Physician Quality and Resource Use." *American Journal of Managed Care* 14 (10): 670–77.

Rosenthal, M. B., and R. A. Dudley. 2007. "Pay-for-Performance: Will the Latest Payment Trend Improve Care?" *Journal of the American Medical Association* 297 (7): 740–44.

Schuster, M. A., E. A. McGlynn, and R. Brook. 1998. "How Good Is the Quality of Healthcare in the United States?" *Milbank Quarterly* 76 (4): 517–63.

Shortell, S. M., and L. P. Casalino. 2008. "Health Care Reform Requires Accountable Care Systems." *Journal of the American Medical Association* 300 (1): 95–97.

Wennberg, J. A. 1999. "Understanding Geographic Variations in Health Care Delivery." *New England Journal of Medicine* 340 (1): 52–53.

READING 5B
THE QUALITY IMPROVEMENT LANDSCAPE

Kimberly D. Acquaviva and Jean E. Johnson
From *The Healthcare Quality Book*, 3rd ed. (2014), Chapter 18, 455–93. Edited by M. S. Joshi, E. R. Ransom, D. B. Nash, and S. B. Ransom. Chicago: Health Administration Press.

The healthcare quality improvement landscape in the United States is dynamic—continuously evolving as both established and new organizations cultivate the seeds of change. Understanding the roles of these organizations is foundational to understanding these quality improvement initiatives and, perhaps more important, to anticipating the future direction of quality improvement in the United States. Public and private entities play significant roles in a complex network of quality improvement efforts, many of which overlap. The means by which these organizations influence quality is varied, with some influencing quality through the accreditation process, others by developing measures of quality, and still others by advocating for the integration of quality improvement into the US healthcare system.

Organizations approach quality improvement from differing perspectives depending on their mission as well as the needs and desires of key stakeholders. Purchasers and insurers strive to link quality and cost containment in an effort to create more value for each dollar spent on healthcare. Healthcare providers work to improve patient care and mitigate risk through internal quality improvement and the use of quality measures. Patients—the ultimate stakeholder of all these organizations—expect (and are beginning to demand) to know more about the quality of care delivered by their providers. Policymakers require data to drive evidence-based policy decisions related to healthcare. This chapter examines the organizations that play a major role in shaping the quality improvement landscape, details important trends in quality improvement, and provides an overview of quality initiatives in specific healthcare settings.

QUALITY IMPROVEMENT ORGANIZATIONS

The quality improvement landscape is complex, with multiple organizations playing overlapping and, at times, divergent roles. The interactions between these organizations may be collegial or contentious depending on the issue under discussion, but almost without exception, the interactions are dynamic. Exhibit 18.1 illustrates the roles of these organizations and demonstrates that consumers are involved in the quality improvement feedback loop and will likely be more involved in the future. The illustration includes organizations that create quality-related incentives through payment; those that are involved in

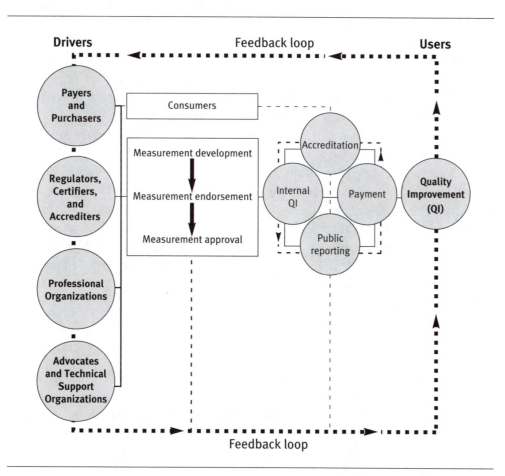

EXHIBIT 18.1
Roles of Organizations in the Quality Improvement Process

the measurement process, including development, review, endorsement, and approval of quality measures; and those that use the measures. While many organizations are involved in quality improvement, Exhibit 18.2 describes the roles of the major organizations that have quality at the center of their mission.

DRIVERS OF QUALITY

Several forces dictate the national quality agenda. These drivers (payers; purchasers; regulators, certifiers, and accreditors; professional organizations; and advocacy and technical support organizations) directly or indirectly shape and advance the national quality agenda.

PAYERS

The entities that have the greatest influence on improving quality are those that pay for care. One of the largest and most powerful of these entities is the Centers for Medicare & Medicaid Services (CMS). With healthcare costs reaching an estimated $2.8 trillion in 2012 and the federal government's share of costs projected to increase almost 14 percent in 2014, CMS is deeply vested in making sure that Medicare and Medicaid enrollees get the best care for each dollar spent (Cuckler et al. 2013).

CMS has driven the accreditation process for all settings and has emerged as a major driver linking financial incentives to improving quality. Because of its role as the largest single healthcare payer in the United States, CMS has the power to catalyze quality improvement through financial incentives, such as the voluntary reporting programs that provide incentives in the form of additional Medicare payment.

As a result of the passage of the Affordable Care Act (ACA), the Center for Medicare & Medicaid Innovation (referred to hereafter as the Innovation Center) was established "to move quickly to identify, test, and spread delivery and payment models to help providers improve care while cutting costs" (CMS 2012b). Because the Innovation Center was established by Congress, its mandate includes both robust financial support and an unprecedented degree of flexibility in testing and evaluating care delivery and payment/reimbursement models (CMS 2013a). In its first year of operation, the Innovation Center launched 16 initiatives (Exhibit 18.3).

PURCHASERS

Businesses (purchasers) and health plans have been able to affect quality through financial incentives similar to those of CMS. As healthcare costs continue to rise, purchasers and health plans are looking to quality improvement to help control costs and maximize return on investment. Coalitions of large businesses that provide health insurance benefits to employees have also provided leverage to improve quality through the development of measures and system changes. Many states, regions, and even cities have business groups on health. The National Business Coalition on Health (2014), an organization of

EXHIBIT 18.2

Organizations with a Major Role in Quality by Type

Type	Name of Organization	Mission	Website
Business groups	National Business Group on Health	• National voice of *Fortune* 500 employers concerned about cost and quality to find solutions to important health issues	www.businessgrouphealth.org
	National Business Coalition on Health	• Organization of employer-based healthcare coalitions to improve quality through value-based purchasing	www.nbch.org
	Pacific Business Group on Health (50 businesses)	• Regional coalition to improve the quality and availability of healthcare, moderate costs through value-based purchasing, use quality measurement and improvement, and engage consumers	www.pbgh.org
	Leapfrog Group	• Mobilizes employer purchasing power to improve care through access to health information, and rewards good care	www.leapfroggroup.org
Federal agencies	Centers for Medicare & Medicaid Services	• Major governmental agency that purchases and pays for care, regulates care through certification and licensure processes for providers receiving Medicare and Medicaid funds, provides consumer information, and conducts demonstration projects	www.cms.gov
	Center for Medicare & Medicaid Innovation (CMS Innovation Center)	• Aims to transform Medicare, Medicaid, and the Children's Health Insurance Program through improvements in the healthcare system	innovation.cms.gov
	Agency for Healthcare Research and Quality	• Improves the quality, safety, efficiency, and effectiveness of healthcare through research and by providing guidelines and other tools to educate and support providers and consumers	www.ahrq.gov
	Institute of Medicine	• Independent, nonprofit organization that works outside of government to provide unbiased and authoritative advice to decision makers and the public	www.iom.edu
	US Preventive Services Task Force	• Makes evidence-based recommendations on clinical preventive services	www.uspreventiveservicestaskforce.org
Accrediting organizations	The Joint Commission	• Supports performance improvement in healthcare organizations	www.jointcommission.org
	National Committee for Quality Assurance	• Accredits health plans and other organizations, develops quality measures, and educates policymakers about quality issues	www.ncqa.org

(Continued)

EXHIBIT 18.2
Organizations with a Major Role in Quality by Type (continued)

Type	Name of Organization		Mission	Website
Alliances	AQA Alliance (formerly known as the Ambulatory Care Quality Alliance)	•	Reviews and approves measures for use in ambulatory care; supports public reporting of measures	www.aqaalliance.org
	Measures Application Partnership	•	Reviews and aligns performance measures in support of public- and private-sector programs as well as federal reporting and rule-making efforts	www.qualityforum.org/map/
	Nursing Alliance for Quality Care	•	Advances the highest quality, safety, and value of consumer-centered healthcare for all individuals—patients, their families, and their communities	www.naqc.org
	Physician Consortium for Performance Improvement	•	American Medical Association–sponsored group that reviews and approves use of measures	www.ama-assn.org/go/PCPI
	Association of American Medical Colleges	•	Supports "the entire spectrum of education, research, and patient care activities conducted by . . . member institutions" (medical schools, health systems, teaching hospitals, and academic and scientific societies)	www.aamc.org
Public–private partnerships	National Quality Forum	•	Sets national priorities and goals for performance improvement, endorses national consensus standards for measuring and publicly reporting on performance, and promotes the attainment of national goals through education and outreach programs	www.qualityforum.org
Professional organizations	Institute for Healthcare Improvement	•	Aims to reduce needless deaths, pain, and waiting; accelerates the measurable and continual progress of healthcare systems throughout the world using the six aims of the IOM	www.ihi.org
	Institute for Patient- and Family-Centered Care	•	Advances the understanding of patient- and family-centered care in healthcare settings	www.ipfcc.org
Foundations	National Patient Safety Foundation	•	Awards small grants, serves as a resource for knowledge and public awareness, and enhances culture of patient safety	www.npsf.org
	Robert Wood Johnson Foundation	•	Supports regional initiatives in quality; supports measure development and communication strategies targeted to communities	www.rwjf.org
	California HealthCare Foundation	•	Aims to improve the care of chronically ill individuals and create incentives to improve care	www.chcf.org
	Commonwealth Fund	•	Supports independent research on healthcare issues and awards grants to improve healthcare practice and policy	www.commonwealthfund.org

Exhibit 18.3

Center for Medicare & Medicaid Innovation Initiatives

Initiative	Description	Start Date	Length	Total Funding
	Primary Care Transformation			
Comprehensive Primary Care Initiative Demonstration	Public–private partnership to enhance primary care services, including 24-hour access, care plans, and care coordination	2012	Four years	$322 million
Federally Qualified Health Center (FQHC) Advanced Primary Care Practice Demonstration	Care coordination payments to FQHCs in support of team-led care, improved access, and enhanced primary care services	November 1, 2011	Three years ending on October 31, 2014	$49.7 million
Multi-payer Advanced Primary Care Practice Demonstration	State-led, multipayer collaborations to help primary care practices transform into medical homes	Phased in starting July 1, 2011	Three years	$283 million
Independence at Home	Home-based care for patients with multiple chronic conditions	Summer 2012	Three years	$15 million
	Bundled Payments for Care Improvement			
Bundled Payment for Care Improvement Initiative	Episodic payments around inpatient hospitalizations to incentivize care redesign	2012	Three years	$118 million
	Accountable Care Organizations			
Pioneer Accountable Care Organization (ACO) Model	Experienced provider organizations taking on financial risk for improving quality and lowering costs for all of their Medicare patients	January 2012	Three years (with optional two-year extension)	$77 million
Accelerated Development Learning Sessions	Public opportunities to learn from leading experts about successful ACO development	June 2011	Three sessions completed	$1.5 million
Advanced Payment Accountable Care Organization Model	Prepayment of expected shared savings to support ACO infrastructure and care coordination	April 1, 2012, or July 1, 2012	Payments end June 2014	$175 million
Physician Group Practice Transition Demonstration	A precursor to the Medicare Shared Savings Program; rewards physician groups for efficient care and high quality	January 1, 2011	Up to three years	$500,000 in administrative costs

(Continued)

EXHIBIT 18.3
Center for Medicare & Medicaid Innovation Initiatives *(continued)*

Initiative	Description	Start Date	Length	Total Funding
Medicare/Medicaid Enrollees				
State Demonstrations to Integrate Care for Medicare-Medicaid Enrollees	Assistance to help states engage stakeholders in redesigning care for Medicare/Medicaid enrollees	April/May 2011	18 months (with extension option)	$15 million
Financial Alignment Model Demonstrations	Opportunity for states to implement new care and payment systems to better coordinate care for Medicare/Medicaid enrollees	January 2013	Three years	To be determined
Capacity to Spread Innovation				
Partnership for Patients	National campaign targeting a 40% reduction in hospital-acquired conditions and a 20% reduction in 30-day readmissions	April 12, 2011	Ongoing	$500 million
Innovation Advisors Program	Training healthcare providers from around the country in achieving the Institute for Healthcare Improvement's Triple Aim	January 2012	Ongoing	$5.9 million
Health Care Innovation Challenge	A broad appeal for innovations with a focus on developing the workforce for new care models	March 30, 2012	Three years	$1 billion
Other				
Medicaid Emergency Psychiatric Demonstration	Expanding access to inpatient psychiatric services for Medicaid beneficiaries	Spring 2012	Three years	$75 million
Medicaid Incentives for Prevention of Chronic Diseases Program	Collaborating with states to test the effectiveness of preventive services in Medicaid	Sites awarded September 13, 2011	Five years	$100 million

SOURCE: CMS (2012b).

52 employer-based healthcare coalitions (representing 7,000 employers and more than 25 million employees), works to enhance value-based purchasing of healthcare services. A similarly named but separate organization, the National Business Group on Health (2013), established the Institute on Health Care Costs and Solutions (and the leadership committees that it comprises) in 2001 to address evidence-based health benefits, consumer engagement, and payment and delivery reform. Business coalitions at the regional level play a significant role in influencing policy to improve health and control costs as well. The Pacific Business Group on Health (2013) represents 60 purchasers that spend a combined $12 billion a year for healthcare coverage for more than 3 million individuals in California.

The Leapfrog Group is another organization representing the business sector's concern about quality and the cost of hospital care. Chartered in 2000, the Leapfrog Group gained considerable attention when it identified four practices that would create a "leap" in quality and patient safety. These practices are "computer physician order entry; evidence-based hospital referral; intensive care unit (ICU) staffing by physicians experienced in critical care medicine; and the Leapfrog Safe Practices Score" (Leapfrog Group 2014). As hospitals improve their quality, the Leapfrog Group members provide financial rewards.

REGULATORS, CERTIFIERS, AND ACCREDITORS

CMS is the executive branch agency that has regulatory control over much of the healthcare system—particularly hospitals, nursing homes, home care, hospice care, and some aspects of outpatient care. Regulations are a powerful tool to influence quality and serve to operationalize legislation. CMS influences quality through the development of standards, survey instruments, and interpretive guidelines (guidance on interpreting regulations). An example of the regulatory influence of CMS is its nursing home survey requirements, which are federally mandated and are conducted by state survey agencies. In addition, through "deemed status" CMS has recognized The Joint Commission as the accreditor of hospitals, with CMS maintaining its regulatory force through the requirements for payment. Accrediting bodies that certify providers as being safe and competent have a significant impact on quality. Several certifying boards are now integrating questions about quality improvement into their exams to highlight the importance of being knowledgeable and engaged in quality improvement.

PROFESSIONAL ORGANIZATIONS

Organizations representing the entire spectrum of health professionals are embracing quality improvement through the development of educational initiatives, tools for providers to use in practice, and certification programs to recognize competence in specific areas. For instance, professional organizations have used seminars, workshops, webinars, and other means to make their members more aware of the need to improve quality. The American Nurses Association (ANA) developed the National Database of Nursing Quality

Indicators, in which more than 2,000 hospitals report nursing-sensitive measures (ANA 2014), and the American Medical Association (AMA) developed measures for ambulatory care through its sponsorship of the Physician Consortium for Performance Improvement (AMA 2014). Professional organizations have also been key partners in consortia that include an array of stakeholders involved in reviewing, endorsing, and approving the use of measures for different settings. Boards of medicine, nursing, and allied health professionals play a major role through certification and licensure programs and by establishing standards for entry into practice as well as continued competence.

ADVOCACY AND TECHNICAL SUPPORT ORGANIZATIONS

Organizations that provide advocacy and technical support related to healthcare quality play an important role in the quality improvement landscape. In fulfillment of its mission to improve the safety of patients, the National Patient Safety Foundation (2013) identifies and creates a core body of knowledge, identifies pathways to apply the knowledge, develops and enhances the culture of receptivity to patient safety, and raises public awareness and fosters communications about patient safety. The Institute for Healthcare Improvement (IHI) has worked to engage healthcare providers, as well as stakeholders and the general public, to improve the quality of care and reduce the number of needless deaths and medical errors. IHI has promoted the Plan-Do-Study-Act (PDSA) method of quality improvement and has created collaboratives to bring providers together to work on projects related to a specific area. (The IHI campaigns are discussed in a case study later in this chapter.)

Quality improvement organizations (QIOs) evolved from the Medicare Utilization and Quality Control Peer Review Program created by statute in 1982. The primary function of QIOs is to improve the quality of care and efficiency of the health system for Medicare beneficiaries. CMS oversees the work of the QIOs and reports annually to Congress on the QIOs' impact. CMS has contracts with QIOs covering all 50 states, the District of Columbia, Puerto Rico, and the US Virgin Islands.

Another group of supporting organizations is philanthropic foundations that focus on quality and provide a catalyst for innovative quality initiatives. For instance, the Robert Wood Johnson Foundation has a team focused on developing and funding programs to improve quality. The foundation has supported initiatives to improve quality, such as Transforming Care at the Bedside, an initiative to reengineer nursing care in medical-surgical units in hospitals. It also funded Rewarding Results, which supported programs providing incentives to improve care, and has invested in regional projects to improve care through Aligning Forces for Quality. The California HealthCare Foundation has funded projects to improve care, such as pay-for-performance initiatives, and has explored ways to improve the quality of chronic illness care. The Commonwealth Fund (2014) sponsors programs that focus on healthcare delivery system reform, tracking health system performance, increasing healthcare access, and identifying practice innovations.

QUALITY MEASURE DEVELOPMENT PROCESS
MEASURE DEVELOPMENT

The major developers of quality measures are the National Committee for Quality Assurance (NCQA), the Agency for Healthcare Research and Quality (AHRQ), the AMA, the ANA, and The Joint Commission. NCQA continues to add and delete measures from the Healthcare Effectiveness Data and Information Set (HEDIS) database, and it develops measures for other programs, such as the Diabetes Recognition Program (NCQA 2013a). In addition, NCQA (2014) has developed measures to recognize patient-centered medical homes (PCMHs). AHRQ (2013) has developed the Consumer Assessment of Healthcare Providers and Systems (CAHPS) survey for hospital, outpatient, nursing home, and home health settings. The AMA (2014) has developed measures as part of the Physician Consortium for Performance Improvement. The ANA (2014) developed the National Database of Nursing Quality Indicators (NDNQI), which comprises measures of hospital nursing care. In 1997, The Joint Commission (2013) developed the ORYX measures, which integrate patient outcome measures into the accreditation process. Other national organizations have developed measures specific to their specialty and stakeholder groups.

MEASURE ENDORSEMENT

The National Quality Forum (NQF) was born from a recommendation in 1998 by the President's Advisory Commission on Consumer Protection and Quality in the Health Care Industry (1998) established by President Clinton. NQF was chartered in 1999 and provides scientific review and endorsement of measures for public reporting purposes. CMS recognizes NQF as a voluntary national consensus standard–setting organization adhering to the guidelines established by the National Technology Transfer and Advancement Act of 1996 and Office of Management and Budget Circular A-119, which allows CMS to use these standards rather than create an entity with a similar function within CMS. NQF is a membership organization with a broad array of stakeholders who participate in the review and endorsement of measures. NQF works to create a coherent approach to measurement and reporting at the national level.

MEASURE APPROVAL

A relatively new phenomenon is the emergence of consortia that bring stakeholders together to review performance measures to ensure that the measures are science-based, important measures of quality. The first consortium formed was the Hospital Quality Alliance (HQA). Founded in 2002 by the Association of American Medical Colleges (AAMC), the American Hospital Association (AHA), and the Federation of American Hospitals (FAH), HQA worked closely with CMS to review and approve measures for hospital reporting. HQA (2011) encompassed a broad array of stakeholders, including consumers, purchasers, health plans, and providers. The consortium continues its efforts today under the name Optional Public Reporting. Another consortium is the AQA alliance, formerly known as the Ambulatory Care Quality Alliance. Initiated in 2004 by the American Academy of Family Physicians, the American College of Physicians, America's Health Insurance Plans, and the AHRQ to work collaboratively on performance measurement and reporting issues in ambulatory care, this consortium includes consumers, purchasers, physicians, health insurance plans, and representatives from more than 100 different organizations. AQA works closely with CMS to adopt appropriate measures for ambulatory care (AQA 2010).

MEASURE USE

Quality measures have four primary uses: (1) for internal quality monitoring and improvement, (2) for accreditation, (3) as a basis for incentive payments to improve care, and (4) for public reporting. The first use primarily enables health professionals to improve care, while the other three uses are primarily related to holding providers accountable.

The first use of quality measures—internal monitoring and improvement—helps providers and institutions track specific measures to improve care and is related to professional and personal commitments to care as well as institutional expectations. Although quality measures have long been used for internal monitoring and reporting, providers have not been able to compare themselves easily to others because the data elements and collection instruments have not been synchronized. Collecting and reporting the same data using the same specifications helps organizations and providers understand how they perform compared to other organizations and enables them to identify opportunities for focused quality improvement efforts. For example, if the rate of preventable falls is significantly higher in Facility X than in similar organizations, the data indicate that Facility X should be able to reduce the number of preventable falls. This example also demonstrates how providers can use quality improvement processes to decrease their exposure to risks as a result of preventable incidents.

The second of these uses—accreditation—is carried out by organizations such as The Joint Commission for hospitals and NCQA for health plans. The Joint Commission accredits nearly all of the hospitals in the United States and has an international accrediting arm, Joint Commission International. The Joint Commission (2013) developed the ORYX system, which consists of a core set of measures used in the hospital accreditation process. NCQA uses the HEDIS measures for accreditation of health plans. Accreditation began in the early 1990s with the initial set of HEDIS measures. HEDIS includes 75 measures representing eight "domains of care" (NCQA 2013b). More than 90 percent of US health plans use HEDIS (NCQA 2013c).

The third use of quality measures—as a basis for incentive payments to improve care—is used by payers to create incentives for the provision of high-quality care. The

CMS pay-for-performance projects, as well as health plans' use of measures to reward the provision of high-quality care, depend on valid and reliable measures as a basis for payment decisions.

The fourth use of quality measures—public reporting—entails reporting of uniform data by provider type (e.g., hospitals), which allows consumers to compare institutions on the basis of the same data. Organizations such as CMS, The Joint Commission, the Leapfrog Group, and NCQA provide the public with information obtained from their quality measures. The Hospital Compare and Nursing Home Compare websites sponsored by CMS are examples of this use. The NCQA Health Plan Report Card is another example. Findings from The Joint Commission accreditation results are also available online.

TRENDS IN QUALITY IMPROVEMENT
IMPACT OF FEDERAL LEGISLATION ON QUALITY

Several pieces of legislation—including the American Recovery and Reinvestment Act, the Health Information Technology for Economic and Clinical Health (HITECH) Act's funding for the Office of the National Coordinator for Health Information Technology to push healthcare providers into the electronic age, and the far-reaching ACA—have greatly influenced quality improvement. These acts have made a significant contribution to improving several important aspects of quality, including value-based purchasing, electronic health records (EHRs), consumer information, and the establishment of a national healthcare quality strategy.

Value-Based Purchasing

The ACA, while having a significant focus on access to healthcare, is largely about value-based purchasing. With the cost of healthcare estimated to increase from $2.6 trillion in 2010 to $4.6 trillion in 2020 and to consume nearly 20 percent of the gross domestic product in 2020, value-based purchasing is viewed as critical to the health of the US economy (Keehan et al. 2011). Preventing the overuse, underuse, and inappropriate use of healthcare is seen as essential for both quality and cost. The federal government has a large stake in cost and quality. A seminal report issued by the US Department of Health & Human Services (HHS) Office of Inspector General (OIG 2010) found that 13.5 percent of Medicare enrollees experienced an adverse event while hospitalized, and an additional 13.5 percent experienced a harmful event during their hospitalization. The report concluded that 44 percent of adverse or harmful events could have been prevented and more than $320 million could have been saved.

Defining value as high-quality healthcare at the lowest cost assumes that the appropriate care is delivered in an efficient and effective manner. The ACA includes requirements for quality measurement coupled with cost controls to stimulate more efficient models of care. While pay for performance is being introduced in many countries, it is a complicated issue. Evidence suggests that pay for performance can have a positive effect on the quality of care in both hospital and outpatient settings. For instance, the CMS Premier Hospital Quality Incentive Demonstration (HQID) project experienced an 18.6 percent increase in its overall quality score over six years (Premier 2012a). In addition, reports have demonstrated improved care of patients with diabetes and those with hypertension (Bernacki et al. 2012; Cheng, Lee, and Chen 2012; Petersen et al. 2009; Petersen et al. 2011).

Even though reports have demonstrated positive effects of pay for performance, particularly in improving care, other reports provide a mixed picture of value-based purchasing (Chen, Lee, and Kuo 2012; Eijkenaar 2012; Petersen et al. 2011; VanLare, Moody-Williams, and Conway 2012). Concerns about pay for performance include several significant issues. One concern is that providers, hospitals, and other healthcare organizations that provide care for largely underserved minority populations and see very ill patients may score lower on reported measures (Jha, Orav, and Epstein 2011; Ryan 2013). Possible adverse effects also include concerns that physicians working in areas with a large minority population may receive reduced payments and that health plans may avoid patients who could cause them to have lower quality scores and poorer outcomes reported to the public (Casalino and Elster 2007). In response to this concern, CMS noted that hospitals and other providers serving minority populations would receive reimbursement based on improvements within the institution or practice rather than in comparison to others (VanLare, Moody-Williams, and Conway 2012). In addition, risk adjustment in reported measures would be needed to avoid penalizing physicians and institutions that care for sicker patients. If providers encounter a financial penalty for taking care of sicker patients, physicians will find it more difficult to accept these patients. While a strong move toward developing aggregated measures of care is in progress, it will take time for these measures to be fully vetted and useful in measuring the quality of care and determining reasonable payment for care of patients with multiple chronic diseases. A final concern is that practices and health organizations may focus their attention on the diseases that are measured, to the exclusion of other important aspects of healthcare.

The mixed results of the impact of value-based purchasing are related to the complex challenge of tailoring the payment to the specific type of care. One size does not fit all. Different payment levels may be effective for different settings and different populations within those settings. Also, sustaining long-term change may be difficult and potentially costly. Practices may become accustomed to getting incentive payments, and if benchmarks are raised and they no longer receive the incentive payment, the program may have a negative effect. While CMS began its focus on value-based purchasing by providing incentives for reporting quality measures, payment incentives in the future will be linked to actual care outcomes based on performance on select measures.

Value-based purchasing is also integrated in the move toward accountable care organizations (ACOs). CMS defines ACOs as "groups of doctors, hospitals, and other health care providers, who come together voluntarily to give coordinated high quality care to their Medicare patients" (CMS 2013b). The focus on ACOs is intended to improve the quality of care as well as to lower costs. The ACO model includes an embedded incentive payment in the form of revenue sharing as part of the savings that can be achieved. However, savings must be accompanied by hitting quality benchmarks. ACOs require providers to share in the financial risk of the plan, rather than place the financial risk on insurers as occurs in a traditional managed care model. CMS has two programs underway: the Shared Savings Program and the Pioneer ACO Model program. The Pioneer program is aimed at high-functioning health systems that can take on great financial risk in exchange for the potential of a greater financial reward. The initial set of Pioneer projects included 32 health systems (CMS 2012c).

While the ACA strongly promotes the ACO model, concerns about the success of ACOs include the challenges inherent in managed care models and the limited incentives available through the revenue-sharing program. Measures will need to be developed to assess the quality of ACOs in addition to the quality of individual participant organizations and individual providers (Devers and Berenson 2009).

In addition to the federal government's focus on value, private insurers are instituting programs that link quality and payment to create more efficient systems of care. An increasing number of private insurers are following CMS's policies on value-based purchasing and are implementing value-based purchasing for physician, hospital, long-term, hospice, and other types of care. No longer can providers expect payment for services from private insurers without accountability. In the time since the AHRQ developed and disseminated information for payers on implementing pay-for-performance and other valued-based approaches (Dudley and Rosenthal 2006), pay-for-performance programs such as Medicare's Premier Hospital Quality Incentive Demonstration have yielded mixed results, with low-performing hospitals realizing slower gains in quality scores than higher-performing hospitals (Ryan, Blustein, and Casalino 2012).

Electronic Health Records

Health systems have been slow to fully adopt EHRs primarily because of cost and complexity. Other industries have far surpassed healthcare in the implementation of electronic systems for data collection, monitoring, and quality improvement. To support the implementation of EHRs, the federal government invested more than $19 billion through the HITECH Act of 2009 to help institutions and outpatient practices adopt EHRs. The reason for the support of EHRs is to improve the quality of care. Regionalized EHRs can provide up-to-date information about patient status regardless of where the patient is, enabling providers to make informed decisions about care, coordinate care across settings, and continually improve care. The HITECH grants funded Regional Extension Centers (RECs) intended to assist primary care providers and institutions providing services to traditionally underserved populations (HHS 2011). The results of these efforts have been impressive: As of November 2013, more than 334,000 healthcare providers were participating in and receiving payment from the Medicare and Medicaid EHR Incentive Programs (CMS 2014b). Institutions that receive federal support must commit to using the EHRs meaningfully—that is, using the EHRs to collect and report data and to use the data to improve care and control costs.

The government supports the use of information technology to create more efficient and effective systems of care. Providers are required to meet several performance standards referred to as *meaningful use criteria*. Meaningful use criteria will be implemented in three stages. The first stage includes the development of the initial measures that providers need to report and processes for implementation of incentive programs. As part of the first stage, 15 core measures and 10 menu measures are being collected, of which 5 measures are required to be reported. In the second stage (launched in 2014), providers must meet either 17 core objectives plus 3 menu objectives or 20 core objectives. When the final stage rolls out in 2016, additional requirements will be added that focus on patient safety, quality, and decision-support tools (ONC 2014).

Consumer Information

Increasingly, efforts are being made to give consumers useful information in making choices about their healthcare. As consumers pick up more healthcare costs by paying a greater share of the cost of health insurance, higher deductibles, and higher copayments, they have more reason to be value conscious. A landmark study supports the contention that consumer sensitivity to costs reduces use of healthcare services with few adverse effects (Brook et al. 1984). In addition, consumers are increasingly using information about quality of services through sources such as Angie's List, *Consumer Reports*, and Consumers' Checkbook. Blogs also serve as sources of information about products and services. Consumers provide ratings when purchasing items online. To make informed decisions, consumers must know about both cost and quality. The reason for informing consumers about quality as well as cost is to have consumers drive demand on the basis of value. While this economic concept is straightforward, providing information about healthcare that is valid and reliable and that consumers find useful in making an informed decision has been a challenge. Consumers rarely know the cost of care before a service is delivered, and only in the last decade has providing information about quality been attempted. The exception in the availability of cost information is in retail clinics, where the costs of visits and procedures are publicly posted.

To support efforts to make information about quality of care available to consumers, CMS has created websites that inform consumers about the quality of care in nursing homes, home care, hospitals, and dialysis facilities (HHS 2013b). The Hospital Compare and Nursing Home Compare sites are informative and widely visited. CMS continues to look for ways of organizing information to make it easy for consumers to interpret. For instance, to help consumers choose a high-quality nursing home, Nursing Home Compare provides a rating of quality using one to five stars, with five stars designating the highest quality (HHS 2013a). Hospital Compare includes general information (including CAHPS results) and information on medical conditions and surgical procedures (Exhibit 18.4). The scores are a numeric rating of the percentage of times that an event happened, such as the percentage of patients who reported that their pain was always well controlled. The website includes regional and national data for comparison.

Determining what information is useful to consumers is an ongoing effort. The AHRQ and others have identified specific recommendations about publicly reported quality information (Hibbard and Sofaer 2010a, 2010b). These findings summarize the key aspects of how reports can be made more useful to consumers, such as by providing meaningful information, illustrative examples, and context for measures. These reports and studies have noted that publicly reported measures are useful but complicated, and many variables go into decisions about where to seek healthcare (Dafny and Dranove 2008; Faber et al. 2009; Hafner et al. 2011; Mazor and Dodd 2009; Mazor et al. 2010). Public reporting of information will continue to move forward in both informing consumer choice and providing incentives for providers to provide better care.

Condition	Measures
Acute myocardial infarction	• Average number of minutes before outpatients with chest pain or possible heart attack who needed specialized care were transferred to another hospital • Average number of minutes before outpatients with chest pain or possible heart attack got an ECG • Outpatients with chest pain or possible heart attack who got drugs to break up blood clots within 30 minutes of arrival • Outpatients with chest pain or possible heart attack who got aspirin within 24 hours of arrival • Heart attack patients given fibrinolytic medication within 30 minutes of arrival • Heart attack patients given PCI within 90 minutes of arrival • Heart attack patients given aspirin at discharge • Heart attack patients given a prescription for a statin at discharge
Heart failure	• Heart failure patients given discharge instructions • Heart failure patients given an evaluation of left ventricular systolic (LVS) function • Heart failure patients given ACE inhibitor or ARB for left ventricular systolic dysfunction (LVSD)
Pneumonia	• Pneumonia patients whose initial emergency room blood culture was performed prior to the administration of the first hospital dose of antibiotics • Pneumonia patients given the most appropriate initial antibiotic(s)

EXHIBIT 18.4
Hospital Compare Measure Set for Timely and Effective Care

(Continued)

Exhibit 18.4

Hospital Compare
Measure Set
for Timely and
Effective Care
(continued)

Condition	Measures
Surgical Care Improvement Project	• Outpatients having surgery who got an antibiotic at the right time (within one hour before surgery) • Surgery patients who were given an antibiotic at the right time (within one hour before surgery) to help prevent infection • Surgery patients whose preventive antibiotics were stopped at the right time (within 24 hours after surgery) • Patients who got treatment at the right time (within 24 hours before or after their surgery) to help prevent blood clots after certain types of surgery • Outpatients having surgery who got the right kind of antibiotic • Surgery patients who were taking heart drugs called beta blockers before coming to the hospital, who were kept on the beta blockers during the period just before and after their surgery • Surgery patients who were given the right kind of antibiotic to help prevent infection • Heart surgery patients whose blood sugar (blood glucose) is kept under good control in the days right after surgery • Surgery patients whose urinary catheters were removed on the first or second day after surgery • Patients having surgery who were actively warmed in the operating room or whose body temperature was near normal by the end of surgery
Emergency department throughput	• Average time patients spent in the emergency department, before they were admitted to the hospital as an inpatient • Average time patients spent in the emergency department, after the doctor decided to admit them as an inpatient before leaving the emergency department for their inpatient room • Average time patients spent in the emergency department before being sent home • Average time patients spent in the emergency department before they were seen by a healthcare professional • Average time patients who came to the emergency department with broken bones had to wait before receiving pain medication • Percentage of patients who left the emergency department before being seen • Percentage of patients who came to the emergency department with stroke symptoms who received brain scan results within 45 minutes of arrival
Preventive care	• Patients assessed and given influenza vaccination • Patients assessed and given pneumonia vaccination
Children's asthma care	• Children who received reliever medication while hospitalized for asthma • Children who received systemic corticosteroid medication (oral and IV medication that reduces inflammation and controls symptoms) while hospitalized for asthma • Children and their caregivers who received a home management plan of care document while hospitalized for asthma

(Continued)

Condition	Measures
Stroke care	• Ischemic stroke patients who got medicine to break up a blood clot within 3 hours after symptoms started • Ischemic stroke patients who received medicine known to prevent complications caused by blood clots within 2 days of arriving at the hospital • Ischemic or hemorrhagic stroke patients who received treatment to keep blood clots from forming anywhere in the body within 2 days of arriving at the hospital • Ischemic stroke patients who received a prescription for medicine known to prevent complications caused by blood clots before discharge • Ischemic stroke patients with a type of irregular heartbeat who were given a prescription for a blood thinner at discharge • Ischemic stroke patients needing medicine to lower cholesterol, who were given a prescription for this medicine before discharge • Ischemic or hemorrhagic stroke patients or caregivers who received written educational materials about stroke care and prevention during the hospital stay • Ischemic or hemorrhagic stroke patients who were evaluated for rehabilitation services
Blood clot prevention and treatment	• Patients who got treatment to prevent blood clots on the day of or day after hospital admission or surgery • Patients who got treatment to prevent blood clots on the day of or day after being admitted to the intensive care unit (ICU) • Patients who developed a blood clot while in the hospital who **did not** get treatment that could have prevented it • Patients with blood clots who got the recommended treatment, which includes using two different blood thinner medicines at the same time • Patients with blood clots who were treated with an intravenous blood thinner, and then were checked to determine if the blood thinner was putting the patient at an increased risk of bleeding • Patients with blood clots who were discharged on a blood thinner medicine and received written instructions about that medicine
Pregnancy and delivery care	• Percent of newborns whose deliveries were scheduled too early (1–3 weeks early), when a scheduled delivery was not medically necessary

EXHIBIT 18.4
Hospital Compare Measure Set for Timely and Effective Care
(continued)

SOURCE: CMS (2014c).

National Quality Strategy

A driving force promoting an integrated approach to improving healthcare quality is the strategic road map for quality that HHS initiated as required under Section 3011 of the ACA. The National Health Care Quality Strategy and Plan requires the inclusion of provisions for: "1) agency-specific plans and benchmarks; 2) coordination among agencies;

3) strategies to align public and private payers; and 4) alignment with meaningful use of health information technology (IT)" (HHS 2010). To achieve these goals, three aims were developed (AHRQ 2014):

1. *Better care:* Improve the overall quality by making healthcare more patient centered, reliable, accessible, and safe.

2. *Healthy people/healthy communities:* Improve the health of the US population by supporting proven interventions to address behavioral, social, and environmental determinants of health in addition to delivering higher-quality care.

3. *Affordable care:* Reduce the cost of quality healthcare for individuals, families, employers, and government.

Toward the fulfillment of these aims, HHS identified six priority areas (AHRQ 2014):

1. Making care safer by reducing harm caused in the delivery of care

2. Ensuring that each person and family is engaged as partners in care

3. Promoting effective communication and coordination of care

4. Promoting the most effective prevention and treatment practices for the leading causes of mortality, starting with cardiovascular disease

5. Working with communities to promote wide use of best practices to enable healthy living

6. Making quality care more affordable for individuals, families, employers, and governments by developing and spreading new healthcare delivery models

AHRQ was charged with implementing the plan, which will require continued involvement of stakeholders including providers, consumers, purchasers, and payers. The implementation of this plan will require active participation of all parties along with continued efforts regarding quality measurement and reporting as well as incentives for providing high-quality care.

TRENDS AND INITIATIVES IN SPECIFIC HEALTHCARE SECTORS
AMBULATORY CARE

Quality improvement efforts have begun to focus more intensely on ambulatory care. Quality improvement in ambulatory care settings has been challenging because of the numerous and varied practices and the inability to obtain critical quality data. The uptake of EHRs in ambulatory care practices has enabled the quality movement to go forward. The Tax Relief and Health Care Act of 2006 mandated CMS to establish the Physician Quality Reporting System (PQRS). Reporting by eligible individual professionals was initially voluntary, with providers receiving incentive payments for reporting. This arrangement will evolve into value-based purchasing, in which providers have to meet certain quality benchmarks to receive incentive payments (CMS 2014f). Some examples of non-physician professionals deemed eligible by CMS are nurse practitioners, physician assistants, clinical social workers, registered dietitians, and physical therapists (CMS 2013c).

Patient care delivery systems have been evolving toward a PCMH model since the 1960s. The American Academy of Pediatrics developed the concept of a "medical home" in 1967 to organize healthcare delivery to meet the needs of chronically ill children (Kilo and Wasson 2010). In the 1990s, the IHI called for the development of primary care models, and the IOM (1996) issued its report on the future of primary care. However, primary care received little attention between the mid-1990s and 2012.

As policymakers, purchasers, and payers look for ways to create efficiencies throughout the system, a strong primary care system continues to be an important part of managing cost and quality. Demonstration projects have shown a variety of benefits of PCMHs, including reduced hospitalizations and readmissions, better management of chronic illnesses, and improved patient satisfaction (Grumbach and Grundy 2010; Reid et al. 2010). Even though the PCMH can improve the quality of care, the National Demonstration Project analyzed data from 36 diverse family practice sites and concluded that the PCMH model would be viable on a large scale only if the healthcare system underwent significant reforms, particularly in regard to financing (Crabtree et al. 2010). The passage of the ACA in 2010 provided numerous elements to support the PCMH movement, including reimbursement strategies, community coordination, innovation, and evidence-based practice and quality improvement initiatives (Safety Net Medical Home Initiative 2010). An example of support provided through the ACA is the Multi-Payer Advanced Primary Care Practice Demonstration intended to evaluate benefits of PCMHs, such as reducing costs, improving the quality of care, increasing patient decision making, and providing better access to underserved populations (CMS 2010).

NCQA has a substantial role in supporting PCMH quality improvement through its recognition program. The program associates scores on the Physician Practice Connection–Patient Centered Medical Home (PPC-PCMH) survey with the assignment of a rating between one and three, with three being the highest achievable (Solberg et al. 2011). PCMH practices have an incentive to secure NCQA PPC-PCMH recognition because it facilitates enhanced reimbursement from public and private payers (NCQA 2014). In 2010, NCQA recognized PCMHs that are led by advanced practice registered nurses (APRNs) in states that allow APRNs to provide the full range of primary care and to practice independently (Scudder 2011).

HOSPITALS

In 2003, CMS and the Premier healthcare alliance initiated the Premier HQID project. The main purpose of the demonstration was to assess the effect on quality of incentive payments to hospitals. This project first required the reporting of data, and then it linked payment to quality (Premier 2012a, 2012b). The reported events became known as "never" events and are now referred to as *serious reportable events*.

Several pieces of legislation have aimed to improve quality and control the costs of hospital care. The Deficit Reduction Act of 2005 created an incentive program for hospitals to report quality measures (CMS 2012a). This program also established the principle that CMS would not pay for treatment of preventable hospital-acquired conditions (CMS 2012a).

The ACA authorized several value-based purchasing policies for hospitals. These provisions followed a significant history of quality improvement efforts and value-based purchasing policies for hospitals. The policies, in general, provide guidance on payment for serious reportable events, institute incentive payments for hitting benchmarks for quality improvement, and establish payment rates related to hospital readmission. For fiscal year 2013, the maximum payment reduction is 1 percent, for FY 2014 it is 2 percent, and for FY 2015 and thereafter it is capped at 3 percent (AAMC 2013). Results from the demonstration showed that hospitals improved performance on the required quality measures for which they received incentive payments (Premier 2012a). The 18.6 percent increase in overall quality score was accompanied by incentive payments of $60 million over six years (Premier 2012a). The measures required for reporting include process, outcome, and Hospital Consumer Assessment of Healthcare Providers and Systems (HCAHPS) measures.

NURSING HOMES

Quality monitoring and improvement in the nursing home industry have been deeply rooted in the regulatory process. Because of the frailty and vulnerability of the population served as well as historic issues related to quality of care, nursing homes have been the target of many sustained efforts to monitor and improve care. In the early 1980s, the nursing home industry developed quality improvement programs such as the Quest for Quality program offered by state nursing home organizations. At the same time, standards for care were established and used as the basis for the survey process. Nursing home quality is monitored by state agencies and includes reporting of data as well as site visits. The survey process includes information about staffing, patient outcomes, and fire safety. A move to focus on outcomes of care has taken place. In the early 2000s, CMS began the national Nursing Home Quality Initiative to provide consumers and providers with information regarding the quality of care in nursing homes through publicly reported data from the nursing home survey. (See the discussion of Nursing Home Compare earlier in

Measure Type	Measure	
Long-Stay Quality Measures	• Percentage of long-stay residents experiencing one or more falls with major injury • Percentage of long-stay residents with a urinary tract infection • Percentage of long-stay residents who self-report moderate to severe pain • Percentage of long-stay high-risk residents with pressure ulcers • Percentage of long-stay low-risk residents who lose control of their bowels or bladder • Percentage of long-stay residents who have/had a catheter inserted and left in their bladder • Percentage of long-stay residents who were physically restrained • Percentage of long-stay residents whose need for help with daily activities has increased • Percentage of long-stay residents who lose too much weight • Percentage of long-stay residents who have depressive symptoms • Percentage of long-stay residents assessed and given, appropriately, the seasonal influenza vaccine • Percentage of long-stay residents assessed and given, appropriately, the pneumococcal vaccine • Percentage of long-stay residents who received an antipsychotic medication	**Exhibit 18.5** Nursing Home Quality Measures
Short-Stay Quality Measures	• Percentage of short-stay residents who self-report moderate to severe pain • Percentage of short-stay residents with pressure ulcers that are new or worsened • Percentage of short-stay residents assessed and given, appropriately, the seasonal influenza vaccine • Percentage of short-stay residents assessed and given, appropriately, the pneumococcal vaccine • Percentage of short-stay residents who are newly administered antipsychotic medications	

SOURCE: CMS (2014d, 2014e).

this chapter.) Exhibit 18.5 provides a list of the measures. In the time since CMS launched the Quality Indicator Survey project using a phased approach in 2005, the initiative has spread nationwide, and surveyors of long-term care programs now use a software program called ASE-Q to carry out computer-assisted surveying (CMS 2014a).

Nursing homes are unique in having a standardized, federally required assessment for every resident in a CMS-certified facility. The Minimum Data Set (MDS) is an instrument that includes information about resident function and major health problems and risks and that generates a plan of care based on the assessment. Every resident in every certified facility undergoes the same assessment, thus providing patient-level data that are useful in monitoring quality of care (CMS 2012d).

As with hospitals and ambulatory care, a push for value-based purchasing is taking place in nursing homes. The Nursing Home Value-Based Purchasing Demonstration project rewards nursing homes that perform well in four areas: nurse staffing, patient outcomes as measured by the MDS, appropriate hospitalizations, and performance on surveys. Nursing homes that score in the top 20 percent on these measures within each state are eligible for bonus payments (CMS 2009).

Home Health Care

Beginning in 1999, CMS (2011b) began to require Medicare-certified home health agencies to complete a standardized health assessment for each client using the Outcome and Assessment Information Set (OASIS). This requirement has evolved, and core measurement elements were revised as clinical and empirical research became available. The objective was to provide home health agencies with essential measurement elements that can be modified on the basis of clinical judgment, rather than produce a comprehensive assessment instrument (CMS 2011b). As with many data collection processes, the information has several uses. OASIS provides aggregate patient data as well as care planning information that links to the patient data. This information provides the basis for quality monitoring and improvement. Exhibit 18.6 provides an overview of the process and outcome measures as well as a list of the potentially avoidable events.

The Home Health Quality Improvement (HHQI) National Campaign was initiated to focus on improving home care. Stakeholders moving the campaign forward include the Visiting Nurse Associations of America, AHRQ, and the National Association for Home Care and Hospice. The campaign's multipronged efforts include disseminating best practices and providing educational resources (HHQI 2013).

Conclusion

The ACA provides the potential for significant impact on healthcare quality strategies for business, accrediting agencies, organizations, and providers across the United States. The momentum of national strategies to improve healthcare quality is sustained by public and private funding and by the development of policies that support measurement, public reporting, and accountability. The enhanced role of consumers in healthcare also represents a substantial societal change. Consumers are positioned at the center of the quality improvement process and are recognized as significant stakeholders in the advancement

Measure Title	Measure Description
Emergent Care for Injury Caused by Fall	Percentage of patients who need urgent, unplanned medical care due to an injury caused by fall
Emergent Care for Wound Infections, Deteriorating Wound Status	Percentage of home health episodes of care during which the patient required emergency medical treatment from a hospital emergency department related to a wound that is new, is worse, or has become infected
Emergent Care for Improper Medication Administration, Medication Side Effects	Percentage of home health episodes of care during which the patient required emergency medical treatment from a hospital emergency department related to improper medication administration or medication side effects
Emergent Care for Hypo/hyperglycemia	Percentage of home health episodes of care during which the patient required emergency medical treatment from a hospital emergency department related to hypo- or hyperglycemia
Development of Urinary Tract Infection	Percentage of home health episodes of care during which patients developed a bladder or urinary tract infection
Increase in Number of Pressure Ulcers	Percentage of home health episodes of care during which the patient had a larger number of pressure ulcers at discharge than at start of care
Substantial Decline in 3 or More Activities of Daily Living	Percentage of home health episodes of care during which the patient became substantially more dependent in at least three out of five activities of daily living
Substantial Decline in Management of Oral Medications	Percentage of home health episodes of care during which the patient's ability to take medicines correctly (by mouth) got much worse
Discharged to the Community Needing Wound Care or Medication Assistance	Percentage of home health episodes of care at the end of which the patient was discharged, with no assistance available, needing wound care or medication assistance
Discharged to the Community Needing Toileting Assistance	Percentage of home health episodes of care at the end of which the patients was discharged, with no assistance available, needing toileting assistance
Discharged to the Community with Behavioral Problems	Percentage of home health episodes of care at the end of which the patient was discharged, with no assistance available, demonstrating behavior problems
Discharged to the Community with an Unhealed Stage II Pressure Ulcer	Percentage of home health episodes of care at the end of which the patient was discharged with a stage II pressure ulcer that has remained unhealed for 30 days or more while a home health patient

SOURCE: CMS (2011a).

NOTE: Measures collected from the Outcome and Assessment Information Set (OASIS).

EXHIBIT 18.6
Home Health Quality Measures—Potentially Avoidable Events

of healthcare delivery systems. Innovation and collaboration will continue to be a priority for quality improvement efforts as new care delivery and value-based purchasing models are explored to support integration across healthcare sectors. The challenge for the future will be to continually incorporate new evidence into quality improvement practice as data emerge from scientific research.

REFERENCES

Agency for Healthcare Research and Quality (AHRQ). 2014. "About the National Quality Strategy." Accessed January 4. www.ahrq.gov/workingforquality/about.htm.

———. 2013. "About CAHPS." Accessed December 20. https://cahps.ahrq.gov/about-cahps/index.html.

Ambulatory Quality Alliance (AQA). 2010. "AQA Strategic Plan." Approved October 28. www.aqaalliance.org/files/AQA_Strategic_Plan_10282010.pdf.

American Medical Association (AMA). 2014. "Physician Consortium for Performance Improvement." Accessed January 4. www.ama-assn.org/ama/pub/physician-resources/physician-consortium-performance-improvement.page.

American Nurses Association (ANA). 2014. "National Database for Nursing Quality Indicators." Accessed January 4. www.nursingquality.org/About-NDNQI#quality-data.

Association of American Medical Colleges (AAMC). 2013. "Selected Medicare Hospital Quality Provisions Under the ACA." Accessed December 19. www.aamc.org/advocacy/medicare/153882/selected_medicare_hospital_quality_provisions_under_the_aca.html.

Bernacki, R. E., D. N. Ko, P. Higgins, S. N. Whitlock, A. Cullinan, R. Wilson, V. Jackson, C. Dahlin, J. Abrahm, E. Mort, K. N. Scheer, S. Block, and J. A. Billings. 2012. "Improving Access to Palliative Care Through an Innovative Quality Improvement Initiative: An Opportunity for Pay-for-Performance." *Journal of Palliative Medicine* 15 (2): 192–99.

Brook, H. R., J. E. Ware, W. H. Rogers, E. B. Keeler, A. R. Davies, C. A. Sherbourne, G. A. Goldberg, K. N. Lohr, P. Camp, and J. P. Newhouse. 1984. *The Effect of Coinsurance on the Health of Adults: Results from the Rand Health Insurance Experiment*. Report No. R-3055-HHS. Santa Monica, CA: The Rand Corporation.

Casalino, L. P., and A. Elster. 2007. "Will Pay-for-Performance and Quality Reporting Affect Health Care Disparities?" *Health Affairs* 26 (3): w405–w414.

Centers for Disease Control and Prevention (CDC). 2012. "Chronic Diseases and Health Promotion." Updated August 13. www.cdc.gov/nccdphp/overview.htm.

Centers for Medicare & Medicaid Services (CMS). 2014a. "CMS Quality Indicator Survey/ASE-Q." Accessed January 4. www.cms.gov/Medicare/Provider-Enrollment-and-Certification/SurveyCertificationGenInfo/Downloads/QIS-Brochure.pdf.

———. 2014b. "EHR Incentive Programs: Data and Program Reports." Accessed January 4. www.cms.gov/Regulations-and-Guidance/Legislation/EHRIncentivePrograms/DataAndReports.html.

———. 2014c. "Measures Displayed on Hospital Compare." Accessed January 4. www.medicare.gov/hospitalcompare/Data/Measures-Displayed.html.

———. 2014d. "Nursing Home Compare: Why Quality Measures Are Important to You (Long-Stay Resident)." Accessed January 4. www.medicare.gov/NursingHomeCompare/Data/Long-Stay-Residents.html.

———. 2014e. "Nursing Home Compare: Why Quality Measures Are Important to You (Short-Stay Resident)." Accessed January 4. www.medicare.gov/NursingHomeCompare/Data/Short-Stay-Residents.html.

———. 2014f. "Physician Quality Reporting System." Accessed January 4. www.cms.gov/Medicare/Quality-Initiatives-Patient-Assessment-Instruments/PQRS/?gclid=CIm4gLfk5bsCFbFxOgod7DQAyQ.

———. 2013a. "About the CMS Innovation Center." Accessed December 19. http://innovation.cms.gov/About/index.html.

———. 2013b. "Accountable Care Organizations (ACO)." Updated March 22. www.cms.gov/ACO/.

———. 2013c. "Physician Quality Reporting System: List of Eligible Professionals." Updated November 14. www.cms.gov/Medicare/Quality-Initiatives-Patient-Assessment-Instruments/PQRS/Downloads/PQRS_List-of-EligibleProfessionals_022813.pdf.

———. 2012a. "Hospital-Acquired Conditions Overview." Updated September 20. www.cms.gov/HospitalAcqCond/.

———. 2012b. "One Year of Innovation: Taking Action to Improve Care and Reduce Costs." Published January 26. http://innovation.cms.gov/Files/reports/Innovation-Center-Year-One-Summary-document.pdf.

———. 2012c. "Pioneer Accountable Care Organization Program: General Fact Sheet." Updated September 12. http://innovation.cms.gov/Files/fact-sheet/Pioneer-ACO-General-Fact-Sheet.pdf.

―――. 2012d. "Research, Statistics, Data and Systems: Minimum Data Sets 2.0 Tool and Public Reports." Updated March 8. www.cms.gov/MinimumDataSets20/.

―――. 2011a. "Home Health Quality Measures—Potentially Avoidable Events." Revised August. www.cms.gov/HomeHealthQualityInits/Downloads/HHQIOutcome-Avoidable Event-Process-Measures.zip.

―――. 2011b. *Outcome and Assessment Information Set (OASIS-C) Process-Based Quality Improvement (PBQI) Manual.* Revised December. www.cms.gov/Medicare/Quality-Initiatives-Patient-Assessment-Instruments/HomeHealthQualityInits/downloads/HHQIProcess-BasedQualityImprovementManual.pdf.

―――. 2010. "CMS Introduces New Center for Medicare and Medicaid Innovation, Initiatives to Better Coordinate Health Care." Press release issued November 16. www.cms.gov/Newsroom/MediaReleaseDatabase/Press-Releases/2010-Press-Releases-Items/2010-11-16.html.

―――. 2009. "Nursing Home Value-Based Purchasing Demonstration: Fact Sheet." Released August. www.cms.gov/DemoProjectsEvalRpts/downloads/NHP4P_FactSheet.pdf.

Chen, P. C., Y. C. Lee, and R. N. Kuo. 2012. "Differences in Patient Reports on the Quality of Care in a Diabetes Pay-for-Performance Program Between 1 Year Enrolled and Newly Enrolled Patients." *International Journal for Quality in Health* Care 24 (2): 189–96.

Cheng, S. H., T. T. Lee, and C. C. Chen. 2012. "A Longitudinal Examination of a Pay-for-Performance Program for Diabetes Care: Evidence from a Natural Experiment." *Medical Care* 50 (2): 109–16.

Commonwealth Fund. 2014. "Programs." Accessed January 4. www.commonwealthfund.org/Grants-and-Programs/Programs.aspx.

Crabtree, B. F., P. A. Nutting, W. L. Miller, K. C. Stange, E. E. Stewart, and C. R. Jean. 2010. "Summary of the National Demonstration Project and Recommendations for the Patient-Centered Medical Home." *Annals of Family Medicine* 8 (Suppl. 1): S80–S90.

Cuckler, G. A., A. M. Sisko, S. P. Keehan, S. D. Smith, A. J. Madison, J. A. Poisal, C. J. Wolfe, J. M. Lizonitz, and D. A. Stone. 2013. "National Health Expenditure Projections, 2012–22:

Slow Growth Until Coverage Expands and Economy Improves." *Health Affairs* 32 (10): 1820–31.

Dafny, L., and D. Dranove. 2008. "Do Report Cards Tell Consumers Anything They Don't Know Already? The Case of Medicare HMOs." *Rand Journal of Economics* 39 (3): 790–821.

Devers, K., and R. A. Berenson. 2009. "Can Accountable Care Organizations Improve the Value of Health Care by Solving the Cost and Quality Quandaries?" Robert Wood Johnson Foundation and Urban Institute. Published October. www.urban.org/uploaded pdf/411975_acountable_care_orgs.pdf.

Dudley, R. A., and M. B. Rosenthal. 2006. *Pay for Performance: A Decision Guide for Purchasers.* AHRQ Publication No. 06-0047. Rockville, MD: Agency for Healthcare Research and Quality.

Eijkenaar, F. 2012. "Pay for Performance in Healthcare: An International Overview of Initiatives." *Medical Care Research and Review* 69 (3): 251–76.

Faber, M., M. Bosch, H. Wollersheim, S. Leatherman, and R. Grol. 2009. "Public Reporting in Healthcare: How Do Consumers Use Quality-of-Care Information? A Systematic Review." *Medical Care* 47 (1): 1–8.

Grumbach, K., and P. Grundy. 2010. *Outcomes of Implementing Patient Centered Medical Home Interventions: A Review of the Evidence from Prospective Evaluation Studies in the United States.* Washington, DC: Patient-Centered Primary Care Collaborative.

Hafner, J. M., S. C. Williams, R. G. Koss, B. A. Tschurtz, S. P. Schmaltz, and J. M. Loeb. 2011. "The Perceived Impact of Public Reporting Hospital Performance Data: Interviews with Hospital Staff." *International Journal for Quality in Health Care* 23 (6): 697–704.

Hibbard, J., and S. Sofaer. 2010a. *Best Practices in Public Reporting No. 1: How to Effectively Present Healthcare Performance Data to Consumers.* AHRQ Publication No. 10-0082-EF. Rockville, MD: Agency for Healthcare Research and Quality.

———. 2010b. *Best Practices in Public Reporting No. 2: Maximizing Consumer Understanding of Comparative Quality Reports: Effective Use of Explanatory Information.* AHRQ Publication No. 10-0082-1-EF. Rockville, MD: Agency for Healthcare Research and Quality.

Home Health Quality Improvement (HHQI). 2013. "Welcome to the HHQI National Campaign." Accessed December 20. www.homehealthquality.org/hh/default.aspx.

Hospital Quality Alliance (HQA). 2011. "Press Release: HQA Recaps Accomplishments, Readies Measures Review Transfer." Press release issued December 13. www.fah.org/fahcms/Documents/On%20The%20Record/Hospital%20Quality%20Alliance/HQA%20Press%20Releases/HQA_Announcement.pdf.

Institute for Healthcare Improvement (IHI). 2013. "Overview: Protecting 5 Million Lives from Harm." Accessed December 20. www.ihi.org/offerings/Initiatives/PastStrategicInitiatives/5MillionLivesCampaign/Pages/default.aspx.

———. 2006. "Overview of the 100,000 Lives Campaign." Accessed December 20, 2013. www.ihi.org/offerings/Initiatives/PastStrategicInitiatives/5MillionLivesCampaign/Documents/Overview%20of%20the%20100K%20Campaign.pdf.

Institute of Medicine (IOM). 1996. *Primary Care: America's Health in a New Era*. Washington, DC: National Academies Press.

Jha, A. K., E. J. Orav, and A. M. Epstein. 2011. "Low-Quality, High-Cost Hospitals, Mainly in South, Care for Sharply Higher Shares of Elderly Black, Hispanic, and Medicaid Patients." *Health Affairs* 30 (10): 1904–11.

Joint Commission. 2013. "Facts About ORYX for Hospitals (National Hospital Quality Measures)." Issued September. www.jointcommission.org/assets/1/6/ORYX_for_Hospitals.pdf.

Keehan, S. P., A. M. Sisko, C. J. Truffer, J. A. Poisal, G. A. Cuckler, A. J. Madison, J. M. Lizonitz, and S. D. Smith. 2011. "National Health Spending Projections Through 2020: Economic Recovery and Reform Drive Faster Spending Growth." *Health Affairs* 30 (8): 1594–605.

Kilo, C. M., and J. H. Wasson. 2010. "Practice Redesign and the Patient-Centered Medical Home: History, Promises, and Challenges." *Health Affairs* 29 (5): 773–78.

Kohn, L. T., J. M. Corrigan, and M. S. Donaldson (eds.). 2000. *To Err Is Human: Building a Safer Health System*. Washington, DC: National Academies Press.

Leapfrog Group. 2014. "Fact Sheet." Accessed January 4. www.leapfroggroup.org/about_leapfrog/leapfrog-factsheet.

Mazor, K. M., J. Calvi, R. Cowan, M. E. Costanza, P. K. Han, S. M. Greene, L. Saccoccio, E. Cove, D. Roblin, and A. Williams. 2010. "Media Messages About Cancer: What Do People Understand?" *Journal of Health Communication* 15 (Suppl. 2): 126–45.

Mazor, K. M., and K. S. Dodd. 2009. "A Qualitative Study of Consumers' Views on Public Reporting of Healthcare-Associated Infections." *American Journal of Medical Quality* 24 (5): 412–18.

McCall, N., J. Cromwell, C. Urato, and D. Rabiner. 2008. *Evaluation of Phase I of the Medicare Health Support Pilot Program Under Traditional Fee-for-Service Medicare: 18-Month Interim Analysis. Report to Congress.* Published October. www.cms.gov/reports/downloads/MHS_Second_Report_to_Congress_October_2008.pdf.

National Business Coalition on Health. 2014. "About NBCH." Accessed January 4. www.nbch.org/About-NBCH.

National Business Group on Health. 2013. "Institute on Health Care Costs and Solutions (IHCCS)." Accessed December 26. www.businessgrouphealth.org/about/hccs.cfm.

National Committee for Quality Assurance (NCQA). 2014. "Patient-Centered Medical Home Recognition." Accessed January 4. www.ncqa.org/Programs/Recognition/PatientCenteredMedicalHomePCMH.aspx.

———. 2013a. "Diabetes Recognition Program (DRP)." Accessed December 26. www.ncqa.org/Programs/Recognition/DiabetesRecognitionProgramDRP.aspx.

———. 2013b. "HEDIS & Performance Measurement." Accessed December 26. www.ncqa.org/HEDISQualityMeasurement.aspx.

———. 2013c. "HEDIS and Quality Compass." Accessed December 26. www.ncqa.org/HEDISQualityMeasurement/WhatisHEDIS.aspx.

National Patient Safety Foundation. 2013. "Mission and Vision." Accessed December 26. www.npsf.org/about-us/mission-and-vision/.

Pacific Business Group on Health. 2013. "About the Pacific Business Group on Health." Accessed December 26. www.pbgh.org/about.

Petersen, L. A., T. Urech, K. Simpson, K. Pietz, S. J. Hysong, J. Profit, D. Conrad, R. A. Dudley, M. Z. Lutschg, R. Petzel, and L. D. Woodard. 2011. "Design, Rationale, and Baseline Characteristics of a Cluster Randomized Controlled Trial of Pay for Performance for Hypertension Treatment: Study Protocol." *Implementation Science: IS* 6 (October 3): 114.

Petersen, L. A., L. D. Woodard, L. M. Henderson, T. H. Urech, and K. Pietz. 2009. "Will Hypertension Performance Measures Used for Pay-for-Performance Programs Penalize Those Who Care for Medically Complex Patients?" *Circulation* 119 (23): 2978–85.

Premier. 2012a. "CMS/Premier Hospital Quality Incentive Demonstration." Accessed February 23. www.premierinc.com/p4p/hqi/.

———. 2012b. "Overview of CMS Hospital Quality Incentive Demonstration Project Payment Method." Accessed February 23. www.premierinc.com/quality-safety/tools-services/p4p/hqi/payment/project-payment-year6.jsp.

President's Advisory Commission on Consumer Protection and Quality in the Health Care Industry. 1998. *Quality First: Better Healthcare for All Americans.* Darby, PA: Diane Publishing.

Reid, R. J., K. Coleman, E. A. Johnson, P. A. Fishman, C. Hsu, M. P. Soman, C. E. Trescott, M. Erikson, and E. B. Larson. 2010. "The Group Health Medical Home at Year Two: Cost Savings, Higher Patient Satisfaction, and Less Burnout for Providers." *Health Affairs* 29 (5): 835–43.

Ryan, A. M. 2013. "Will Value-Based Purchasing Increase Disparities in Care?" *New England Journal of Medicine* 369 (26): 2472–74.

Ryan, A. M., J. Blustein, and L. P. Casalino. 2012. "Medicare's Flagship Test of Pay-for-Performance Did Not Spur More Rapid Quality Improvement Among Low-Performing Hospitals." *Health Affairs* 31 (4): 797–805.

Safety Net Medical Home Initiative. 2010. *Health Reform and the Patient-Centered Medical Home: Policy Provisions and Expectations of the Patient Protection and Affordable Care Act.* Published October. www.safetynetmedicalhome.org/sites/default/files/Policy-Brief-2.pdf.

Scudder, L. 2011. "Nurse-Led Medical Homes: Current Status and Future Plans." *Medscape News.* Published May 27. www.medscape.com/viewarticle/743197.

Solberg, L., S. Asche, P. Fontaine, T. Flottemesch, L. Pawlson, and S. Scholle. 2011. "Relationship of Clinic Medical Home Scores to Quality and Patient Experience." *Journal of Ambulatory Care Management* 34 (1): 57–66.

US Department of Health & Human Services (HHS). 2013a. "Nursing Home Compare." Accessed January 15. www.medicare.gov/nursinghomecompare/.

———. 2013b. "Quality Care Finder." www.medicare.gov/Quality-Care-Finder/.

———. 2011. "Over 100,000 Primary Care Providers Sign Up to Adopt Electronic Health Records Through Their Regional Extension Centers." News release issued November 17. www.hhs.gov/news/press/2011pres/11/20111117a.html.

———. 2010. *National Health Care Quality Strategy and Plan*. Issued September 9. www.hhs.gov/news/reports/quality/nationalhealthcarequalitystrategy.pdf.

US Department of Health & Human Services Office of Inspector General (OIG). 2010. *Adverse Events in Hospitals: National Incidence Among Medicare Beneficiaries*. Published November. http://oig.hhs.gov/oei/reports/oei-06-09-00090.pdf.

US Department of Health & Human Services Office of the National Coordinator for Health Information Technology (ONC). 2014. "How to Attain Meaningful Use." Accessed January 4. www.healthit.gov/providers-professionals/how-attain-meaningful-use.

VanLare, J. M., J. Moody-Williams, and P. H. Conway. 2012. "Value-Based Purchasing for Hospitals." *Health Affairs* 31 (1): 249.

Wachter, R. M., and P. J. Pronovost. 2006. "The 100,000 Lives Campaign: A Scientific and Policy Review." *Joint Commission Journal on Quality and Patient Safety* 32 (11): 621–27.

CHAPTER 6

PAYMENT INCENTIVES

Another major theory that underlies the Affordable Care Act (ACA) is the use of payment incentives to drive behavior. Payment policies in the ACA were projected to save significant Medicare expenditures from otherwise expected cost increases. This "bending of the cost curve" is demonstrated in Exhibit 6.1. The payment policies that accomplish these savings can be broadly grouped into four areas:

1. Reduced total cost of care through improved chronic care management

2. Reduced inpatient use and cost per admission

3. Reduced fraud and abuse

4. Reduced payment to providers

Medicare policy drives almost all other payer policy, and therefore the Medicare (and Medicaid) payment incentives contained in the ACA will change all healthcare delivery in the United States.

Although private payers will experiment with different payment systems, most providers design their operations to maximize payment from Medicare and Medicaid. Designing and improving patient care systems that provide quality care and maximize payment for one payment system is difficult; trying to create different patient care processes for multiple payers is nearly impossible.

However, a few exceptions to this rule are worth noting.

◆ Formularies are devised by private health plans to optimize costs and quality of pharmaceuticals, whereas the Medicare Part D networks continue to be very broad.

◆ Reference pricing is a tool used by the California Public Employees' Retirement System (CalPERS) as an incentive to its members to use low-cost providers for selected services.

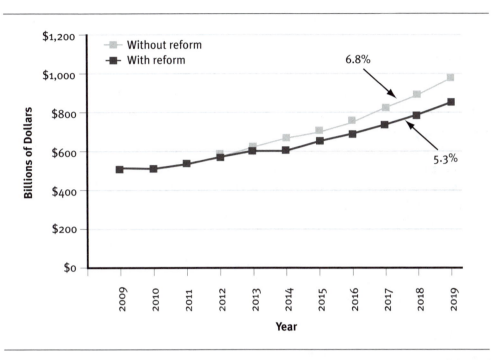

EXHIBIT 6.1
Medicare
Spending with and
Without Reform

SOURCE: Analysis based on data from the CMS Office of the Actuary's April 22, 2010, report "Estimated Financial Effects of the Patient Protection and Affordable Care Act, as Amended." www.cms.gov/ActuarialStudies/05_HealthCareReform.asp

CalPERS pays the reference price, and the member pays the difference. After this system was instituted, the average prices charged to CalPERS members declined by 5.6 percent at low-price facilities and by 34.3 percent at high-price providers (Robinson and Brown 2013).

◆ Narrow provider networks have grown in order for health plans to be price-competitive in the health exchanges (see Chapter 8). These networks are constructed with low-cost providers.

◆ Centers of Excellence have been identified by large employers to provide high-quality, low-cost services (e.g., heart surgery, transplants). These employers then provide financial incentives and free transportation to employees to receive healthcare services at these centers.

Many areas of the United States deliver higher-quality and lower-cost care than others because of their more efficient use of healthcare services. The ACA was crafted with the belief that the whole system can be made more effective and efficient by encouraging the spread of these more efficient practices throughout the nation. However, some policymakers have raised concerns that policies that provide incentives for efficiency can lead to rationing. The experiences with tightly managed HMOs in the 1980s and 1990s provided some highly public examples of patients being denied care because of the financial incentives inherent in health plan management (Blendon et al. 1998; Bodenheimer and Pham 2010).

The antidote to this problem is quality reporting. Quality measurement and public reporting have matured significantly in the past 20 years. The federal website Healthcare.gov provides patients and providers with numerous metrics to evaluate performance in three spheres: clinical quality, safety, and patient experience. In addition, state-based quality reporting organizations are becoming more widespread and useful to consumers (see Wisconsin Collaborative for Healthcare Quality 2014; MN Community Measurement 2014; and the Commonwealth of Massachusetts Health Care Quality and Cost Council 2014). Quality reporting systems have matured to the point that the authors of the ACA felt comfortable including payment incentives in the final law.

Payment policies can be characterized as incentives (carrots) and penalties (sticks). Unfortunately, fraud continues to plague the Medicare system, and therefore a number of new policies in the ACA give an incentive to providers to fully comply with Medicare payment rules.

In addition to specific payment policies, the ACA contains more general features to improve payment in the future (i.e., Center for Medicare and Medicaid Innovation) or take a stronger hand to control costs (i.e., Independent Payment Advisory Board). These payment polices are explored in the following sections.

INCENTIVES: THE CARROTS

ACCOUNTABLE CARE ORGANIZATIONS

One of the more highly publicized portions of the ACA is the shared savings program for Medicare: the accountable care organization (ACO) (§3022). (The ACA also includes an ACO for pediatric Medicaid patients in §2706.) The ACO concept was based on proposals from Fisher and colleagues (2009) at Dartmouth and by the results of the Medicare Group Practice Demonstration Project (MedPAC 2009).

The basic principle of an ACO is that a group of providers becomes accountable for the care—including quality and cost—of a specific population. If the quality goals are met and the cost is less than the target set by the payer, the savings are shared, hence the name *shared savings*. Three advantages for providers are inherent in the ACA version of ACOs. First, the capitation risk is removed as providers receive their normal fee-for-service payments plus a bonus if cost and quality targets are met. Second, patients need not enroll, as Medicare automatically includes them as part of a specific ACO based on their choice of providers. Third, ACOs need not be fully integrated healthcare systems, as more loosely structured organizations can be used (e.g., physician hospital organizations [PHOs]). Thorpe and Ogden (2010) have called these looser structures "virtual integrated systems." ACOs have specific requirements (Fisher et al. 2009):

◆ ACOs must have a formal legal structure to receive and distribute shared savings to participating providers.

◆ Each ACO must employ enough primary care professionals to treat its beneficiary population (minimum of 5,000 beneficiaries). The Centers for Medicare & Medicaid Services (CMS) decides how many professionals is sufficient.

◆ Each ACO must agree to participate at least three years in the program.

◆ Each ACO will develop sufficient information about its participating healthcare professionals to support beneficiary assignment and for the determination of payments for shared savings.

◆ ACOs will be expected to have a leadership and management structure that includes clinical and administrative systems.

◆ Each ACO will be expected to have defined processes to promote evidence-based medicine, report on quality and cost measures, and coordinate care.

◆ ACOs will be required to produce reports demonstrating the adoption of patient-centered care.

An interesting addition to §3022 is the ability of HHS to provide partial capitation to selected ACOs. Partial capitation could be for ambulatory care only or other selected services. This provides an interesting entry for ACOs into areas previously reserved for health plans.

Implementing ACOs includes some challenges:

◆ ACOs will only succeed with chronic disease management that minimizes preventable conditions, acute care episodes, and complicated inpatient admissions.

◆ Legal structures need to be developed to allow full participation and cooperation by all providers in an ACO.

◆ The shared savings model does not provide up-front funding, so initial capital must be found to fund the systems (people and health information technology) needed to perform well in chronic disease management.

◆ The leadership of newly formed ACOs must be exceptionally skilled to bring together providers who have not had a history of effectively working together.

The Marshfield Clinic was one of the most successful participants in the Physician Group Practice (PGP) Demonstration, which was sponsored by CMS and was the precursor to the structures and financing of ACOs in the ACA. By year three of the PGP Demonstration, Marshfield had met greater than 98 percent of the 32 quality measures (measures regarding diabetes, heart failure, coronary artery disease, hypertension, and preventive services) and received a performance payment of $13.8 million. Savings to Medicare in that year were $23.49 million (Praxel 2009).

Marshfield Clinic staff attribute much of their success to their mature health information technology (HIT) and electronic health record systems. As the *New York Times* reported (Lohr 2008):

> The Medicare pilot prompted Marshfield to take a fresh look at how it cares for various chronic conditions, including heart disease and hypertension. That led to a new software tool, called the iList, which has proved a big help, said Dr. Theodore A. Praxel, Marshfield's medical director of quality improvement and care management. The iList (for "intervention list") culls the patient records of a primary care physician and ranks and flags patients by conditions not met, including uncontrolled blood pressure and cholesterol, overdue lab tests and vaccinations. Nurses and medical assistants then "work the iList," calling patients with reminders and scheduling them for exams and lab work.
>
> In medicine, the computer is to memory what the X-ray machine is to vision—a technology that vastly surpasses human limitations. The benefits of a computer-helper, doctors say, become quickly evident in everyday practice.

Bard and Nugent provide a detailed overview of creating and operating an effective ACO in **Reading 6A**.

The current CMS regulations regarding Medicare ACOs are found here: http://bit. ly/Reform6_1

BUNDLED PAYMENTS

Bundled payments are another mechanism for making providers accountable for care. Bundled payments are included in the ACA in §3023. In this payment pilot, an organization takes on the responsibility for costs and quality for an episode of inpatient care.

The bundled payment policy is based on the positive results of the Medicare Acute Care Episode (ACE) Demonstration (CMS 2011). The ACE program pays a flat bundled rate for 9 orthopedic and 28 cardiac procedures. This fee includes hospital care, physician fees, and outpatient follow-up and rehabilitation. Twenty-two quality measures are reported each quarter to CMS. Physician payments can be increased by 25 percent if certain cost reduction targets and quality goals are met. Interestingly, patients are also paid a bonus of up to $1,157 to participate in the ACE project, but this payment is not part of ACA §3023 and §2704. The Baptist Health system in Texas participated in the ACE project and received gain-sharing payments from Medicare that ranged from $65 to $6,000 per admission (Finley 2009).

The ACA significantly expands the number of conditions that will be part of the bundled payment project. These include a mix of chronic and acute conditions—surgical and medical—and will have an opportunity for quality improvement and reduced expenditures. The conditions chosen vary in the number of readmissions, the amount of expenditures for post–acute care spending, and whether the condition is amenable to bundling across the spectrum of care.

Organizations that can participate are composed of providers of services and suppliers, including hospitals, physician groups, skilled nursing facilities, and home health agencies. Because these organizations can be structured in numerous ways, they face the same organizational and funding challenges of ACOs.

An overview and details for the Bundled Payments for Care Improvement Initiative can be found here: http://bit.ly/Reform6_2.

PENALTIES: THE STICK

The ACA also contains sections intended to reduce unwanted behaviors or results.

In 2007 MedPAC reported that 17.6 percent of hospital admissions resulted in readmissions within 30 days of discharge, 11.3 percent within 15 days, and 6.2 percent within 7 days. MedPAC found that Medicare spends about $12 billion annually on potentially preventable readmissions. In addition, variation in readmission rates by hospital and geographic region suggests that some hospitals and geographic areas are better than others at containing readmission rates (MedPAC 2007).

Therefore, §3025 contains a new and complex payment adjustment to provide incentives for hospitals to reduce the rate of unnecessary readmission. Hospitals with "excessive" 30-day readmissions for specified conditions will incur financial penalties.

The complex rules for readmission penalties are found here: http://bit.ly/Reform6_3.

MedPAC suggests a number of ways hospitals can reduce readmissions based on best practices of leading hospitals (MedPAC 2007, 111):

◆ Provide better, safer care during the inpatient stay.

◆ Attend to the patient's medication needs at discharge.

◆ Improve communication with patients before and after discharge.

◆ Improve communications with other providers.

◆ Review and improve practice patterns.

The industry has responded, and progress is occurring. The all-cause 30-day hospital readmission rate among Medicare fee-for-service beneficiaries was reduced to approximately 17.5 percent in 2013, translating into an estimated 150,000 fewer hospital readmissions between January 2012 and December 2013. This represents an 8 percent reduction in the Medicare all-cause 30-day readmissions rate (CMS 2014).

HOSPITAL-ACQUIRED CONDITIONS

Unfortunately, approximately 1 in 20 patients admitted to a hospital for routine surgery or other treatment pick up serious infections that they did not have at the time of admission. These infections can lengthen stays and may cause death. In a survey of the problem, policy analyst Ramanan Laxminarayan (2010) found that

> [i]n 2006 alone, some 290,000 people contracted bloodstream infections (sepsis) and another 200,000 caught pneumonia while in US hospitals. Their hospital stays were extended by 2.3 million patient-days. The cost: $8.1 billion and 48,000 deaths, all preventable.
>
> One reason for the high mortality rate is that common infections have become resistant to some antibiotics. *Staphylococcus aureus,* especially methicillin-resistant *S. aureus* (MRSA), is the primary cause of lower respiratory tract infections and surgical site infections. MRSA is now endemic, and even epidemic, in many US hospitals, but it is not the only problematic pathogen. Increasingly, resistant strains of enterococci and gram-negative bacteria such as *Pseudomonas aeruginosa* and *Klebsiella pneumoniae* are infecting hospital patients. Resistant pathogens persist in hospitals because of excessive antibiotic use, high susceptibility of patients, and colonization of hospital staff or the hospital environment. They are then carried to other facilities by colonized patients.
>
> The root cause of the problem is the lack of infection control, which in turn is caused by the lack of incentives to do something about it. Hospitals don't pay the full costs of treating cases of infection because they can charge third-party payers for infections regardless of their origin. (Reprinted with permission from rrf.org.)

The ACA addresses this problem in §3008 by reducing Medicare payment to some hospitals. Hospitals are first ranked on the number of hospital-acquired conditions per discharge. For hospitals in the top quartile of this ranking, their Medicare payment rate is reduced by 1 percent. The ACA also prohibits Medicaid payments completely for hospital-acquired conditions (HACs) in §2702.

The policies and regulations regarding hospital-acquired conditions are available at http://bit.ly/Reform6_4.

FRAUD AND ABUSE: THE BIG STICK

Medicare and Medicaid fraud is the unfortunate consequence of a complex and occasionally vulnerable payment system. Through FY 2011, 2,690 healthcare fraud cases were investigated by the FBI, resulting in 1,676 indictments and 736 convictions. The FBI also achieved: $1.2 billion in restitutions; $1 billion in fines; $96 million in seizures; $320 million in civil restitution; and over $1 billion in civil settlements in 2011 (FBI 2011).

Many new policies are included in Title V of the ACA to combat this problem. They are too numerous to list in this book, but a few will cause notable disruptions in some administrative and care processes. New provider screening rules are enacted in §6401 to prevent fraudulent providers from receiving payments; §6402 authorizes the use of advanced data mining techniques to uncover patterns of billing that may be fraudulent; §6406 requires that physician and other suppliers maintain documentation relating to written orders or requests for payment for durable medical equipment, certifications for home health services, or referrals to suppliers.

Section 6407 mandates a face-to-face encounter with a patient before physicians can certify eligibility for home health services or durable medical equipment, changing a simple phone call into a clinic visit that will clearly reduce fraud but may also reduce the use of needed services.

Recovery Audit Contractors (RAC)

In 2008 CMS reported that it had identified nearly $1.03 billion in improper Medicare payments since the Recovery Audit Contractors (RAC) program began in 2005. Approximately 96 percent of the improper payments ($992.7 million) identified by the RACs were overpayments collected from healthcare providers; the remaining 4 percent ($37.8 million) were underpayments repaid to healthcare providers. Most overpayments occur when providers do not comply with Medicare's coding or medical necessity policies (CMS 2008). This program is expanded to Medicaid in §6411.

Reading 6B presents an overview of RACs from the provider perspective. CMS provides detailed information regarding the RAC program at http://bit.ly/Reform6_5.

The most successful solution to fraud is not contained in this title of the ACA but rather in portions of the ACA that reward "systems-based care." When providers are organized to provide coordinated care and have transparent systems to monitor funds flow in their systems, the opportunities for fraud are significantly diminished.

The Backup Plans

Because the ACA was enacted in an intense political environment, not every payment policy strategy could be included. Therefore, two new organizations were included to improve the ACA in the future.

Center for Medicare & Medicaid Innovation

Although CMS has initiated a number of pilots and demonstration projects in the past, it has encountered two problems. First, the programs must be budget neutral, which is challenging in that some concepts take many years before they can achieve this goal. Second, for demonstrations to become a permanent part of CMS policy, they need to be enacted by Congress. These obstacles are removed with the creation of the Center for Medicare & Medicaid Innovation (CMI) (§3021), where budget neutrality is not required and the CMI can move successful pilots directly into permanent CMS policy.

The purpose of the CMI is to test innovative payment and service delivery models to reduce Medicare and Medicaid expenditures while preserving or enhancing the quality of care. The CMI will give preference to models that also improve the coordination, quality, and efficiency of healthcare services. The ACA contains 20 initial ideas, ranging from using geriatric assessments for care coordination to moving payment systems away from fee-for-service to salary models to state-based all-payer systems.

Creative healthcare leaders should consider submitting delivery system innovations to the CMI for possible pilot projects.

The Innovation Center can be found at http://bit.ly/Reform6_6.

INDEPENDENT PAYMENT ADVISORY BOARD

In stark contrast to the creativity and intricate changes supported by the CMI, the blunt tool of cost control is enacted in §3403 with the creation of the Independent Payment Advisory Board (IPAB). Its purpose is to reduce the per capita rate of growth in Medicare spending to the per capita gross domestic product plus one percentage point by 2018. Its recommendations become Medicare policy unless changed by Congress.

The 15-member independent panel to be appointed by the president and confirmed by the Senate will likely be composed of talented healthcare and policy professionals but is strictly limited in what it can recommend and implement. For example, the board can't change cost sharing for covered Medicare services. The only policy tool available is to cut Medicare payment rates for providers. The IPAB is one of the most controversial sections of the ACA, and Congress deleted funding for this board in 2011. Because this section of the ACA transfers significant policy power from Congress to the White House, change is likely. Chapter 10 examines this and a number of other features of the ACA that have a high probability of modification in the future.

AFFORDABILITY

A clear goal of the ACA is affordability. All of the policies discussed above are targeted at reaching this goal.

In **Reading 6C**, Tyson identifies four trends that will be important for healthcare systems in achieving affordability in coming years:

◆ Providers will shift from fee-for-service to capitation models of payment.

◆ Hospitals will decrease unnecessary admissions and develop financial models to succeed with lower inpatient volumes.

◆ Hospitals will invest in new, nonhospital modes of care delivery.

◆ Hospitals will increase their investments in technology and HIT.

These changes all must be made in the context of the historical fee-for-service structure, which will continue to provide the majority of funding for many healthcare systems in the near future. These legacy systems will require ongoing emphasis and funding, and **Reading 6D** provides an analysis of the need to continue to optimize payments from these increasingly complex systems.

STRUCTURE

The current American healthcare system is fragmented, with many small organizations or individuals providing services. The ACA has a clear policy direction to increase "systemness" as a way of reducing costs and improving quality. The policies outlined in this chapter are all directed at this goal. However, a key question is to how to achieve systems of care—does it require complete vertical integration, or can it be achieved by networks of providers? Shay and Mick deliver a comprehensive analysis of these two alternative strategies in **Reading 6E**.

HEALTHCARE INFLATION TODAY

Healthcare cost inflation has declined recently, but there are numerous explanations beyond the ACA, including the recession of 2008, the increase in high-deductible health plans, and restrained wages in the healthcare employment sector. However, the Obama administration argues that the ACA structural reforms discussed in this chapter are a major part of this decline (Office of the President 2013). In addition it also suggests that even though most of the ACA reforms are targeted at Medicare and Medicaid, these policy changes also spill over into the private sector, which helps to restrain the total costs of the US healthcare system. Exhibit 6.2 provides an overview of this trend.

If healthcare inflation rises about the general inflation rate in the future, the challenge to policymakers will be to develop new tools beyond those contained in the ACA to more effectively constrain costs.

SUMMARY

The second major theory of the ACA is that payment policy can provide incentives for providers to increase desired behaviors and improve outcomes. Payment policy can also be used to reduce unwanted behaviors.

Accountable care organizations and bundled payments provide positive financial incentives for providers. However, the ACA also imposes penalties for high rates of

EXHIBIT 6.2
Real Per Capita
Growth in
National Health
Expenditures

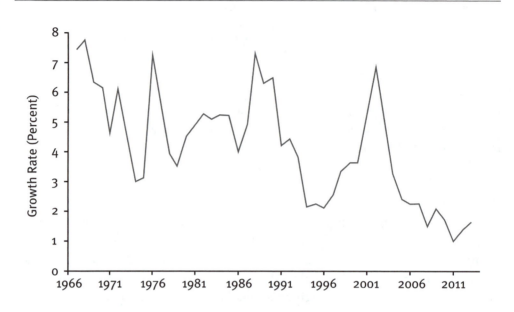

inpatient readmissions and hospital-acquired conditions. The ACA also contains a much expanded set of tools to fight fraud, including the expansion of the Recovery Audit Contractors program to Medicaid.

Future payment changes are enabled through the Center for Medicare & Medicaid Innovation. However, if the cost of Medicare continues to grow beyond inflation, the new Independent Payment Advisory Board can unilaterally reduce payments to providers.

Providers are restructuring to meet these new policies in the context of the existing fee-for-service system. However, if healthcare inflation again rises significantly above inflation, the IPAB or other new policy innovations will need to be implemented.

APPLICATIONS: DISCUSSION AND RESEARCH

1. What are the challenges in implementing an ACO inside a healthcare organization whose revenue is predominately fee-for-service? Interview a hospital or clinic manager to understand how they are handling this transition.

2. Can an ACO become a Medicare Advantage health plan? If so, how? Search journals such as the *Journal of Healthcare Financial Management* or *Health Affairs* on *Medicare Advantage*. Also review the CMS website on Medicare Advantage at www.cms.gov/Medicare/Health-Plans/HealthPlansGenInfo.

3. What are alternatives to the use of Recovery Audit Contractors? Search journals such as *Health Affairs*, *JAMA*, *New England Journal of Medicine* and the general Internet on *healthcare fraud*.

4. Compare the two models suggested by Mick and Shay (**Reading 6E**): transaction cost economics (TCE) and network theory. Which is better for each of the following goals, and why?

   • ACO development

   • Market share increases

   • Cost management

   • Fraud prevention

REFERENCES

Blendon, R. J., M. Brodie, J. M. Benson, D. E. Altman, L. Levitt, T. Hoff, and L. Hugick. 1998. "Understanding the Managed Care Backlash." *Health Affairs* 17 (4): 80.

Bodenheimer, T., and H. H. Pham. 2010. "Primary Care: Current Problems and Proposed Solutions." *Health Affairs* 29 (5): 799.

Centers for Medicare & Medicaid Services (CMS). 2014. "New HHS Data Shows Major Strides Made in Patient Safety, Leading to Improved Care and Savings." Published May 7. http://innovation.cms.gov/Files/reports/patient-safety-results.pdf.

———. 2011. "Medicare Acute Care Episode (ACE) Demonstration." Accessed August 5, 2014. http://innovation.cms.gov/initiatives/ACE.

———. 2008. "The Medicare Recovery Audit Contractor (RAC) Program: An Evaluation of the 3-Year Demonstration." Accessed August 5, 2014. www.cms.gov/Research-Statistics-Data-and-Systems/Monitoring-Programs/recovery-audit-program/downloads/RACEvaluationReport.pdf.

Commonwealth of Massachusetts Health Care Quality and Cost Council. 2014. "My Health Care Options." http://hcqcc.hcf.state.ma.us.

CMS/Office of Legislation. 2011. "Medicare 'Accountable Care Organizations' Shared Savings Program—New Section 1899 of Title XVIII. Preliminary Questions and Answers."

Online white paper; Accessed August 5, 2014. https://www.aace.com/files/cmsprem-limqa.pdf.

Federal Bureau of Investigation (FBI). 2011. "Financial Crimes Report to the Public, Fiscal Years 2010-2011 (October 1, 2009 – September 30, 2011)." Accessed July 30, 2014. www.fbi.gov/stats-services/publications/financial-crimes-report-2010-2011/financial-crimes-report-2010-2011#Health.

Finley, D. 2009. "Providers Nationwide Watch Medicare Experiment Here." *My San Antonio*. Published October 12. www.mysanantonio.com/default/article/Providers-nationwide watch-Medicare-experiment-844486.php#page-1.

Fisher, E. S., M. B. McClellan, J. Bertko, S. M. Lieberman, J. J. Lee, J. L. Lewis, and J. S. Skinner. 2009. "Fostering Accountable Health Care: Moving Forward in Medicare." *Health Affairs* 28 (2): w219.

Laxminarayan, R. 2010. "Avoiding the Unnecessary Costs of Hospital-Acquired Infections." *Resources for the Future*. Published March 19. www.rff.org/Publications/WPC/Pages/Avoiding-the-Unnecessary-Costs-of-Hospital-Acquired-Infections.aspx.

Lohr, S. 2008. "Health Care That Puts a Computer on the Team." *New York Times*. Published December 26. www.nytimes.com/2008/12/27/business/27record.html?page wanted=1&_r=2&sq=Marshfieldclinic&st=cse&scp=1.

Medicare Payment Advisory Commission (MedPAC). 2009. *June 2009 Report to the Congress: Improving Incentives in the Medicare Program*, p. 49. www.medpac.gov/documents/jun09_entirereport.pdf.

———. 2007. *June 2007 Report to the Congress: Promoting Greater Efficiency in Medicare*, Chapter 5. www.medpac.gov/documents/jun07_entirereport.pdf.

MN Community Measurement. 2014. www.mncm.org.

Office of the President of the United States. 2013. "Trends in Health Care Cost Growth and the Affordable Care Act." Accessed July 30, 2014. www.whitehouse.gov/sites/default/files/docs/healthcostreport_final_noembargo_v2.pdf.

Praxel, T. A. 2009. "Quality Improvement in the Marshfield Clinic." Presentation at the Institute for Clinical Systems Improvement Annual Meeting, October 26.

Robinson, J. C., and T. K. Brown. 2013. "Increases in Consumer Cost Sharing Redirect Patient Volumes and Reduce Hospital Prices for Orthopedic Surgery." *Health Affairs* 32 (8): 1392–97.

Thorpe, K. E., and L. L. Ogden. 2010. "Analysis & Commentary: The Foundation That Health Reform Lays for Improved Payment, Care Coordination, and Prevention." *Health Affairs* 29 (6): 1183.

Wisconsin Collaborative for Healthcare Quality. 2014. www.wchq.org.

CHAPTER 6

ADDITIONAL READINGS

READING 6A

THE ACCOUNTABLE CARE ORGANIZATION

Marc Bard and Mike Nugent

From *Accountable Care Organizations: Your Guide to Strategy, Design, and Implementation* (2011), Chapter 2, 29–69. Chicago: Health Administration Press.

This has been a journey that has required an "all-in" leadership commitment. No dabbling in an ACO.... This model fundamentally changes the way we do business. This journey is not for the timid; it is full of risk and potential obstacles, but it is the necessary path for us to fulfill our core mission of providing exemplary healthcare with access for all in our community. It puts us into a full partnership with our medical staff.

—Judy Rich, President and Chief Executive Officer
Tucson Medical Center/TMC Healthcare, ACO Pilot Site

Only a few pages—four to be precise—of the Patient Protection and Affordable Care Act of 2010 (PPACA) are devoted to the development and deployment of the accountable care organization (ACO). Other than Medicare rate regulation, no other issue within the PPACA has stirred more interest, passion, and imagination among healthcare providers than the ACO.

But what exactly is an ACO? It's hard to say. There are three ACO pilot projects in development, but none is fully operational at this time. Many feel that describing an ACO is like the familiar parable about the three blind people and the elephant. One touches the trunk and says the elephant is a snake. Another touches a leg and says the elephant is a pillar. And another touches the ear and says it is a fan. Of course, they are all right. And they are also all wrong.

It's much easier to say what an ACO is not.

Contrary to common perception, an ACO is not an entity. Calling it an *organization* is, in many respects, a misnomer. It is really a *system*. The actual entity is the integrated delivery system (IDS), whether it is traditional or a new model. The IDS enters into an agreement with the Centers for Medicare & Medicaid Services (CMS) and, presumably in the future, with other non-government payers to deliver care to a population of patients. Then, as long as the IDS achieves predetermined quality outcomes, it shares in any savings generated by its clinical effectiveness and operating efficiencies. So the ACO is really an umbrella financial and clinical care delivery redesign *strategy* that uses fee-for-service, pay-for-performance, bundled payments, and partial or full-risk capitation tactics to improve quality and efficiency.

VARIOUS ACO PERSPECTIVES AND INTERPRETATIONS

Those looking at the ACO today can only see part of the whole, because many of the requirements, regulations, and policies that govern the ACO have not yet been established. And many project what they want to see onto the four ambiguous pages of the PPACA (2010):

◆ Those passionate about clinical quality improvement see the ACO as a means to achieve their goals.

◆ Those driven by the need for greater efficiency and cost management see the ACO as a potential pathway to that end.

◆ Those seeking improvements in population management see the ACO as a potential step in the right direction.

◆ Those focused on physician development and alignment see the ACO as an opportunity to achieve those goals.

The ACO lives at the complicated intersection of all four of these perspectives. The ACO will eventually succeed through the successful integration of all four.

Three different strategies to adopt the ACO are emerging for provider organizations interested in learning more about ACO opportunities or already committed to the new approach. Each strategy is based on an interpretation of the ACO.

1. The first interpretation places the emphasis on *accountable* and sees the ACO as a movement or way of being, just as the environmentally minded do in trying to reduce their carbon footprints. For these interpreters—either healthcare organizations or their leaders—accountability is imminently supportable and far superior to the current healthcare system, which fails to link payment to performance in any meaningful way. For many of these interpreters, there is enough clarity about what the ACO will be that they support it emotionally. But there is not enough clarity to make the investment and take meaningful action. In short, these interpreters are *interested* but far from committed.

2. The second interpretation places the emphasis on *care* and uses the ACO to set the organization's compass. The ACO sets a direction for a journey without a clear end. While still not completely tangible, the current understanding on the part of these interpreters is that accountable care focuses primarily on clinical integration and coordination. For them, the linkages to value-based purchasing of care are clear enough to be able to set a general direction and start the journey. If the first category of interpretation describes those who are interested, this second category describes those who are *engaged* in making the ACO a reality. Those who support this interpretation appreciate the value proposition of care integration across all dimensions. Ultimately, the laboratory for innovation will be in the overall integration and coordination of care and how that integration gets translated into new reimbursement strategies. For those who set their compasses, the driving motivation appears to be a desire to be in the pole position when the initial ACO implementation rules and regulations are finally promulgated by the federal government. This could happen anytime before 2012. For many of these interpreters, the designated CMS Center for Innovation will be the real pot of innovative "gold" at the end of the ACO rainbow.

3. The third interpretation places the emphasis on *organization*. Those who interpret the ACO in this way see the new care delivery and financing model as a life raft amid a rising tide of real and immediate financial, competitive, and operational threats. For these interpreters, the ACO is a true competitive destination and one to which they are *committed* before the system takes on any more water. Many of our nation's safety net and public hospitals, particularly those that provide relatively lower acuity care, face financial and operational challenges that cannot be solved operating in the current healthcare ecosystem, where reimbursement depends almost exclusively on independent, disconnected transactions. Like Cambridge Health Alliance, they cannot survive under the current fee-for-service reimbursement system.

THE CMS STRATEGY

Despite the fact that the entirety of the ACO description is limited to pages 277–281 of the PPACA, CMS has adopted a relatively clear strategy for creating the first ACO. CMS is promoting a series of noble experiments by well-intentioned and thoughtful people and organizations. Transforming the "nonsystem" into a system of care is fraught with complexity, resistance, trade-offs, and likely missteps along the way. But CMS understands that to accomplish this through the establishment of policy is like trying to perform delicate vascular surgery using a carving knife. By sponsoring pilots and promoting experiments, CMS will tease out the elements of success as the ACO strategy is adopted more widely.

To date, CMS has specified a limited number of design principles for the ACO. It appears as if CMS's intention is to rely on the innovative potential present in local, regional, and national healthcare delivery systems to design organized systems of care around those principles. At the present time, CMS is debating whether to establish regulations that will make only those with a high likelihood of success eligible to play or regulations that will enable many others to enter the fray as well. In similar fashion, CMS is debating the merits and liabilities of regulations to ensure that all those who participate "win," none of those who participate "lose," or some balance between the two.

We believe that the strategy is best served by ensuring that all the emerging ACO systems be based on a common set of principles, a common DNA. If designed around common core principles, emerging ACOs will have enough similarities to better evaluate what it takes to make an organized system of care work. There will also be enough differences to learn what elements offer greater or lesser benefit. In brief, it appears that CMS is supporting an experimental process in which the elements that make an ACO succeed are derived from creative but bounded experimentation. Over time, systems should gravitate toward common successful elements of a system of care without any one party (governments, health plans, or others) being forced to take full ownership of the process.

TRANSFORMING THE CURRENT HEALTHCARE NONSYSTEM

T. R. Reid's (2009) examination of alternative national healthcare systems reinforces the observation that there is no perfect or best national healthcare model. Each system is an imperfect work in progress based on a rational and supportable set of principles, trade-offs, and choices. The challenge is in transforming an existing system to another. Still, the fact remains that several industrialized nations have successfully achieved that transformation. The most striking point in Reid's book is that what *most* differentiates the US healthcare system from those in other industrialized nations is the complete absence of anything resembling an organized system. The other striking point is that the United States is the only industrialized nation that does not recognize access to healthcare as a right of citizenship but rather sees it as a privilege of wealth.

Similarly, Atul Gawande (2009), in his recent article in *The New Yorker*, shows how Great Britain, France, Switzerland, and the United States all developed their unique healthcare systems by building on the circumstances at hand—something that social scientists call *path dependence.* The ACO is an attempt to free the US healthcare nonsystem from some of the burdens it carries because it took shape largely as a result of historical accidents. The ACO is intended to create an organized system of care that can, over time, evolve to provide a high level of care to every American as a right rather than as a privilege. The challenge is that it is much harder to modify a system that is already treating a population than to start from scratch. Unlike a restaurant that can close overnight for renovations, American healthcare cannot temporarily shut its doors during its renovation process.

What Is an ACO?

The term *ACO* is attributed to Glenn Hackbarth, chair of MedPAC, and Elliott Fisher, director of The Center for Health Policy Research at Dartmouth College. One of the first descriptions of the ACO appeared in the *New England Journal of Medicine* in 2009. In that article, the ACO was described as "a provider-led organization whose mission is to manage the full continuum of care and be accountable for the overall costs and quality of care for a defined population" (Rittenhouse, Shortell, and Fisher 2009).

Expanding on that definition, an ACO is a high-performing, organized system of care and financing that can provide the full continuum of care to a specific population over an event, an episode, or a lifetime while assuming accountability for clinical and financial outcomes.

For CMS, the emphasis is on a system of care that can hold itself accountable not only for the resources used and the cost of delivery but also for the outcomes produced. For healthcare delivery systems, the emphasis shifts from looking at one patient at a time to being accountable for a defined population of patients through all of their healthcare needs.

There is a common misconception about how the first ACOs will be reimbursed. Many of those who envision the ACO today are equating payment reform with capitation or a global payment mechanism. The reality is that only highly developed models will be using capitation as the payment model. CMS's initial programs are currently designed around Medicare fee-for-service reimbursement rather than partial or complete capitation. This will challenge the delivery system because it will need to provide a strong enough culture and set of incentives for teamwork to overcome the economic self-interests of those who provide care within the ACO.

In brief, the ACO is not really an entity as much as it is a contractual relationship that consists of delivery and financing tactics between an organized healthcare delivery system and CMS or another payer to provide measurably high quality care efficiently and to share the benefits of efficient delivery with CMS (and possibly with patients).

The Early Stages of ACO Implementation: An Overview

Currently, healthcare leaders and consultants assume that CMS will be sanctioning or designating delivery systems as "ACO approved." This will mean those systems are authorized to accept ACO payment strategies, at least from CMS. As with any assessment criteria, the requirements and standards can be expected to be refined and become increasingly rigorous over time. The PPACA specifies only a small number of requirements. Those requirements will certainly be expanded on the basis of experience from the initial pilots under way in 2010 and from the programs slated to begin in January 2012. Even with the evolving requirements, PPACA is never expected to be one size fits all. There will be a natural maturing process in which developing or evolving systems will be authorized to participate in low-risk, low-reward, shared-savings reimbursement strategies while fully integrated delivery systems will be authorized to participate in higher-risk, higher-reward savings models.

In the meantime, those organizations that choose to participate in the program will be able to choose at what level they wish to compete—novice, intermediate, or expert, each of which will have its own level of risk and reward. CMS and some delivery systems are concerned that the low-risk/low-reward model will not be attractive enough to encourage participation. For some, "the juice may not be worth the squeeze." We predict that, over time, if the experiment appears promising, the risk/reward systems will get richer, offering better paybacks for those with the most advanced ACO strategies.

It is not clear whether ACOs will be ranked for the purposes of determining which economic model will be used by CMS for contracting purposes. For example, delivery systems with a history of success managing risk contracts could be considered for a higher risk/reward model, while delivery systems without a history of successful risk management could be considered for a more modest shared savings model. But regardless of the economic model, common elements will likely be present in all ACO models.

Medicare is currently debating a number of different methodologies for enrolling patients in ACOs. We discuss these later in this chapter. Primary care, in turn, will be linked to a core group of clinical specialists and subspecialists, hospitals, and other institutions and programs that provide specific services. They will span the full spectrum of care, including urgent care, emergency care, acute inpatient care, rehabilitation, psychiatric treatment, subacute and long-term care, specialty care, ambulatory surgical care, home care, diagnostic evaluation, alternative therapy, and nutritional services, to name but a few. They could also include pharmacy networks, pharmacy benefits managers, and durable medical equipment suppliers. All of these institutions, programs, and caregivers will be linked to one another and their patients through an electronic health platform, medical record, and information exchange.

The question of ACO stratification will ultimately be determined by how tightly integrated the system is. There will be different formulas for assumption of risk and distribution of shared savings depending on the systems' level of integration and other capabilities. This will be further explored in the upcoming chapters on ACO anatomy, physiology, and sociology and economics, as the linkages are structural, operational, cultural, and financial.

ACO Requirements

In those four pages in the PPACA (2010), CMS manages to spell out a lot of details about what these local "microsystems" of care will look like. Under the requirements, the ACO must operate under the joint leadership of clinicians and professional managers working collaboratively. They must design and deliver a system of care based on the fundamental principles of efficiency and effectiveness. Efficiency targets resource utilization. Effectiveness targets clinical outcomes. Section 3022 of the PPACA, titled "Shared Savings Program," directs the US secretary of health and human services to establish a "shared savings program that promotes accountability for a patient population and coordinates items and services under [Medicare] parts A and B, and encourages investment in infrastructure and redesigned care processes for high quality and efficient service delivery." These stated PPACA requirements apply only to CMS's initial 2012 ACO programs. Exhibit 2.1 details the basic requirements.

Ultimately, the requirements that are spelled out seem to have been determined by political realities. Noncontroversial, politically safe attributes are spelled out in great detail. Politically charged areas have been deliberately left vague. (For more details on the requirements in the law, see the sidebar.) For example, the requirement that ACOs cover only 5,000 beneficiaries is unrealistic with regard to the required infrastructure investment. Moreover, 5,000 lives is too small a number for a healthcare provider to accept actuarial risk or be able to determine whether measured outcomes are causal or simply accidental.

Must an ACO Contain a Hospital?

At first glance, a highly integrated, 400-physician group practice that generates excellent clinical outcomes would be a logical choice for an ACO. Unfortunately, such a physician practice may well be one of the higher-cost delivery systems in its market, and it may have

EXHIBIT 2.1

PPACA's Basic Requirements for ACO Programs

- ACOs must have a mechanism for shared governance; governance here is broadly defined as governance, management, and contracts that link the participants to one another.

- The following providers are eligible:
  - ACO professionals in group practice arrangements,
  - Networks of individual practices of ACO professionals,
  - Partnerships or joint-venture arrangements between hospitals and ACO professionals,
  - Hospitals that employ ACO professionals, and
  - Other groups of service providers and suppliers as the US secretary of health and human services determines appropriate.

- The ACO must be willing to become accountable for the quality, cost, and overall care of the Medicare fee-for-service beneficiaries assigned to it.

- The ACO must have a formal legal structure, including clinical and administrative leadership, that allows the organization to receive and distribute payments and shared savings to participating service providers and suppliers. (Though, surprisingly, in a recent confidential conversation, a MedPac official indicated that a contractual arrangement would meet the criteria of a "formal legal structure.")

- The ACO must have a minimum of 5,000 beneficiaries assigned to it for at least three years.

- The ACO must provide full transparency with regard to quality.

SOURCE: PPACA (2010).

ACO Provisions in the PPACA

The anatomy of organizations that contract for Medicare accountable care reimbursement is described more in Chapter 3, but here is a brief list of the required elements:

- A shared program governance (not necessarily organizational governance) that includes, at a minimum, hospital leadership and physician leadership* and may also include the payer
- A collection of physicians who operate with sufficient integrity to pass, as a minimum standard, the Federal Trade Commission definition of "clinical integration"
- Agreement to cover 5,000 patients for a minimum of three years
- Enough integration with at least one hospital and other care facilities to operate as a system; such facilities may include skilled nursing facilities, long-term acute care hospitals, nursing homes, or ambulatory surgical centers (Practically speaking, we believe that the hospital or healthcare system needs to be a full partner in the endeavor, as described in Chapter 3.)
- An advanced medical home model for primary care
- Innovative payer strategies, beginning with CMS
- Comprehensive information technology framework, fully linked across the system
- Comprehensive medical management system, including patient registries
- Internal systemwide education
- Patient education for those who elect to receive care within the ACO (assuming a formal enrollment rather than an attribution process)
- Committed leadership
- Supportive culture

Each of these elements is described in the forthcoming chapters. At present, what is abundantly clear is that inclusion of only 5,000 members is grossly insufficient to adequately serve the goals of the program.

*While Section 3022 of the PPACA suggests that a large multispecialty group practice can operate as an ACO, the practice will require a tightly integrated relationship with a hospital to operate as an ACO.

only middle-of-the-road performance in its risk contracts, partly because of its relationship with a very high-cost/highly reimbursed hospital for inpatient services. Is this "system" well suited for ACO contracting? Until this practice has a full hospital partner with real skin in the game—one that will win or lose on the basis of the shared savings all partners can achieve—it is unlikely to drive enough savings to thrive under a shared savings ACO model.

The more vexing question is whether a physician group practice can operate independently as an ACO. The answer must be considered within three planes. At a regulatory level, the answer is unequivocally "yes"; there is nothing in the statute that prevents it from doing so. At a theoretical level, the answer is "occasionally." This might be possible where a large, mature, and high-performing multispecialty group has enough market presence to effectively manage care along the continuum and has a well-developed infrastructure that requires little capital investment. At a practical level, however, the answer is "unlikely." Only a few group practices have the management expertise, strategic insights, span of influence, or capital to develop an ACO without a hospital partner. Therefore, in Chapter 3 we focus on the more common circumstances where a physician organization partners with a hospital as the two "anchor tenants" for the ACO "mall."

An even larger unanswered question at this time is whether the system can be created in such a way that the anticipated payoff is worth the effort. As noted earlier, will the "formula" for shared savings—where the first dollar goes back to the US Treasury and "above-threshold" savings are shared between CMS and the delivery system—create a large enough incentive for high-performing delivery systems to participate? Because the formulas are just now being considered, it is possible that the system will fail to create sufficient incentives to attract delivery systems to participate. We will all have to wait for the answer to this looming question.

THE SIX GOALS OF THE ACO

The ACO, with its roots among academics and policy leaders, emerged out of growing frustration with the lack of "systemness" and organization in American healthcare delivery. This lack of systemness certainly contributes significantly to disappointing US healthcare outcomes. While the United States ranked highest in overall per capita spending ($7,290 in 2007 compared with an estimated $3,387 in the Netherlands) (OECD 2010), it came in seventh out of seven in the outcomes ranking. World Health Organization rankings demonstrate similar relative performance, despite the fact that the United States spends more than $2.1 trillion a year on healthcare, or more than the entire gross domestic product of all but seven industrialized nations (Anderson et al. 2005).

The ACO model has six underlying principles and goals. These six goals are efficiency, quality, effectiveness, timeliness, patient-centeredness, and equitability.

1. The first goal is based on the belief that improved alignment of the structures, organizations, professionals, and functional systems will improve the *efficiency* of care, including reductions in avoidable costs. The rationale for this assumption comes from the demonstrated efficiencies produced by IDSs such as Kaiser Permanente, Intermountain Health Care, and Geisinger Health System.

2. The second goal is based on mounting data that support the positive correlation between integration and *quality*. Integration refers to an

unspecified but commonly accepted standard of systemness across delivery settings, providers, specialties, disciplines, programs, delivery systems, and time. It was based largely on this growing body of data that the Federal Trade Commission created the standard of "clinical integration" to enable more closely integrated physician associations and health systems to negotiate as clinical delivery systems without running afoul of federal restrictions on collective bargaining. Common sense and experience support the notion that better clinical outcomes, greater employee and patient satisfaction, and improved efficiency result from better-integrated care.

3.   The third goal is intended to address *effectiveness*—delivering the appropriate care in the safest and least resource-intense setting. The critical step in improving effectiveness is reducing treatment variations that simply don't add value. It is well known that orthopedic surgeons who standardize total hip-replacement processes can perform more surgeries in a given day than those who do not. The point was strongly underscored in Atul Gawande's (2007) *New Yorker* article that shows how standardized procedures for inserting central intravenous lines resulted in sharp drops in avoidable infections. He followed up that article with the best-selling book *Checklist Manifesto*, which argues for standardization across a variety of clinical practices.

Loosely coupled systems lack the capacity to reduce unnecessary variation; therefore, one of the core qualifications for becoming an ACO is demonstrating a level of structural integrity and a commitment and capacity for standardizing practices that will benefit from reductions in variation. This principle is the driving force behind Geisinger Health System's ProvenCare model, an approach to care in which standardization enables greater predictability of outcomes for patients, providers, and payers.

4.   The fourth goal is access to healthcare. The Massachusetts healthcare reform law, enacted in 2006, shows that access to health insurance should not be confused with access to healthcare. Access to insurance may be a necessary prerequisite, but it is not a guarantor of access to care. For instance, in Massachusetts a severe shortage of primary care physicians meant that even residents with new subsidized or free healthcare policies still frequently showed up in the emergency department for routine treatment. Nevertheless, the ACO, along with the health insurance reform specified in the PPACA, is an attempt to address the problem of *timeliness*, an area in which American healthcare falls far short of that in other industrialized nations.

5.   The fifth goal is envisioned to address the growing need for patient-centeredness in all clinical process design. David Hanna of RBL Group famously stated in 1988 that "All organizations are perfectly designed to get the results they get" (Hanna 1988). In American healthcare, most processes

are designed around the needs and interests of those who deliver and finance care. Few follow the guiding principle of *patient-centeredness*. Doctors and other caregivers need to create proactive patient care plans and work with patients in a cooperative way to improve their overall health. This is considerably more than a marketing gimmick or an advertising slogan.

6. The sixth goal, with its emphasis on standardization and provision of the full continuum of care for a designated population, is envisioned as one response to the challenge of *equitability*—that is, turning healthcare into a right of citizenship rather than a privilege of status or wealth.

The shocking realization is that these are the same exact goals outlined by the Institute of Medicine's (IOM's) 2001 report *Crossing the Quality Chasm*. Though more than a decade separates the IOM report and the healthcare reform statute, the shortcomings of US healthcare haven't changed. The mere fact that it has taken more than a decade to meaningfully respond to the initial IOM report is testimony to the flagrant absence of a national system of care. While the problems are the same, the ACO strategy outlined in the PPACA at least provides a new way to try to address these long-standing problems.

The ACO model is also an attempt to integrate the many schools of thought regarding how to fix healthcare in the United States. One school believes in the power of markets and that the answer lies in increasing consumerism—that is, making patients pay more for healthcare so that they respond to price signals and treat healthcare like other services they purchase. Another school believes that the answer lies in technology, and another believes that the solution rests in quality. Another school believes strongly that payment reform is the ultimate answer, and yet another believes that management and organizational design can lead healthcare out of the morass. The ACO strategy is an attempt to combine all these approaches into a single, comprehensive solution.

Moreover, the concept of the ACO seems to be filling an unmet professional and psychological need for a large number of physicians and hospital leaders. It reminds them why they went into medicine or healthcare in the first place. It wipes away the cynicism that develops from being exposed to the corrupting and perverse financial incentives prevalent in today's ecosystem. The ACO has hit a nerve. It's no surprise that there is more interest in developing this new delivery strategy than in almost anything in healthcare today.

Definitely Not a Slam Dunk

ACOs will face many challenges. Here are just a few:

◆ Will enough providers want to integrate sufficiently to participate in this program?

◆ Will enough patients participate?

◆ How will participants pay for the massive infrastructure required to become functioning ACOs?

◆ If patients are not locked into ACO delivery systems, can costs really be managed over time?

◆ Will provider systems lose interest and drop out of the program?

◆ What quality measures and standards will ultimately be used to determine eligibility for shared-savings distribution?

Unless these questions are effectively addressed, there is (and should be) much concern over the viability of the approach. In late October 2010 the National Committee for Quality Assurance (NCQA) released its first set of quality-measure recommendations for public commentary. These initial measures provide some insight into the answer to the last question listed above. The NCQA's initial recommendations include measures directed at the following specific areas:

◆ Structure

◆ Resource stewardship

◆ Health services contracting

◆ Access availability

◆ Practice capabilities

◆ Data collection

◆ Initial health assessment

◆ Population management

◆ Practice support

◆ Information exchange

◆ Patient rights and responsibilities

◆ Performance reporting

Further details of the initial measures and standards and the assessment methodology can be found on NCQA's website at www.ncqa.org.

What is clear to everyone, however, is that setting too lofty a bar for eligibility, such that only highly evolved IDSs qualify, won't really advance the dial of healthcare improvement needed across America.

ACO's Roots in History

The ACO is neither radical nor entirely innovative. As a system of healthcare delivery, the ACO will bear many similarities to the more advanced health maintenance organization (HMO) of the 1970s, 1980s, and 1990s. The HMO was a system that successfully achieved care integration but was severely limited by a lack of information technology and evidence-based medical standards. Today's ACO will be supported by contemporary information and technology systems and exchanges along with quality metrics that were unavailable during the HMO heyday.

A number of programs have served as early pilots for ACOs. One pilot is the Physician Group Practice Demonstration, a project that was established at many different locations, including the Billings Clinic, Dartmouth-Hitchcock Clinic, Everett Clinic, Forsyth Medical Group, Geisinger Health System, Marshfield Clinic, Middlesex Health System, Park Nicollet Health Services, St. John's Health System, and University of Michigan Faculty Group Practice. Another pilot is the Brookings-Dartmouth ACO Collaborative, which includes, among others, private-sector groups in Irvine and Torrance, California. Others are the ACO pilot sites in Roanoke, Virginia; Louisville, Kentucky; and Tucson, Arizona. These pilot sites were selected to experiment with large and small group practices, different competitive environments, and different practice models that range from fully integrated systems to multiple independent provider groups. A pilot under way is the Medicare "646" Demonstration in Indianapolis, Indiana, and North Carolina.

The Physician Group Practice Demonstration, initiated by Medicare in 2005 to test the impact of efficiency and quality performance payment incentives and rewards within 10 selected provider organizations, has reported extensively on its results. McClellan and colleagues (2010) report that through the third year of the program, all 10 participating sites achieved success on most quality measures. The groups demonstrated cost reductions of $32 million, more than $25 million of which was distributed by CMS to the groups as incentives (McClellan et al. 2010).

The data from the Physician Group Practice Demonstration and the ACO pilot programs support the fundamental thesis that improved systemness demonstrably increases the efficiency and effectiveness of clinical care. Further support is provided by numerous other reports of pilot or demonstration programs that show a positive correlation between improved systemness of care and rational economic incentives, lowered costs of care, and better clinical outcomes.

A Disputable Assumption About Systems of Care

One of the core assumptions underlying the conceptualization of the ACO is that while IDSs in America are relatively rare, "virtual" delivery systems composed of community hospitals and their medical staffs are ubiquitous. But this is flawed thinking. To call a community hospital with its medical staff a system of care is akin to referring to US healthcare as a system. Having all the components of a system does not make a system or does not make it spontaneously generate the benefits of integrated care.

MEASURING EFFECTIVENESS AND EFFICIENCY: THE CORE ACO TENETS

The first cornerstone of the ACO is the belief that optimal clinical outcomes and resource utilization are achievable only within an organized system of care. The second cornerstone is the observation that there is no single best model for that system of care. A growing body of quality standards enables CMS to feel reasonably secure in establishing clinical outcome standards, and increasingly sophisticated technology enables accurate reporting of results. Efficiency, however, is more elusive, and does not easily fit into a set of national standards. For this reason, CMS has set the benchmark for measuring efficiency as *showing improvement over current performance.*

Here's how it will work: Based on analysis of historic resource utilization, mix, and costs, CMS is able to extrapolate costs over the next period of time for defined populations. Currently available systems and controls will enable CMS to recalibrate those projections, thereby "bending the trend" downward. This recalibrated projection will become the benchmark for the shared-savings calculations. The difference between total cost of care to a defined population and the recalibrated benchmark represents the shared-savings pool, some of which will be shared between CMS and the delivery system using yet-to-be-determined formulas.

What is known at this time is that first dollars will go to CMS. Once a performance threshold is reached, additional shared savings will be distributed between CMS and the ACO. Those formulas will ultimately be adjusted on the basis of the ACO's appetite for risk: The greater the potential loss the ACO is willing to assume, the greater the reward within the shared-savings program. See Exhibit 2.2 for an illustration.

It is unlikely that any two systems will be satisfied with the same distribution formula, so it is expected that each ACO governing body will take on the responsibility of establishing and managing its own redistribution/funds flow formula. Clearly, internal checks and balances will need to be established and approved by CMS or the authorizing agency to ensure appropriate avoidance of underutilization and avoidance of adverse patient selection.

Underutilization—often because of rejection of physicians' and patients' requests—was one of the unforgiveable sins of the HMOs of the 1980s. It gave managed care a bad name. So there must be checks and balances to prevent underutilization in the ACO. To a certain extent, clinical quality standards ensure that adequate care will be provided.

EXHIBIT 2.2
Bending the Trend

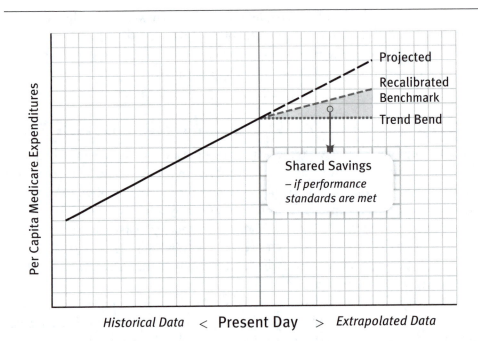

EXHIBIT 2.2

Bending the Trend

Moreover, underutilization becomes a self-defeating strategy when it prevents providers from meeting stated quality thresholds. The need to achieve excellent clinical outcomes will be a powerful balance against the impulse to single-mindedly pursue cost reductions.

Overutilization has its own internal implications and has to be managed internally through peer accountability. If a particular physician is ordering too many tests or performing too many procedures, the transparency of reporting using electronic health records will bring that behavior to light. The more sinister issue is the avoidance of adverse patient selection. Here the answer is not as clear. At first pass the assignment of "healthy" 65-year-olds to the ACO would seem advantageous. But if CMS risk- or cost-stratifies patients, older patients with multisystem diseases and higher projected costs that can be managed through better integration might prove strategically advantageous to the ACO.

THE FIVE AND ONE-HALF CORE COMPETENCIES OF THE ACO

We fully acknowledge that no single approach or organizational model will achieve the outcomes necessary for success in the ACO. But, it is clear that success will require the demonstration of five and one-half core competencies, as shown in Exhibit 2.3.

1. *Leadership and culture.* Leadership commitment is clearly critical for success. The laws of physics tell us that objects in motion will stay in motion while objects at rest will stay at rest unless energy is applied to change the present

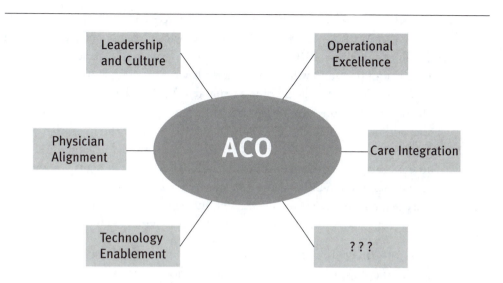

EXHIBIT 2.3
Core
Competencies of
an ACO

state. Organizational behavior is based largely on the results of a complex set of organizational habits that developed over years as a result of direct and indirect reinforcement. Without that internal reinforcement, the habits would be extinguished. Declaration of an intention for change will initially produce resistance, because most in the system have learned to adapt to and therefore enjoyed success in the current system. Often, the *most* resistant are those who have "risen" highest within the current system. If these leaders do not support this strategy, it is doomed to failure. The real test of leadership commitment is whether leaders can acknowledge and respond rationally to the resistance while remaining true to their change goals.

Because culture ultimately trumps strategy, the most effective strategy implementation requires a supportive culture. This, in turn, requires clarification of values and consistency in adhering to those values as manifested in expectations, incentives, rewards, performance management, and group behavioral norms. Any dissonance between what the organization espouses and what is observed will ultimately lead to the staff's cynicism and deep resignation—the two powerful toxins to organizational performance and change. Taking the bold leap of redesigning incentives and rewards is often the most difficult transition for executive leadership to make, because it requires letting go of something that has been working long before there is any proof that the new strategy will work better. A culture of trust, optimism, and confidence is ultimately the only tool available for overcoming the lack of evidentiary basis for the proposed changes. This requires an investment in building social capital throughout all elements of the enterprise.

2. *Operational excellence.* Healthcare waste—resources consumed without added value—in America has been estimated at 30 percent or more of total spending (Skinner and Fisher 2010). Reduction in that number will challenge many core assumptions and will threaten sacred cows. Some sacred cows need to be fed; others ignored; and still others slaughtered, particularly if top line growth slows. Organizations need to become intolerant of steps, resources, and habits that add no measurable value—those that are based on beliefs, assumptions, former realities, habits, or rumors. Excellence must extend beyond the clinic to the strategic management suite. Operational expertise in managing the economics of the ACO must be developed, including revenue and expense management tactics, capital investment, managed care contracting, risk management, and funds flow/incentive design activities.

3. *Care integration.* This critical competency extends across the system and across key partnerships with providers and organizations, such as subacute or long-term-care settings that may be only contractually related to the ACO. This requires a patient-centered focus and vigilance in the adherence to evidence-based care. It also requires incorporation of some core design principles commonly ascribed to "concierge medicine" within everyday practice. The principles associated with concierge medicine will vastly improve information transfer, direct communication, and coordination of care. It will require a high degree of physician–physician and physician–organization teamwork in design and delivery.

    To balance performance with innovation, the entire system has to operate using simultaneous loose–tight properties, in which the system as a whole is tightly managed while the local components of the system operate with great flexibility. If the system is too loose, it threatens organizational integrity. If it's too tight, caregivers and patients will feel constricted and innovation will be stifled.

    What are needed are well-defined systems and processes that can be customized according to the unique needs of the caregivers and an individual patient or patient's family. Care providers are always quick to demand the ability to invoke exceptions to rules, but remember that there cannot be exceptions to rules unless there are rules first.

4. *Physician alignment.* Physician alignment is difficult to describe and also difficult to achieve. Simply put, alignment represents the degree to which physicians, acting out of enlightened self-interest, operate with a common vision, mutual goals, balanced accountability and authority, and the

acceptance of a shared destiny. Physician–physician alignment is often more difficult to achieve than alignment between the physicians and the hospital. While over the past 25 years hospitals and physicians have competed vigorously, more recent advances in science and technology have significantly intensified competition among procedural-based physicians. Those tensions require appropriate forums and processes for resolution; they cannot be addressed one conflict at a time. Care integration requires strong physician–physician alignment in order to assess, design, implement, and adhere to standardized care processes. Population management, in which the ACO uses information technology and standardized care to improve outcomes for the entire population covered by the organization, raises the bar and makes this even more important.

5. *Technology enablement.* A robust electronic health record system is the central nervous system that links together care processes and resource utilization to engineer care. Information technology (IT) must be substantial and sophisticated enough to integrate clinical effectiveness with operational efficiency. The growing belief is that common IT platforms are not the only option; IT "exoskeletons" or "umbrellas" are currently being piloted that can be superimposed to integrate disparate platforms and enable them to operate as a virtual common platform. In addition, information exchanges are also being developed to allow information to be shared across institutions and practices. That option makes the investment in electronic medical records more manageable for many health systems.

And the final one-half core competency? We will reveal it at the end of this chapter.

ORGANIZATION OF THE ACO

Many hospitals and healthcare systems are looking for an ACO template. It does not yet exist. Washington policymakers are steeped in efforts to craft policy to produce intended outcomes and, as noted, are recognizing that trying to achieve a set of outcomes using policy as the only tool is a bit like trying to sculpt a delicate piece of alabaster with a dull chisel and a 10-pound mallet. Policy is powerful and potentially destructive. If it is too restrictive, innovation is stifled. If it is too broad, gamesmanship and chaos ensue. This delicate balance is yet another "edge of chaos" (see sidebar) for healthcare reform.

While this ambiguity is unsettling and paralyzing to some organizations, it is conversely energizing to others for whom it represents opportunity. These empowered organizations are reassured that the successful formula will be built around their own strengths, their culture, and their leadership. Despite the looseness of the current requirements, a

The Edge of Chaos Concept Applied to ACOs

There is no single or best model for organizing the components of an ACO. Whatever model is selected must include a legal structure that defines how the ACO relates to its external environment and an organizational structure that defines how the ACO's components relate to one another. More important, both external and internal elements of structure must enable the entity to operate according to the description of "the edge of chaos," a concept created and defined by author Michael Crichton (1995) in *The Lost World*:

a zone of conflict and upheaval, where the old and the new are constantly at war. Finding the balance point must be a delicate matter—if a living system drifts too close, it risks falling over into incoherence and dissolution; but if the system moves too far away from the edge, it becomes rigid, frozen, totalitarian. Both conditions lead to extinction. Too much change is as destructive as too little. Only at the edge of chaos can complex systems flourish. And, by implication, extinction is the inevitable result of one or the other strategy—too much change, or too little.

Successful ACOs will need to operate in a zone of constructive tension between the forces of local control that support innovation and the systemwide standardization that supports efficiency, efficacy, and predictability. Both forces are vital to the success of the ACO. At times the forces of innovation must prevail; at other times, the forces of stability must prevail. Either way, the ACO structure must be designed to enable the healthy tension between the forces to be exposed, debated, analyzed, and managed. Too much innovation will be as destructive as too much standardization. Each of the structural elements can be designed in a way that either enables or limits the ability of the organization to manage the tension in a healthy and constructive way within the ACO's "edges of chaos."

limited set of elements and attributes will be common to most ACOs. They include the following:

1. Effective, collaborative, and enlightened leadership made up of both physicians and professional administrators

2. A culture that supports clinical and operational integration, care redesign, operating efficiency, innovation, and systemness

3. A medical home model for primary care providers able to provide care management, coordination, integration, and patient navigation

4. Comprehensive patient registries to identify high-risk patients and offer services to mitigate risk

5. A broad array of clinical specialists within or in relationship with the ACO

6. One or more acute care hospitals, including associated ambulatory care sites, even though this is not required in the legislation

7. Affiliations, partnerships, joint ventures, or joint operating agreements with subacute care facilities with well-developed management that links and coordinates care across settings

8. Medical risk-management functions that have previously been the purview of the payers

9. Supportive compensation, incentive, and reward systems that align with what the market values and is willing to pay for

10. Systems and processes to encourage, manage, and reward patient "stickiness"—the propensity of patients to choose to stay within the system for all their care. (This point is further discussed in the next section.)

WHICH PATIENTS JOIN AND WHICH STAY?

A key factor for ACO success will be patient "stickiness," also referred to as customer loyalty. In the initial Medicare pilot programs, beneficiaries have been attributed retroactively to ACOs using evaluation and management codes. At present, CMS is debating whether to formally enroll members, rely on physicians to enroll members, or continue with the "double blind" methodology to minimize the potential for elimination of high-risk or high-cost patients. We believe strongly that patients should be full partners in the program, and that can only be achieved by a formal up-front enrollment process. Additionally, basing results on annual retroactive analysis limits organizational learning and the ability to influence real-time results. Few students would find acceptable a system that provided little or no feedback during the course of studies and awarded grades only at the time of graduation.

There is another issue with enrollment methodology. Systems could seek to avoid high-cost patients who will need a lot of care—called "high utilizers." Providers would be skeptical of patients assigned to them by Medicare, fearing a large number of high utilizers. If providers enroll the patients, the risk is at the other end. However, as noted, to the degree possible that Medicare could risk-adjust or calculate predicted expenses based on previous expenses for the patients enrolled, the ACO would desire to receive a "balanced portfolio" of patients. Having a certain number of heavy utilizers within the ACO leaves room for improvement. If an organization only enrolls healthy, low utilizers, there is very little room for improvement and shared savings. There's mutual incentive to have a mixed portfolio of members.

As the policy is currently crafted, however, patients will not be captive to the ACO program and will be free to receive care wherever they want. This is a clear reaction to the restrictions imposed by managed care in the 1990s, which consumers soundly rejected. It will be up to the ACO program to create "stickiness" for patients so that they voluntarily choose to stay within the system of care. There will be no formal agreements that bind patients to that system or its partners.

Many who study the HMOs of the 1970s and 1980s think that patient and employer demands for greater choice ultimately led to the HMOs' demise. Employees who felt forced by their employers to join restrictive HMO networks and had no other coverage options demanded more choice. They felt the restrictive networks disrupted relationships they had with existing physicians and hospitals. For these reasons, we believe voluntary enrollment is the preferred attribution option. We have already learned that patients don't like being forced into care relationships that they may not know or trust. Still, keep in mind that some patients were happier with the HMO provider networks. Those who valued "systemness" over "choice" were often highly satisfied, while those who favored choice over systemness often were not.

PHYSICIAN EMPLOYMENT AND PHYSICIAN ALIGNMENT ARE NOT SYNONYMS

Many healthcare organizations equate "alignment" with employment, assuming that as long as physicians are employed by the system, their interests are aligned with the system or the hospital. This is a common and often costly error. For some workers, employment is the straightest path to alignment, but there are no guarantees that employment will lead to alignment. Many system leaders, for example, observe significant out-of-system "leakage" from employed physicians. This raises clear questions about how closely aligned the employed physicians actually are with their system. Why are they sending patients elsewhere? The inverse is often also true: Many healthcare systems enjoy high degrees of alignment with private physicians who are not employed and receive little or no direct compensation from the system.

At the most basic level, physician–hospital alignment represents the degree to which physicians and hospitals, each acting out of enlightened self-interest, operate with a shared vision, mutual goals, balanced accountability and authority, and the recognition of a common destiny. Employment is not a precondition for alignment.

In many hospital-based systems, the hospital's relationship with physician "employees" mirrors the relationship it has with other employed caregivers, such as respiratory therapists, radiology technicians, or dieticians—these are the individuals under employment agreements with the hospital or system. But unlike what it gives to other skilled workers, the hospital often does not provide the physicians with leadership, performance management, or support systems necessary to ensure their success as employees in a traditional sense. Hospitals often rely on the physicians to provide that for themselves. Aggregating a collection of independent specialists without common context or shared vision and then assuming that self-governance and management will occur is an optimistic delusion. This is a developmental need for many system-employed practices. The physicians will need to develop those supports before they can function fully in an ACO partnership.

To further accentuate the problem, many of the employment agreements represent past deals developed between individual physicians or small group practices and for potentially rational reasons. Often the affiliation was part of the hospital's larger defensive strategy, which is no longer relevant to the ACO going forward. Employment agreements are often created without the benefit of a strategic framework, common design principles, or shared values. Any sense of teamwork engendered by this kind of relationship is purely accidental. The members of these employed practices resemble a track team rather than a soccer team: Each member of the track team competes individually rather than as part of an organized group. But the nature of healthcare requires that the delivery team operate more like a World Cup soccer team, with each player simultaneously supporting the common goal (pun fully intended) of care integration and efficiency optimization.

These physician groups with "leftover" agreements typically fall short of the level of alignment and integration required for success in an ACO. Therefore, the first step toward more effective physician–hospital alignment must focus on physician–physician alignment: Design and help the physicians build the level of professional relationships required for optimal efficiency and clinical care outcomes.

PAYMENT MODELS WITHIN THE ACO

Many health systems have concluded that CMS's preferred or intended payment methodology for the ACO is global capitation. This is a widespread belief, and it is incorrect. Both CMS and commercial payers fully acknowledge that capitation is only supportable for those systems with more advanced clinical and operational integration.

As already noted, simply designing a payment system in which the Geisingers, Mayo Clinics, and Kaiser Permanentes operate as ACOs will not advance healthcare in America one iota. These advanced healthcare systems are already integrated, and their patients are already reaping the benefits of that model. Rewarding these organizations doesn't help change the larger healthcare crisis in the United States. It's the other 99 percent of healthcare in America that needs to be influenced by the PPACA.

The Medicare programs are initially intended to operate using a fee-for-service model and organized around shared savings within an asymmetric risk model that provides potential upside for the delivery system and with little or no downside risk for the providers. CMS understands that no interests are served by encouraging health systems to assume any risk until they have demonstrated the capacity to generate intended clinical and economic outcomes. Rather than help to improve the US healthcare system, this model would only put it in even greater jeopardy. Consequently, the payment model will likely evolve over time from traditional fee for service to selective capitation, bundling, and other arrangements.

Fully integrated delivery systems, such as those mentioned, can accept risk because they have demonstrated the capacity to manage it and achieve predictable quality outcomes without falling into the traps of overutilization or underutilization of services. But most delivery systems will use alternative integrative models, such as co-management agreements, independent practice associations, physician organizations, physician hospital organizations, or foundations as the functional physician alignment vehicle. In general, the more integrated and experienced the medical organization, the higher the level of risk it can safely assume, as shown in Exhibit 2.4a. The same two parameters—risk tolerance and level of integration—can be used to profile reimbursement strategies that might be considered by organizations with different levels of integration, as shown in Exhibit 2.4b.

Pay-for-performance (P4P) strategies yield mixed quality and efficiency improvements in systems with relatively low levels of integration. Where P4P metrics have focused on process improvements, process has arguably improved although costs have not.

EXHIBIT 2.4A
Practice Type and
Risk Tolerance

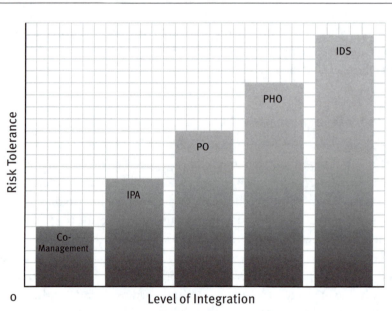

The higher the level of integration, the higher the level
of risk that can safely be assumed

NOTE: IPA = independent practice assoc.; PO = physician organization; PHO = physician hospital organ.;
IDS = integrated delivery system

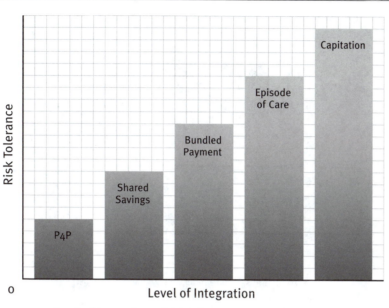

EXHIBIT 2.4B
Reimbursement
Strategy and Risk
Tolerance

Levels of integration and risk indicate reimbursement strategies

*The higher the level of integration, the higher the level
of risk that can safely be assumed*

Consequently, ACOs need to think hard about linking P4P bonuses, specific cost-savings opportunities, and shared savings *together* with the "bundling" approach that is used.

Here's how it works (see Exhibit 2.5). Payers and providers start by distinguishing between core, evidence-based, and avoidable costs within the hospital (e.g., heart bypass surgery) or even across the care continuum "bundle" (e.g., diabetes). They subsequently agree to reduce avoidable costs (e.g., infection, emergency department visit rate) over time. To hold providers whole, both sides agree to share in the savings, as calculated by the actual versus expected performance on prior period's cost savings. That way, new P4P bonus or shared-savings payments (black) are partly funded by actual avoidable cost savings. In this way, P4P bonuses and shared-savings arrangements are evolving from a "no-risk" model to one in which providers have at least some skin in the game.

Bundled and episodic payment methods are essentially different ways to aggregate resources into packages/products that patients buy. The resources and actors that are bundled together influence the cost and quality improvement potential. Emerging examples include a 30-day hospital and physician bundle that pays for the initial admission and associated readmissions within 30 days. In this model, hospitals and physicians could retain any variable or fixed cost savings associated with avoidable readmissions, similar to the cost savings hospitals achieved from reduced length of stay when prospective DRG (diagnosis-related group) payments were implemented in the early 1980s. Furthermore,

EXHIBIT 2.5
Bending the Cost
Curve and the
Integration of P4P,
Shared Savings,
and Bundles

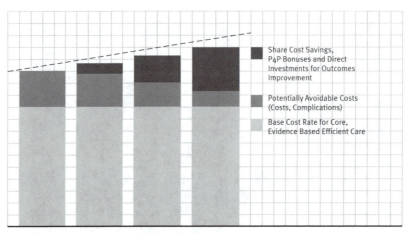

Keys to Success

1. Agree to fair, evidence based costs
2. Tie bonus payment for actual versus expected avoidable costs
3. Share cost savings for better outcomes
4. Resulting in lower yearly cost increases than the past

providers could even get an additional P4P bonus for satisfying additional quality and efficiency standards. These additional payments could be manifested as a P4P "value-based multiplier" on top of a negotiated, 30-day DRG case rate-based fee schedule.

Finally, capitation (PM/PM or PM/PY) assumes full risk for a "covered life" over a defined period of time (one year) and, for all practical purposes, assumes full financial risk for the Medicare beneficiary. Payments would certainly need to be risk adjusted, as is the case with some of the bundling approaches profiled earlier.

Capitation, of course, also carries potential reward: Innovation, preventive care, and coordination can all contribute significantly to potential cost savings and improved outcomes. The level of clinical and systems integration required for full capitation reimbursement is typically greater than that required for bundled payment because bundled payments can be limited to a select group of services, physicians, and staff. Consequently, global capitation requires the full commitment of the system, but it is not necessarily the end game for all ACOs.

POTENTIAL LEGAL IMPEDIMENTS

The perverse incentives in the US healthcare system have led, over time, to a number of outrages: self-referrals, kickbacks, and other forms of self-serving and financial abuse. Many responses have been implemented over the past 25 years, including the Stark law, antikickback regulations, and other consumer protections. But do these legal and regulatory rules now threaten the nascent ACO movement, which requires greater integration among disparate economic entities?

It is safe to assume that, over time, enforcement of the legal protections will remain roughly proportional to the perceived need. But it is also safe to assume that, in the short run, inspectors general, attorneys general, and US attorneys will be required to continue to enforce the existing legislation.

On October 5, 2010, the Federal Trade Commission, CMS, and the Office of Inspector General hosted a public workshop featuring panel discussions on antitrust issues related to ACOs. Within 24 hours of that meeting, the Federal Trade Commission issued an announcement that it will develop antitrust safe harbors for ACOs as well as an expedited review process for ACOs that do not qualify for those safe harbors. At the conference, CMS administrator Donald M. Berwick sought to reassure participants that his agency was not looking to trip up well-intentioned ACO innovators: "We have underlying statutory requirements. For example, CMS will have to enforce Stark provisions. But, we can interpret those statutes wisely and in a manner that, while still consistent with the plain language and intent of the applicable statutes, does not unnecessarily impede the development of ACOs" (Berwick 2010).

Fundamental antitrust principles will continue to apply to the formation and operation of ACOs. More specifically, ACOs developed and operated to improve quality and reduce healthcare costs that do not create undue market concentration will be considered "pro-competitive," while ACOs formed by independent, competing providers solely to raise prices will not be considered favorably.

LONG-TERM VERSUS SHORT-TERM SOLUTION

Albert Einstein is often quoted as having said, "The significant problems we face today cannot be solved at the same level of thinking we were at when we created them." This applies to the current healthcare system. Today's system is a highly developed transactional framework designed to favor the interests of those who deliver and finance care over those who receive it. Reversal of that highly evolved system will take time and patience. Success will be marked by a series of rational, bounded, and responsible experiments that, over time, will coalesce into a new system of care. The ultimate goal of the ACO strategy is to organize care rather than to create a true national system of care, or to create microsystems of care rather than a national health system. Promotion of a national health system would be folly in today's divisive and politically charged environment.

CMS recognizes that a Big Bang approach is doomed to failure. Healthcare systems in every developed nation have supporters and critics. The American healthcare system will continue to have both as it transforms itself, though the ACO strategy is clearly intended to create a little more balance between the supporters and the critics. No one expects to achieve universal satisfaction. More achievable will be a set of healthcare outcomes that demonstrates improvement in the health of our population, access to reasonable care for every American as a right of citizenship, and the provision of care at a cost that is affordable and sustainable.

Even in its most optimistic form, the ACO strategy is imperfect, making trade-offs that will be hailed by some and lambasted by others. That is the nature of democracy and the natural history of change. The ACO represents a rational system of care delivery and financing that unites purchasers, payers, and providers (and, here's hoping, patients as well) in a system that can, over time, evolve and improve. Therefore, the ACO must be seen as a long-term solution rather than as a short-term fix. It will certainly emerge as the result of countless experiments and approximations based on a limited common set of principles set forth in the PPACA. It is not for everyone—not for all purchasers, payers, providers, or patients. As such, it is not *the* solution but rather one of many solutions to the crisis of America's fractured health system. And like any change process, it will be adopted by the innovators first, the early adopters next, and the late adopters last.

ACO Pilot Site: Tucson Medical Center

Describing the innovative process is best left to the voice of one innovator—Judy Rich, president and CEO of Tucson Medical Center/TMC Healthcare, which was selected as an ACO pilot site by the Engelberg Center for Health Care Reform at the Brookings Institution and the Dartmouth Institute for Health Policy and Clinical Practice. Here is Rich (2010) discussing the project in her own words:

At Tucson Medical Center (TMC) we have created the TMC Accountable Care Organization, LLC. The ACO earns a bonus pool from payors that is based on lowered costs and improved quality. The ACO Steering Committee, composed of both hospital and physician representation, is responsible for setting the quality measures to be used in determining the distribution of the bonus pool. TMC's ACO is unique in that the overwhelming number of participants are community, non-hospital-employed physicians. Physicians have been invited into the ACO based on the value that their respective practices bring to the goal. We have settled upon a patient attribution model that will assign the practice's patients to the ACO, and the data collection will track improvement over time. Physician willingness to participate in the ACO has far exceeded our initial expectations. The next step in the process will be to develop an MSO (management services organization) that will sell services to the ACO. These services will improve the primary care of patients through case management and data throughout the continuum of care. This requires a robust electronic medical record with the ability to share data.

(continued)

> *(continued from previous page)*
>
> *At TMC we have embraced the ACO as an alignment strategy with our physicians and as a means to improve the health of our community through coordinated care. Unlike models in the past this one is not designed to produce volume for the hospital. This model keeps patients out of the hospital. We have learned that our physicians value a partnership that is focused on the patient and "doing the right thing." It has been a journey that has required an "all in" leadership commitment. No dabbling in an ACO...this model fundamentally changes the way we do business. It put us into a partnership with our medical staff that is supporting their autonomy and expertise as managers of patient care. It lowers the costs of care by reducing repetitive, unnecessary care, lowering length of stay and utilization of expensive resources. TMC's ACO is a model for the future of healthcare in Southern Arizona, which I am sure will evolve in its appearance and makeup over the next few years. This journey is not for the timid. It is full of risk and potential obstacles, but it is the necessary path for us at TMC to fulfill our core mission of providing exemplary healthcare with access for all in our community.*

BUILDING ACO READINESS

Because there is no ACO template, there is no right formula for building ACO readiness. Exhibit 2.6 outlines the five steps that are serving a number of organizations well today as they prepare to apply for ACO status in 2012.

1. *Envision and educate.* Step 1 is envisioning the overall ACO delivery model that will work best within the primary organization and educating those within the organization, including their governing bodies, about the intention, rationale, vision, and requirements and competencies. Some providers also use this step to educate and engage external organizations that are likely to become partners within the ACO system.

2. *Assess and analyze.* Step 2 concentrates on assessment and analysis to determine which resources and programs currently exist within the organization and whether they are configured in a manner that improves quality and efficiency. This step underscores the Stockdale Paradox discussed in Jim Collins's book *Good to Great*: Organizational leaders must remain confident in their vision but at the same time face the brutal facts of their current reality. As we visit more health systems, we find that many seem to want to believe they are more advanced than they really are. The Stockdale

Exhibit 2.6

Five Steps to an
ACO

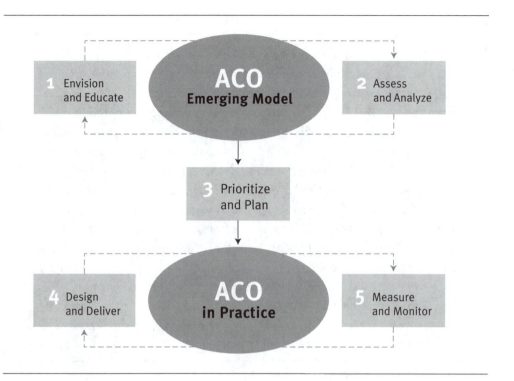

Paradox posits that an organization won't truly advance until it recognizes the reality of where it is, regardless of how brutal those facts are.

3. *Prioritize and plan.* Step 3 is used for establishing priorities and developing a plan. Given finite tangible and intangible resources, especially capital and leadership, each organization must determine which areas to concentrate on first. The important outcome of this step is momentum. Many organizations may not have made the decision to contract as an ACO. But they have already determined that clinical integration and improved operating efficiency are crucial competencies. They are actively engaged in initiatives to improve clinical effectiveness, care integration, and operating efficiencies, which can only be beneficial regardless of their ultimate ACO strategy.

4. *Design and deliver.* Step 4 is detailed design and delivery. While some design elements can be borrowed from other systems, many must be crafted around the particular strengths and weaknesses of the current delivery system. That process, by definition, will generate a series of repetitive experiments. It is wise to remember that today's Mayo Clinic is Version 10.0 of the Mayo brothers' initial vision, just as Geisinger is Version 10.0 of Abigail Geisinger's vision. Few organizations can design and deliver Version 10.0 in the first round. This leads us to our final step.

5. *Measure and monitor.* Step 5 is measuring and monitoring, which is how to track progress and improve over time. The key to success in this step lies in the ability to translate data into information, information into knowledge, and knowledge into action. Through sequential actions, Version 1.0 will transform itself into Version 1.1 and so on.

THE FINAL ONE-HALF CORE COMPETENCY OF THE ACO

We listed five core competencies earlier in this chapter, though we promised five and one-half. The final half core competency is the most difficult to describe and arguably the most difficult to achieve. The current activities-based transactional delivery model with activities-based reimbursement is not going to be terminated one weekend and replaced with a new care delivery, organizational, and economic model by the next weekend. The transition will be gradual, and, for some period of time, organizations that pursue this strategy will be living a paradox in which they will be asked to simultaneously support two opposing and even contradictory realities. Short-term reality must acknowledge that success in today's competitive delivery and economic model requires behaviors that are antithetical to those required for success in the future model. Leaders and key participants in ACO experiments will have to live with one foot in each world.

Ignoring this paradox will only produce organizational anxiety, confusion, and cynicism, given that both truths simultaneously exist. Trying to *resolve* the paradox is an exercise in futility for the same reason. Instead, the paradox must be *acknowledged directly* and *managed sensitively in the context of your competitive market.* This is the most important role and the most difficult challenge for leaders who are pursuing this strategy. There is no proven recipe for managing the paradox, but the first step is clear: Acknowledge that it exists.

ORGANIZATIONAL QUESTIONS

The organizational questions raised in this chapter include the following:

◆ What do we believe about the future of healthcare delivery in our community?

◆ What do we want our future to look like?

◆ How is our future likely to be most different from our present?

◆ How should we be engaging those within our organization about our future?

◆ What questions do we need to answer in order to select the best strategic course for us?

Category of Readers	Key Concepts	Actions to Consider
Category A (interested)	• What is an ACO?	• Educational forums on ACOs for board, managers, and physicians
	• Requirements for an ACO	• Executive, board, and physician leadership strategic retreat
	• Core ACO tenets: effectiveness and efficiency	• Attend national ACO meeting with other system leaders
Category B (engaged)	• 6 goals of an ACO	• Executive, board, and physician leadership strategic retreat
	• 5½ ACO core competencies	• Outreach to system physician leaders
	• Physician employment vs. alignment	• Initiate high-level ACO assessment
Category C (committed)	• 10 ACO elements and attributes	• Initiate a conversation with other external entities regarding interest in ACO
	• ACO payment and delivery strategies, mindful of market dynamics	• Initiate a detailed ACO status assessment
	• Steps for building an ACO (see Chapter 9)	• Begin to develop a physician organization or physician hospital organization

REFERENCES

Anderson, G., P. Hussey, B. Frogner, and H. Waters. 2005. "Health Spending in the United States and the Rest of the Industrialized World." *Health Affairs*, 24 (4): 903–14.

Berwick, D. 2010. "Workshop Regarding Accountable Care Organizations, and Implications Regarding Antitrust, Physician Self-Referral, Anti-Kickback, and Civil Monetary Penalty

Laws." Transcript of meeting sponsored by the Office of Inspector General, Department of Health and Human Services, 10/5/10. [Online information; retrieved 12/28/10.] http://oig.hhs.gov/fraud/docs/workshop/10-5-10ACO-WorkshopAMSessionTranscript.pdf.

Crichton, M. 1995. *The Lost World*. New York: Alfred A. Knopf.

Gawande, A. 2009. "Getting There from Here." *The New Yorker*, January 26.

———. 2007. "The Checklist." *The New Yorker*, December 10.

Hanna, D. P. 1988. *Designing Organizations for High Performance*. Upper Saddle River, NJ: FT Press.

Institute of Medicine. 2001. *Crossing the Quality Chasm: A New Health System for the 21st Century*. Washington, DC: National Academies Press.

McClellan, M., A. McKethan, J. Lewis, J. Roski, and E. Fisher. 2010. "A National Strategy to Put Accountable Care into Practice." *Health Affairs* 29 (5); 982–90.

Organisation for Economic Co-operation and Development (OECD). 2010. "OECD Health Data 2010: Statistics and Indicators." [Online information; retrieved 6/1/10.] www.oecd.org/document/30/0,3343,en_2649_37407_12968734_1_1_1_37407,00.html.

Patient Protection and Affordable Care Act of 2010. [Online information; retrieved 8/1/10.] http://democrats.senate.gov/reform/.

Reid, T. R. 2009. *The Healing of America: A Global Quest for Better, Cheaper, and Fairer Health Care*, 1st ed. New York: Penguin Press.

Rich, J. 2010. Personal e-mail with the author. October 3.

Rittenhouse, D. R., S. M. Shortell, and E. S. Fisher. 2009. "Primary Care and Accountable Care: Two Essential Elements of Delivery-System Reform." *New England Journal of Medicine*, October 28 (published online).

Skinner, J., and E. Fisher. 2010. "Reflections on Geographic Variations in U.S. Health Care." The Dartmouth Institute for Health Policy & Clinical Practice. [Online information; retrieved 12/28/10.] www.dartmouthatlas.org/downloads/press/Skinner_Fisher_DA_05_10.pdf.

READING 6B

WHAT EVERY CEO SHOULD KNOW ABOUT MEDICARE'S RECOVERY AUDIT CONTRACTOR PROGRAM

Alan J. Goldberg and Linda M. Young

From *Journal of Healthcare Management* 56 (3): 157–61.

Under the Affordable Care Act, President Obama expressed his support for the use of "high-tech bounty hunters" to help fight healthcare fraud in the Medicare and Medicaid programs (US Government 2010). President Obama was referring to the recovery audit contractors (RACs) employed by Medicare, tasked to identify and correct improper Medicare payments. Contractors are highly incentivized to identify payment errors as a result of their contingency-based compensation arrangements. RACs' contingency rates range from 9 to 12.5 percent and are based on the principal amount recouped from or refunded to the provider or supplier.

The fiscal landscape in healthcare today is severely overburdened by a litany of varying payment schemes, preadmission certification criterion, and regulatory mandates. In keeping up with these requirements, providers manage the deluge of third-party audits, all simultaneously requesting information (Blue Cross Blue Shield of Massachusetts 2009). The RAC can request up to 10 percent of Medicare discharges, but never more than 300 medical records (in certain cases, up to 500) every 45 days. Keeping abreast of the various cycles of audit and deadlines required to preserve the right of appeal is an arduous task, and while Medicare RACs continue to ramp up, providers prepare for a new wave of Medicaid and insurance company RAC audits.

The RAC audit program began as a demonstration project under the Medicare Modernization Act of 2003 (MMA) (42 CFR §1395dd 2003). The intent of the project charged the RACs with identification of provider underpayments and overpayments due to payment errors (CMS 2004). RAC audits began in 2005, focused on overpayments, in the three states with the highest Medicare expenditures: California, Florida, and New York. The program was expanded in 2007 to Massachusetts, South Carolina, and Arizona. In June 2010, the Centers for Medicare & Medicaid Services (CMS) reported an astounding $693.6 million net return from those first six states over a period of three years to Medicare trust funds, with 85 percent from acute care hospitals (CMS 2010). During the demonstration project, providers appealed only 12.7 percent of denials, of which 64.4 percent were decided in the providers' favor (CMS 2008). On the cusp of what was considered a huge success by CMS, the project became permanent under section 302 of the Federal Tax Relief and Healthcare Act of 2006.

Under Section 935 of the MMA and the RAC Statement of Work (CMS 2004, 6), RACs must use proprietary data analysis techniques to perform a targeted review to predict the claims likely to contain overpayments. RACs perform two types of claim reviews: automated and complex. An automated review is a review of claims data only. When data are extrapolated from a small number of claims, such as with duplicate services or once-in-a-lifetime procedures, into a much larger universe of claims, the projected results can be staggering. Complex reviews include scrutinizing the medical record to uncover medically unnecessary services and DRG miscoding.

Prevention is the axiom we all know and respect, yet the harsh reality is that while the RACs collect contingency *payments* for their success, providers need to *plan* to counter. Providers who strive for coding precision for clinical and payment accuracy on the front end should construct appeal plans as a must to mitigate overall impact on the back end.

Much national debate is ongoing in anticipation of the Medicaid RACs. While CMS has taken a top-down approach to the administration of the Medicare RACs, the states will maintain control over the rollout of the Medicaid RACs. Power over healthcare as a whole is presently shifting to the federal level, obscuring the degree of autonomy the states will truly retain with administration of Medicaid. Yet uncertainty remains. Health-care reform has received criticism in terms of the federal power and individual rights as to health insurance, an issue that we believe is headed for the Supreme Court. The *New York Times* (Pear 2011) reported that the House Republicans said that they would pass discrete bills to achieve some of the same goals, but with more restraint in the use of federal power. Federal power over healthcare today stretches from clinical documentation and privacy to payment of claims and retrospective audit, traveling far beyond state borders. However, because the states have historically maintained administration of the Medicaid program, the Medicaid RAC appeal procedure will be up to the discretion of each state. In terms of the struggle over the states' desire to retain control of Medicaid, a lack of uniform appeals procedures between the Medicare and Medicaid RACs will be problematic for providers. A good analogy here is the difference between filing annual federal tax returns and state tax returns. Every state is different and filing in each state requires unique work and effort.

Likewise, providers must keep track of multiple audit cycles each with individual time lines or else risk technical denials in order to preserve the right of appeal. For example, failure to supply a medical record within the required time frame results in a technical denial. Once this occurs without good cause, the provider appeal rights under the RAC are permanently waived. Payment denials can be generalized into three categories:

1. Provider agrees with the RAC or case value is low; no appeal

2. Provider disagrees with the RAC and case has value; will appeal

3. Provider and RAC disagree on interpretation of regulation; may appeal

The ICD-9-CM Official Guidelines for Coding and Reporting are the framework of rules that providers use to assign the proper codes to each claim for billing. In some instances, coding rules are not clear. These gray areas in the rules can sometimes lead to code assignment based on one interpretation of the rules versus another, which in turn can result in payment denial. Coders are charged with the delicate balance of choosing between two legitimate codes in order to collect the most appropriate reimbursement. When the RAC disagrees with the code assignment, a Review Results Letter is generated. The letter provides notice to the provider of the basis to the denial, which the provider can then use to determine whether an appeal is indicated. Evaluation of cases for appeal requires a two-pronged approach:

1.   Whether the documentation justifies the code assignment(s)

2.   If the documentation does not justify the assignment, whether the case should be appealed on legal grounds

Appeal statistics show that hospitals rarely appeal their denials at all (Pear 2011), and of the cases that are not appealed, in many instances that lack of appeal is because of a failure to evaluate beyond the first prong. Failure to evaluate each case under the second prong is a mistake providers routinely make. When the coding staff agrees with the RAC auditor, the provider should always evaluate the case again to determine whether there are any legal grounds for appeal.

Other issues to take into consideration before appeal include the option to re-bill (CMS 2011a) for Part B services and whether the provider would benefit from the MMA limitation on recoupment (CMS 2011b), which allows the provider to avoid refunding the overpayment during appeal. The right to rebill for Part B services exists only when the ordinary filing limits have not expired.

Several theories can be invoked in order to lodge a valid appeal, such as waiver of liability (42 CFR §405 1996), provider without fault (Social Security Act §1879(a)), due process (Montilla v. INS 1991, Clemente 2010), treating physician rule (20 CFR §404.1527(d)(2)) 2006), and the Medicare act's prohibition against federal interference (42 USC §1395 2010). Appeals can be time-consuming and complicated, but the rate of reversal in the demonstration project suggests appeals are worth the effort.

Expert testimony, along with a concise and organized legal brief asserting the background of facts and legal argument in support of each claim, places the provider in the best possible position to effectively advocate the merits of a disputed claim. The appeal levels are as follows:

◆   **Level 1**: The provider must appeal for redetermination to the Medicare Administrative Contractor within 120 days of the RAC's initial decision. If the appeal is made within 30 days, there is no automatic recoupment of funds. Otherwise, funds are taken back on day 41.

◆   **Level 2**: Reconsideration is submitted to the Qualified Independent Contractor (QIC) within 180 days of the redetermination or 60 days to avoid recoupment on day 61. The regulations require providers and suppliers to *present all evidence*, allegations of fact, or law related to the issues in dispute at this stage.

◆ **Level 3**: Cases may be bundled in this stage for efficiency. The Administrative Law Judge (ALJ) hearing can be requested if the amount in controversy is at least $130 and requests for an ALJ hearing must be received within 60 days of the provider's notice of the reconsideration outcome.

◆ **Level 4**: Medicare Appeals Council (MAC) request for review of the ALJ's decision may be submitted to the Departmental Appeals Board (DAB)/ (MAC) within 60 days of the ALJ decision and meet an amount-in-controversy requirement of $130. CMS or any CMS contractor can refer a case to the MAC within 60 days on an ALJ decision or dismissal if in their opinion there was an error.

◆ **Level 5**: U.S. District Court Review may be requested within 60 days of the MAC's decision, and the amount in controversy must be at least $1,300.

Bear in mind that if the provider fails to prevail on appeal at the QIC, the entire amount plus interest becomes due. This also works in reverse should the provider prevail on appeal (MMA §935 2003).

The best advice: Position your facility to manage results efficiently at an early stage, evaluate each case thoroughly, avoid technical denials at all costs, and preserve the right of appeal. Once Medicaid reviews are in full swing, a well-organized appeal management process will be vital. This is an emerging part of the revenue cycle and should be part of the CEO's dashboard of critical items to monitor.

REFERENCES

20 CFR §404.1527(d)(2) (2006).
 The treating physician is in the best position to determine the best course of treatment for the patient than the RAC auditor can conclude in hindsight.

42 CFR §405 (1996).
 Under 42 CFR 405.355(a) and 405.358(a)(b)(2), even if it is found that an inpatient admission was not appropriate, the provider of services or such other person as the case may be did not know and could not reasonably have expected to know that payment would not be made for such items or services.

42 USC §1395 (2010).
 "Nothing in this title shall be construed to authorize any Federal officer or employee to exercise any supervision or control over the practice of medicine or the manner in which medical services are provided."

Blue Cross Blue Shield of Massachusetts. 2009. "Blue Medicare PFFS Medicare Advantage Private Fee-for-Service Plan Terms and Conditions of Payment." Published January 1. www.bluecrossma.com/staticcontent/medicare_pffs/PFFS_Terms_and_Conditions.pdf.

Centers for Medicare & Medicaid Services. 2011a. *Medicare Claims Processing Manual. Rebilling for any service will only be allowed if all claim processing rules and claim timeliness rules are met. The time limit for rebilling claims is 15 to 27 months from the date of service. These filing rules can be found in Chapter 1, Section 70.*

———. 2011b. "Publication 100-02 Medicare Benefit Policy." http://www.cms.gov/transmittals/ downloads/R141FM.pdf.
CMS issued Transmittal 141, which addresses a provider's ability to appeal early under Levels 1 and 2 in order to prevent the automatic recoupment.

———. 2010. "Update to the RAC Demonstration Report."

———. 2008. "The Medicare Recovery Audit Contractor Program: An Evaluation of the Three-Year Demonstration." www.cms.gov/RAC/Downloads/RACEvaluationReport.pdf.

Centers for Medicare & Medicaid Services. 2005. "MMA Section 306 Audit Recovery Contracts." www.fbo.gov/index?s=opportunity&mode=form&id=1889cc7b8672a9e2c1cbe 5a007b9dceb& tab=core&_cview=1.

———. 2004. "Draft SOW and Information Meeting for MMA Section 306." Posted August 4. www.fbo.gov/index?s=opportunity&mode=form&id=1889cc7b8672a9e2c1cbe5a007 b9dceb&tab= core&_cview=1.
The "appropriate remedy for the refusal of an agency to follow its own regulations may be injunctive relief, reversal of the agency action, or reversal and remand with an order requiring the agency to follow its own procedures."

Medicare Modernization Act 42 CFR §1395dd (2003).
Section 935 of the Medicare Modernization Act limitation on recoupment must be carefully considered as interest continues to accrue when the provider exercises this option.

Montilla v. INS, 926 F.2d at 167 (1991).
"The Accardi doctrine is premised on fundamental notions of fair play underlying the concept of due process." The Supreme Court has recognized a rule of federal administrative law which requires agencies to follow their own procedures. "Due process requires that the procedures by which laws are applied must be evenhanded, so that individuals are not subjected to the arbitrary exercise of government power."

Social Security Act §1879(a).

Under Section 1879(a) of the Social Security Act, Provider deemed to be without fault if the Secretary of Health and Human Services determination that more than such correct amount was paid was made subsequent to the third year following the year in which notice was sent to such individual that such amount had been paid; except that the Secretary may reduce such three-year period to not less than one year if she finds such reduction is consistent with the objectives of this title.

Pear, R. 2011. "House Republicans Plan Their Own Health Bills." *New York Times.* Published January 20. www.nytimes.com/2011/01/21/health/policy/21health.html.

US Government. 2010. "Finding and Recapturing Improper Payments." *Federal Register* 75 (49): 12119–12120, paragraph 2. www.whitehouse.gov/sites/default/files/omb/assets/financial_improper/03102010_improper_payments.pdf.

READING 6C
THE QUEST FOR AFFORDABILITY IN HEALTHCARE
Bernard J. Tyson

From *Futurescan 2014: Healthcare Trends and Implications 2014–2019* (2014), Chapter 5, 27–31. Chicago: Society for Healthcare Strategy & Market Development of the American Hospital Association and Health Administration Press, a division of the Foundation of the American College of Healthcare Executives.

Healthcare in the United States is at a critical inflection point.

With healthcare costs expected to reach an unsustainable 20 percent of the country's gross domestic product by 2020, the entire industry is, rightfully, under intense scrutiny. The resulting transformation of the healthcare industry will require healthcare leaders to carefully consider revenue growth and cost management amid declining reimbursement for care.

There has never been a more exciting time to be in healthcare—or a more challenging one. We must look closely at one of our country's biggest and most pressing problems—the affordability of healthcare—and lead the way to solutions. Whether we approach the next decade with confidence or trepidation, one thing is certain: This is no time for business as usual.

The collective view of consumers, employers, and the government is that the cost of care is too high. As an industry, healthcare and its leaders need to be motivated to actively reduce costs and be prepared to face lower reimbursement rates that are intended to drive costs down.

Affordability will certainly be the dominant force for change in the healthcare market over the next decade and is one of the biggest drivers of the reimbursement trends discussed in this article. How we manage costs and continue to evolve our business models—while still delivering high-quality patient care—will determine our viability as we look ahead at the changing healthcare landscape.

Clearly, the new focus on costs will be long-term. Both in theory and in practice, organizations that own more pieces of the healthcare dollar can more effectively manage costs while maintaining high-quality standards of care. Certainly, moving to a bundled-payment approach—sharing more risk along the continuum—is intended to create greater efficiency and drive down the cost of care.

Other powerful currents of change offer potential solutions. Technology is mobilizing healthcare as never before, and the expectations of a younger, more diverse, and more sophisticated workforce demand innovation. We can harness this momentum to create a profoundly different healthcare delivery and financing system. But our true north should be our patients and customers, who deserve real value from new or revised ways of providing healthcare and services.

We must navigate to sustained improvement in healthcare in the United States, and I see the following trends shaping that journey.

Trends

Providers will shift from fee-for-service and volume-based measures to a provider capitation model, where risk and patient populations are managed differently than costs are. The current fee-for-service model, which rewards more use with more revenue, will go away in many markets. Enrollment in managed care plans has increased steadily since the 1990s, and this shift away from fee-for-service will accelerate as patients and purchasers recognize that more healthcare services do not equate with better health outcomes (Kaiser Family Foundation 2012). The *Futurescan* survey results show that nearly 90 percent of hospital CEOs believe that by 2019 their hospital will have arrangements in place with physicians in their area to support bundled payments.

The rise of accountable care organizations and other pay-for-performance strategies is creating a demand for more transparency and is driving hospitals and physician groups to align and take on more risk as they struggle to improve performance and compete for market share. As a result, the healthcare industry continues to bustle with mergers and acquisitions, showing a 15 percent increase in activity in the first half of 2013 (de la Merced 2013). This receptivity to greater acquisition activity and partnership opportunities is reflected in the *Futurescan* survey data.

But managing costs is different from managing care, as we saw in the late 1980s and early 1990s when HMOs experienced tremendous public backlash because some plans were incentivizing physicians to restrict care and withhold services. Hundreds of plans either closed or were acquired by competitors (Christianson, Wholey, and Sanchez 1991).

Successful risk-based models will keep central what is best for patients and will align payment incentives to promote value instead of volume of care. The *Futurescan* survey results indicate support for a provider capitation model by 2019.

Hospitals and healthcare systems will develop greater specificity around appropriate admissions. Hospital admissions for both government-sponsored and commercial populations have dropped significantly in many markets and are projected to drop in all markets over the next five to ten years (Grube, Kaufman, and York 2013). The trend of declining admissions is likely here to stay, as hospitals and healthcare systems adjust to declining reimbursement rates and revenue for inpatient services as well as new reform regulations that do not pay for hospital readmissions (for certain diagnoses).

Of the CEOs responding to the *Futurescan* survey, 82 percent predict that by 2019 their hospital will be financially sustainable with reduced inpatient admissions. And almost all (96 percent) believe that their organization's strategic plan will, by 2019, include goals for decreasing unnecessary admissions.

Hospital leaders will focus on wellness and prevention to further reduce preventable hospitalizations and to direct care to the right settings. Inpatient care will not be the default choice for care. Hospital leaders will have to provide more oversight of the appropriateness of care and apply care standards according to evidence-based medicine.

The treatment of routine back pain is a perfect example of how hospital leaders can influence adherence to best practices. According to a recent Harvard University study, many doctors are not following the established guidelines for care, which stress a less-is-more approach that includes core exercises, increased activity, and physical therapy (Mafi et al. 2013). Instead, physicians are exposing patients with back pain to unnecessary X-rays and potentially addictive prescription pain medication. They are also referring greater numbers of patients to specialists who are likely to perform spine surgery, despite little evidence that surgery is an appropriate first-line treatment for low back pain. If physicians consistently followed the established guidelines, patients would receive better and safer care, and hospitals could save payors a significant portion of the $86 billion annual cost of treating low back pain.

Hospitals will invest in alternative sites of care delivery and will develop a financial model that is sustainable with fewer inpatient admissions. Technology is changing the traditional footprint of care delivery so rapidly that it is hard to predict what the delivery model might look like in even five years.

Technology is making healthcare increasingly mobile and enabling patients to access care in convenient and customized locations, such as work sites and retail centers, as well as on mobile devices. As care becomes more mobile, patients' expectations around care and service will become more sophisticated. Savvier consumers mean increased expectations

Futurescan Survey Results: Reimbursement and Cost Management

How likely is it that the following will be seen in your hospital's area by 2019?

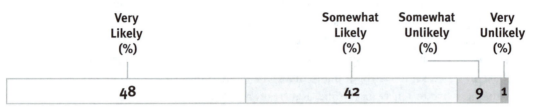

Very Likely (%)	Somewhat Likely (%)	Somewhat Unlikely (%)	Very Unlikely (%)
48	42	9	1

Your hospital will have financial arrangements in place with physicians to support bundled payments.

How likely is it that the following will be seen in <u>your hospital</u> by 2019?

ACHE

27	38	27	7

SHSMD

40	43	15	2

Both

31	40	24	6

Your hospital will support a provider capitation model (receiving a set payment for members of the covered population for a period of time).

32	42	21	4

At least 15 percent of your hospital's patients will be under an at-risk (capitated) contract.

53	30	13	4

Your hospital will have made greater investments in alternate sites of care delivery (e.g., satellite outpatient facilities).

33	49	15	3

Your hospital will be financially sustainable with fewer inpatient admissions.

74	22	4	1

Your hospital's strategic plan will have a goal of reducing unnecessary admissions.

NOTE: Percentages may not total to exactly 100% due to rounding.

(continued)

Futurescan Survey Results: Reimbursement and Cost Management *(continued)*

What Practitioners Predict

Organizations will support bundled payments. Nearly 90 percent of respondents think it likely that by 2019 their hospital will have arrangements in place with physicians in their area to support receiving bundled payments.

Hospitals will support a capitation model. Most survey respondents (66 percent of ACHE respondents and 83 percent of SHSMD respondents) predict that by 2019 their hospital will support a provider capitation model. Further, about three-quarters of survey respondents predict that at least 15 percent of their hospital's patients will be under an at-risk contract by that time.

Hospitals will invest in alternate care delivery sites. Most (83 percent) of the CEOs surveyed believe that by 2019 their hospital will have increased its investment in alternate sites of care delivery, such as satellite outpatient facilities.

Hospitals will be financially sustainable with decreased inpatient admissions. Among CEOs responding to the survey, 82 percent predict that by 2019 their hospitals will be financially sustainable with reduced inpatient admissions.

Strategic plans will target reducing unnecessary admissions. Almost all practitioners (96 percent) believe that their organization's strategic plan will, by 2019, include goals for decreasing unnecessary admissions.

for connectivity and access. Decisions about where care is provided will be made from the patient's perspective instead of the provider's. New delivery configurations will have profound effects on hospitals' staffing and workflows. Consequently, hospital and healthcare leaders will have to champion new staffing and scheduling models that turn the old provider-centric paradigm on its head.

The acute care hospital will become the care setting for only the most critically ill, while outpatient care settings—enabled by technology—will provide preventive care and wellness, ambulatory, and post-acute care services in comfortable, customized, and convenient environments.

Hospitals will invest in technology, specifically electronic medical records (EMRs), to reduce the cost of care. Hospitals will invest in EMR systems to manage care for their patient populations, especially high-risk patients. In addition, hospitals will leverage EMRs to coordinate patient care—among the physician's office, hospital, laboratory, pharmacy, and patient's home—and to eliminate the pitfalls of incomplete, missing, or unreadable paper charts.

EMR technology offers caregivers immediate access to patients' critical medical information, resulting in better care. It also provides patients with access to convenient, time-saving features such as online scheduling, prescription filling, and connecting with their doctors via secure e-mail.

IMPLICATIONS FOR HOSPITAL LEADERS

No matter where one lands on the payment continuum—bundled payments, shared risk, partial capitation, or full risk—assuming more risk will require healthcare organizations to invest substantially up front in the infrastructure for preventive care and care management and to tolerate longer payback periods on investments. This up-front financing could prove to be a barrier to infrastructure investment for small- to medium-sized healthcare providers.

Successful hospitals will empower physicians to manage care decisions and coordinate care throughout the continuum, including pharmacy, outside medical, post-acute, and end-of-life care and prevention and wellness services. Physicians will use real-time data to understand and manage the care of individuals, clinical cohorts, and communities. And they will practice evidence-based medicine, using proven clinical protocols to consistently yield the best care.

The increased emphasis on care management and quality will require leaders and organizations to be more interdependent than ever before. Vigilant oversight of transitional care is critical, and coordination of care will extend into the community as hospitals increasingly partner with community health advocates and other services to reduce admissions and address the social, economic, and behavioral drivers of hospital use.

With such phenomenal changes in the healthcare market, hospital and healthcare leaders have no choice but to seek new opportunities for growth while also driving greater affordability for consumers and patients. We will have to reinvent ourselves and develop new markets and niche industries to meet our patients' expectations for quality care that is also affordable. It will not be the biggest among us who will survive; it will be the most creative and resourceful. Bringing value to patients—focusing on our mission and not our margins—will drive innovation that leads to sustainable business in healthcare. As hospital leaders, we can be the solution that America deserves.

References

Christianson, J.B., D.R. Wholey, and S.M. Sanchez. 1991. "State Responses to HMO Failures." *Health Affairs* 10 (4): 78–92.

De la Merced, M.J. 2013. "Merger Activity Was Down but Not Out in First Half." *The New York Times DealBook*. Published July 1. http://dealbook.nytimes.com/2013/07/01/merger-activity-was-down-but-not-out-in-first-half/.

Grube, M., K. Kaufman, and R. York. 2013. "Decline in Utilization Signals a Change in the Inpatient Business Model." *Health Affairs Blog*. Posted March 8. http://healthaffairs.org/blog/2013/03/08/decline-in-utilization-rates-signals-a-change-in-the-inpatient-business-model/.

Kaiser Family Foundation. 2012. "State Health Facts: Total HMO Enrollment." Published June. http://kff.org/other/state-indicator/total-hmo-enrollment/.

Mafi, J., E. McCarthy, R. Davis, and B. Landon. 2013. "Worsening Trends in the Management and Treatment of Back Pain." *JAMA Internal Medicine* 173 (17): 1573–81.

READING 6D
THE MEDICARE HOSPITAL PAYMENT UPDATE
Daniel B. McLaughlin
From *Healthcare Executive* November/December 2013, 56–59.

PPS will continue to be an important payment source for many years.

Every organization has various kinds of legacy systems. It could be a billing system written in an old computer programming language or a building on the hospital campus that was built in 1890 and is now used for storage. Legacy systems are expensive, and unfortunately the hospital industry must continue to maintain a payment system that was first devised 30 years ago.

The Medicare prospective payment system (PPS) is once again being "improved," and the Centers for Medicare & Medicaid Services released its final regulations in August 2013. Although the Affordable Care Act initiated many new payment policies, it is likely that the current PPS will be a significant source of hospital revenue for the foreseeable future; therefore, hospital leaders will need to continue to focus on details of the current fee-for-service Medicare system while simultaneously developing new systems to optimize financial returns from bundled payments, value-based purchasing, accountable care organizations and many other payment models.

THE PPS UPDATE: A MIX OF FINANCING AND POLICY

Medicare has had a consistent but evolving approach to its payment policy. These payment policies are based on Medicare staff's own experience, demonstration projects, The Medicare Payment Advisory Commission (MedPac) recommendations, and comments and concerns from the provider community. These policies are continued in the rule and include the following:

Pay enough to keep providers in the system. Concerns are frequently raised that Medicare pays below costs and Medicare beneficiaries will be unable to access a doctor or hospital. MedPac takes this issue very seriously and does a number of surveys each year to assess the health of hospitals and other clinical services. Its 2013 report found the number of hospitals in the United States was increasing as were services provided to beneficiaries. MedPac asserts that this continued growth in hospital services demonstrates there is not an access problem today.

The final rule provides a 1.1 percent increase for hospitals and a 21.5 percent increase for long-term care hospitals; however, in the rule Medicare also states its actuaries have calculated a needed 9.7 percent reduction in rates due to prior years' CMS-DRGs coding that "does not reflect real changes in case mix." Medicare did not attempt to recoup this amount this year, but hospitals can expect continued rate pressure from this issue during the next four years.

Encourage efficiency. One of MedPac's key indicators is hospital margins (as calculated from Medicare cost reports). Although the average Medicare margin for 2011 was in the red 5.8 percent, MedPac has identified a set of "efficient providers" who have a Medicare margin of 2 percent on the plus side. These hospitals represent about 10 percent of hospitals in the U.S., and they perform well on cost, mortality and readmission measures. The fact that some hospitals can do well at Medicare payment levels means Medicare will assume current payment levels are adequate for the foreseeable future.

Encourage and pay for quality. A major policy objective of the Affordable Care Act is to move from paying for volume to paying for results, and the proposed rule supports this direction. For example, Medicare is reducing DRG payments to increase the funds available in the value-based purchasing pool. The final rule continues to increase the sophistication of the value-based purchasing program with the addition of an efficiency measure. For instance, maximum penalties for readmissions rise to 2 percent, and hospitals that rank in the lowest-performing quartile of hospital acquired conditions could see a 1 percent penalty in 2015.

Prevent fraud and discourage payment errors. Another high priority for Medicare has been fraud prevention. They have a number of ongoing initiatives to prevent fraud, including outright fraud (e.g., billing for services not delivered), billing errors (e.g., wrong codes used) and professional judgment (e.g., procedures unsupported by medical record documentation).

The ongoing concern about billing errors and inappropriate professional judgment resulted in the creation of the Recovery Audit Contractor program, and the proposed payment rule takes this initiative to another level. Called the "two midnight" rule, it is one of the most controversial policies proposed by Medicare. This policy creates a presumption that an inpatient admission is reasonable and necessary if the admitting physician expects the patient to require a stay spanning at least two midnights or if the patient requires a procedure on the inpatient-only list.

As the AHA stated in its comments regarding the proposed rule "Our member hospitals tell us that the medical judgment of treating physicians is all too often second guessed by RACs, which are able to evaluate a beneficiary's admission in hindsight, looking at the entire medical record rather than only the information that was known to the physician at the time of the admission."

Although Medicare received many strong comments from providers on this rule, it will nonetheless go into effect. However, because of industry concerns Medicare will delay enforcement of the rule until at least January 1, 2014, to assure that it is working properly. The line between inpatient and observation status will continue to be debated, particularly by hospitals and RACs.

Make policy payments. The proposed rule continues payments for medical education, community access hospitals and disproportionate share hospitals—all payments based in the policy that Medicare should fund certain aspects of the American healthcare system that are critical to the system's well-being.

The DSH formula is detailed in the rule and is designed to reduce DSH payments as more individuals gain health insurance through the exchanges. The effective payment of DSH is particularly difficult to forecast as it will be based on a hospital's base DSH payment, "reduced for changes in the percentage of individuals that are uninsured." This calculation will be complex and complicated as a result of the one-year delay in the employer mandate.

THE HEALTHCARE COMPLEXITY INDUSTRY

U.S. healthcare policy vacillates between market based solutions—Medicare Part D—and detailed payment control from the government—inpatient PPS. Detailed payment control is based on the viewpoint that some providers will exploit the federal government because it is distant, bureaucratic and slow.

To minimize overpayments, Medicare continues to refine the details of its payment system, and this is well demonstrated in the final rule. Third-party vendors to Medicare identified in the rule include contractors that specialize in the following:

◆ Recovery audits

◆ Medicare administration

◆ Long-term care hospital payment research

◆ ICD-9-CM

- Local claims payment

- Rates of the uninsured

- Total hospital-acquired condition scores

- Comprehensive error rate testing

- Medicare specific groups and payment software contractors

LOOKING FORWARD

Although one can question the value of the highly complex payment systems, it is incumbent on hospitals to develop appropriate and cost-effective responses. Because PPS will continue to be an important payment source for many years, a continued focus on its functioning is critical, even in the face of other new reimbursement systems coming on line.

The legacy prospective payment system has lasted 30 years—it may last for 30 more.

READING 6E

POST-ACUTE CARE AND VERTICAL INTEGRATION AFTER THE PATIENT PROTECTION AND AFFORDABLE CARE ACT

Patrick D. Shay and Stephen S. Mick
From *Journal of Healthcare Management* 58 (1): 15–27.

EXECUTIVE SUMMARY

The anticipated changes resulting from the passage of the Patient Protection and Affordable Care Act—including the proposed adoption of bundled payment systems and the promotion of accountable care organizations—have generated considerable controversy as U.S. healthcare industry observers debate whether such changes will motivate vertical integration activity. Using examples of accountable care organizations and bundled payment systems in the American post-acute healthcare sector, this article applies economic and sociological perspectives from organization theory to predict that as acute care organizations vary in the degree to which they experience environmental uncertainty, asset specificity, and network embeddedness, their motivation to integrate post-acute care services will also vary, resulting in a spectrum of integrative behavior.

INTRODUCTION

Will acute care organizations integrate vertically with post-acute care providers as a result of the changes ushered in by the Patient Protection and Affordable Care Act of 2010 (ACA)? This prospect may be facilitated by the promotion of accountable care organizations (ACOs) and bundled payment systems in the post-acute healthcare sector. We elaborate on this possibility on the basis of contrasting conceptual schemes, providing two avenues that highly differentiated organizations may pursue when facing an integration decision. Our argument is that an acute care organization's motivation to integrate post-acute services will vary commensurate with the degree to which it is embedded in a network of related organizations given an environment of heightened uncertainty and asset specificity.

The ACA ushered in a series of reforms and changes that have begun to alter the American healthcare landscape. We examine two aspects of the ACA—ACOs and bundled payment programs—as changes that may have a dramatic impact on healthcare organizations and the post-acute care sector. Of the many provisions included in the ACA, we focus on these two reforms given their shared purpose of promoting quality while controlling spending—needs prescribed for the post-acute care sector in light of its rampant growth and fragmented nature—and their identity as the two prominent payment reform provisions demanding heightened coordination of services between acute and post-acute providers (e.g., Dresevic & Kalmowitz, 2011; Taft, 2010). Some industry observers expect healthcare organizations to consolidate in response to these changes (Goldsmith, 2011; Zigmond, 2010; Greis, rawlings, & Jackson, 2009; Welch, 1998), with vertical integration comprising a major form of consolidation. Vertical integration is commonly reduced to "make or buy" arrangements in which organizations decide to internalize their production and distribution procedures rather than purchase materials or services from the market (Diana, 2009; Harrigan, 1985). Applying such arrangements to patient care, this article defines vertical integration as the provision of a continuum of office-based primary care, acute care, and post-acute services within a single organization or joint ownership structure, allowing for a coordinated progression of services across the patient care spectrum. Although the acute care hospital need not necessarily be the focal organization involved in vertically integrating other health services units, it is the most common strategic business unit among the continuum of health services units, with the human and financial resources required for such ambitious organizational change (Mick & Conrad, 1988). Therefore, we study the question of vertical integration of post-acute care services from the perspective of the acute care facility. Following the promotion of ACOs and bundled payment programs as ACA provisions, most observers have focused on the potential for integration between hospitals and physician practices (e.g., Keckley & Hoffmann, 2010; Shortell, Casalino, & Fisher, 2010; Weinstock, 2010), with trends already pointing to an increase in hospital–physician integration activity (Tocknell, 2012). However, little attention has been devoted to examining post-acute care as a potential area for vertical integration, and to address this gap, we focus on acute care hospitals' integration of post-acute care services.

WHY THE VERTICAL INTEGRATION CHOICE IS IMPORTANT

Does it really matter whether or not acute care organizations increasingly integrate with post-acute care organizations following ACA reforms? Proponents of vertical integration suggest that vertically integrated organizations enjoy enhanced efficiencies and reduced expenses through economies of scale (Walston, Kimberly, & Burns, 1996; Conrad, 1992). Thus, vertical integration is valued for its perceived ability to enable better continuity of care while economizing on administrative expenses (Conrad, 1992). To such advocates of vertical integration, the aspects of the ACA that promote integration activity may be viewed as beneficial to the healthcare system in their ability to promote greater efficiency, quality, and effectiveness among providers.

On the other hand, critics of vertical integration point to lessons learned in the healthcare industry during the end of the 20th century as many integrated organizations experienced increased costs and failed to realize anticipated benefits, including prominent organizations such as Humana and Allina (Luke, Walston, & Plummer, 2004; Walston et al., 1996). The potential costs of vertical integration, including increased start-up and learning costs, competitive backlash, and a "lack of attention to community and social goals," may outweigh any anticipated benefits (Clement, 1992, p. 104). additionally, and often not recognized, *internal* transaction costs develop inside organizations, especially in vertically integrated organizations (Mick, 1990; Mick & Conrad, 1988). In the burst of vertical integration that accompanied the managed care and integrated delivery system revolution of the 1990s, administrative costs skyrocketed due to a lack of experience and poor management of these increasingly complicated organizational arrangements, including the confusion and expense stemming from the implementation of effective electronic management and clinical control systems.

Furthermore, the consolidation of providers as a result of integration bears significant consequences within local healthcare markets, specifically in regard to the concentration of market power. evidence suggests that consolidation of healthcare organizations leads to higher prices (Town, Wholey, Feldman, & Burns, 2006), although this verdict is not unanimous (Moriya, Vogt, & Gaynor, 2010). Robinson (1996b, p. 166) argues that, in times of "rapid technological and market change," vertically integrated organizations sacrifice the flexibility and autonomy gained through contractual relationships and embedded networks, thereby exacerbating expenses and inefficiencies among healthcare organizations. Elsewhere, he concludes that, at the worst, vertical integration may lead to "managerial arrogance at the top, a civil service mentality among physicians, and a corporate culture of growth, merger, and acquisitions as ends in themselves" (Robinson, 1997, p. 8). Those who are skeptical of the benefits of vertical integration suggest that the aspects of the ACA that promote integration activity may actually yield unintended consequences in the forms of heightened expenses and inefficiencies—the same problems that such reform aims to address—to the detriment of the healthcare industry and the communities it serves (Robinson, 1997). Thus, the prospect of vertical integration following healthcare reform is one that needs to be carefully evaluated given the diversity of views about the performance possibilities that might ensue.

BACKGROUND

The post-acute care sector is a substantial element of the U.S. healthcare system, providing a range of services for patients following their acute care hospitalizations. Post-acute service providers include home health agencies, inpatient rehabilitation facilities, long-term acute care hospitals, skilled nursing facilities, and outpatient rehabilitation clinics, all of which seek to expedite the recovery process of patients, ease their transition back into the community, and restore them to their previous level of functioning (Buntin, Colla, & Escarce, 2009; CPS, 2009). Over the past 30 years, demand and utilization of post-acute care services in the United States have increased significantly, yielding tremendous growth and development of post-acute care providers and, with them, significant problems within the post-acute care sector (Buntin et al., 2009; Yip, Wilber, & Myrtle, 2002). Recent attempts by the U.S. Congress to rein in soaring post-acute care expenses and promote greater efficiency include the gradual introduction of individual prospective payment systems (PPSs) for each post-acute care setting, starting with the Balanced Budget Act of 1997 (BBA). However, post-acute care facilities have learned to manage patient costs and profit margins under newly fixed reimbursements by accelerating patient discharges to other segments of the post-acute care sector providing substitutable services.

The substitutability of post-acute services is traced to the mid-1980s, when acute care facilities began a pattern of discharging patients more quickly than in the past. This trend led to increased demand for post-acute services, and post-acute settings responded by expanding their offerings to treat patients with higher acuity levels, often resulting in overlapping services (Zinn, Mor, Feng, & Itrator, 2007; Banks, Parker, & Wendel, 2001). As separate PPSs for each post-acute setting were introduced following the BBA, post-acute care sites were motivated to accelerate patient discharges, and providers took advantage of the substitutability of post-acute services by shifting patients between settings (Welch, 1998). Today, the post-acute care industry expects more than one half of its patients to bounce back and forth between two or more types of post-acute sites during a single episode of care, thereby encouraging overutilization while requiring redundant treatments, assessments, and documentation for patients (CPS, 2009). In light of such redundant services and an increase in patient acuity, post-acute providers display general confusion and a "lack of clinical consensus" in determining the appropriate setting for patients (Buntin et al., 2009, p. 1190). The post-acute care sector is also criticized for being fragmented or siloed—a term used in post-acute care to refer to the separate identities, cultures, and standards maintained by each setting. The separate payment systems and regulatory standards recently introduced for each post-acute setting have further reinforced their individual identities and fostered strong competition among them for the same patients and resources (AMRPA, 2009; CPS, 2009; Currie, 1996). Aware of the redundant, fragmented, inefficient, and expensive state of the post-acute care sector, U.S. healthcare policy experts recently focused on ways to improve patient care while reducing expenses through Medicare payment system reform (Galewitz, 2009). Concepts that have received growing interest and endorsements over the past five years include two elements incorporated into the ACA: bundled payment systems and ACOs (Berenson, 2010; CPS, 2009; Devers & Berenson, 2009; Lubell, 2009).[1]

BUNDLED PAYMENTS

The concept of bundled payments is admired for its seeming simplicity and promotion of a holistic approach. Rather than pay each provider for separate services provided to a patient during an episode of care, the bundled payment system defined in the ACA would pay one provider a single payment for all services the patient received during the entire episode, including post-acute services received within 30 days of an acute care hospital discharge. The entity receiving the bundled payment would then divide the reimbursement to pay each contributing provider the amount deemed appropriate for the services rendered. Healthcare facilities would realize no payment incentive to shift patients between post-acute settings, thereby addressing problems of inefficiency and redundancy that substitutable care has created (Welch, 1998).

Section 3023 of the ACA requires the secretary of the U.S. Department of Health and Human Services (HHS) to establish the National Pilot Program on Payment Bundling by January 1, 2013, to include expenditures related to acute care inpatient services, physician services, outpatient hospital services, and post-acute care services provided to Medicare beneficiaries. Should the project succeed, Medicare will likely expand the bundled payments concept to all post-acute care providers and services (Galewitz, 2009). Although no decision has been made regarding how a bundled payment system ultimately will be implemented, many observers suggest that acute care facilities will be the most likely recipients of bundled payments (Galewitz, 2009; Greis et al., 2009; Lubell, 2009; Murer, 2009), citing recommendations by the Congressional Budget Office (CBO, 2008, p. 62). Thus, for purposes of this article, we assume that bundled payments will be directed to acute care hospitals, which will be responsible for disbursing reimbursements to contributing providers.

ACCOUNTABLE CARE ORGANIZATIONS

Section 3022 of the ACA requires the secretary of HHS to have created the Medicare Shared Savings Program (MSSP) by January 1, 2012, for providers participating as ACOs; this program was established on November 2, 2011, as a final rule in the *Federal Register*.

The concept of ACOs has been recently promoted as a means to pair cost reduction reform with efforts to improve quality (Devers & Berenson, 2009). ACOs are provider-led organizations that are responsible for a defined population and that manage the full continuum of care for participating patients, overseeing the overall cost and quality of care (Keckley & Hoffmann, 2010; Shortell et al., 2010; Devers & Berenson, 2009; Rittenhouse, Shortell, & Fisher, 2009). ACO participants in the MSSP can share a portion of Medicare's realized savings—essentially receiving bonus payments—by meeting quality benchmarks and reducing expenditures below spending projections. Although guidelines for participation are fairly general, organizations seeking to comply with Section 3022 of the ACA and participate as ACOs must be able to either provide or arrange for the provision of the full continuum of care for at least 5,000 Medicare beneficiaries.

Many policy experts and representatives of the post-acute care sector expect bundled payments and ACOs to improve efficiency, coordination, and cost-effectiveness, mitigating some of the unintended consequences of past post-acute payment systems (DeVore & Champion, 2011; Craver, 2010; CPS, 2009; Galewitz, 2009; Terry, 2009; Welch, 1998). However, despite general support among them for ACOs and bundled payments, many involved remain uncertain regarding the effects of such reimbursement changes. As acute care hospitals become responsible for the coordination and payment of all patient care following the introduction of bundled payments, they will face the make-or-buy decision of whether to provide post-acute services directly to patients or develop contractual arrangements with post-acute care providers to allow patients to receive post-acute services outside of the acute care facility (Murer, 2009; Banks et al., 2001; Welch, 1998). Considering this scenario, some scholars anticipate that the implementation of bundled payments will encourage acute care and post-acute care organizations to integrate vertically to realize production efficiencies and ensure survival (Greis et al., 2009; Banks et al., 2001; Byrne & Ashton, 1999). Similarly, organizations considering the ACO model must choose whether to develop long-term relationships with external entities (including post-acute care providers) to form an ACO or make the "commitment to 'make' rather than 'buy'" (Keckley & Hoffmann, 2010, p. 18).

Two Distinct Strategies

In response to the question of whether organizations are likely to pursue vertical integration, two prominent organizational theories—transaction cost economics (TCE) and network theory—suggest two distinct strategies firms may pursue following ACA reforms.[2]

Transaction Costs

Proponents of TCE claim that, under uncertain market circumstances in which the asset specificity of transactions is both idiosyncratic and recurring, vertical integration is preferred over market exchanges because the former produces lower transaction costs than the latter does (Mick & Conrad, 1988; Williamson, 1975). *Asset specificity* is the phenomenon of an organization being "locked in" to a relationship with another organization because the resources it invested in the relationship would be of lesser value if they were invested in other relationships (Scott & Davis, 2007). Examples of asset specificity related to transactions between acute care and post-acute care organizations are physical and human capital, brand names, and time. The promotion of ACOs and bundled payments may heighten such forms of asset specificity in exchange relationships between acute care and post-acute care organizations. For example, as acute care facilities invest in equipment, personnel, and "infrastructure for effective care coordination" with post-acute organizations participating in their ACO or as bundled payment partners (CMS, 2011, p. 19638), the levels of physical and human asset specificity in their exchange relationship may increase. As organizations consider forming or joining ACOs, providers with valuable brand names must decide whether they approve of associating their brand with other ACO participants. Furthermore, as ACOs and bundled payments increase pressure for providers to attend quickly and carefully to beneficiaries' transitions across settings, acute care hospitals may integrate vertically with post-acute care providers to address high temporal asset specificity, allowing them to "evaluate admissions and discharges from the perspective of the integrated organization" rather than that of an independent care provider (Robinson, 1996a, p. 361).

In the presence of asset specificity, TCE maintains that an increase in uncertainty creates a primary motivation to integrate (Joskow, 2008). Within today's complex post-acute care sector, an environment perceived to be chaotic and confusing (AMRPA, 2009), the implementation of ACOs and bundled payment systems is likely to engender an even greater sense of uncertainty among providers, motivating increased consolidation for the next several years (Harris, Grauman, & Hemnani, 2010; Zigmond, 2010; Zuckerman, 2009). Acute care entities may pursue vertical integration with post-acute care organizations to gain competitive advantage, control patient flow through service offerings, and offer a full continuum of services that meet a patient's needs for an entire care episode. Vertical integration may also address increased uncertainty in the form of opportunistic behavior among acute care and post-acute care facilities that participate together in ACOs or share bundled payments.

To limit opportunistic behavior, bundled payments and ACOs will require the development of a high level of infrastructure to address system needs and contingencies, including legal, technical, and financial arrangements (DeVore & Champion, 2011; Keckley & Hoffmann, 2010; Shortell et al., 2010; CPS, 2009; Lubell, 2009). Such infrastructure demands time and resources that will increase transaction costs for participating providers. By integrating vertically, the transaction costs associated with continuous negotiating and monitoring efforts may be reduced. Vertical integration may also address the heightened uncertainty resulting from providers' exposure to various risks following the adoption of bundled payment systems or ACO models. Before bundled payment schemes emerged, acute care facilities did not assume financial risk for the future costs and potential complications of patients following their discharge to post-acute settings.

However, by tying reimbursements together for an entire episode of care, increased patient costs or future complications in post-acute settings create an increase in the overall costs for a patient's episode of care. Therefore, an acute care facility sharing a bundled payment with external post-acute care facilities assumes the financial risk that patient costs may exceed expectations following acute care discharge despite their best efforts (Jackson, Greis, & Rawlings, 2009). As the acute care and post-acute care facilities look to divide the bundled payment, increased overall patient costs may take away from the acute care facility's portion of the bundled payment. Similarly, acute care providers participating in ACOs may face considerable challenges in the event they must manage beneficiaries' care received from post-acute care providers outside of the ACO (CMS, 2011). For example, post-acute care providers operating outside of an ACO may adopt patient care philosophies or treatment decisions that conflict with the ACO's preferences, and the ACO may lack the ability to enforce its preferences on independent post-acute care providers. Such post-acute care providers would not be obligated to support the ACO and would be able to operate under a presumption of autonomous interests. For these risks, vertical integration may address providers' uncertainties by aligning the interests of the acute care and post-acute care facilities as a single organization.

Thus, we suggest that an overall effect of ACO and bundled payment policies will be to increase uncertainty throughout the healthcare industry, particularly within the post-acute care sector. When combined with exchanges of high asset specificity, this overall increase in uncertainty will pressure many organizations to integrate vertically in response.

Proposition *Following the implementation of ACOs and bundled payments in the post-acute care sector, vertical integration between acute and post-acute care organizations will increase as a result of increased environmental uncertainty and asset specificity.*

NETWORK EMBEDDEDNESS

In contrast to the predictions of vertical integration promoted by TCE, network theory suggests that organizations embedded within networks enjoy economic opportunities that do not require a vertically integrated organizational form (Uzzi, 1997). Networks are "the informal connections" among organizations "that often arise out of work patterns but can have a large influence beyond them" (Scott & Davis, 2007, p. 23). In that context, embeddedness is defined as the degree to which an organization maintains links or relational ties with other organizations throughout its network, thereby influencing organizations' economic activities through consideration of social factors and relations (Dacin, Ventresca, & Beal, 1999). As opposed to the distant and impersonal arms-length ties that characterize transactions within ideal markets, embeddedness leads to close and personal exchanges among independent organizational entities that do not require complicated organizational systems but are characterized by high levels of trust, information transfer, and joint problem-solving arrangements (Uzzi, 1997). As a result, asset specificity and environmental uncertainty are less problematic than they would be otherwise because opportunism and deception by one organization are much more difficult to conceal from another embedded organization in its network (Robinson, 1997; Uzzi, 1997). In addition to discouraging opportunism, embedded network relationships foster ethical values and mutual support among exchange partners (Podolny & Page, 1998). Each organization's success depends on the success of the network, motivating members to develop the trust necessary to share access to privileged resources in order to enhance the overall competitiveness of the network.

An examination of how embedded organizations may react to ACA reforms highlights the ways in which such organizations are uniquely positioned to meet the challenges of uncertainty and asset specificity without requiring vertical integration. For embedded healthcare organizations, the introduction of bundled payments and ACOs will not produce fears of opportunistic behavior, as acute care organizations will trust that cooperating post-acute care facilities will continually seek to advance the network's competitive standing. Transactional details and monitoring activities are no longer needed to protect against opportunism and behavioral uncertainty, as embedded organizations find little strategic motivation to behave opportunistically and instead operate on conditions of trust (Podolny & Page, 1998; Uzzi, 1997; Provan, 1993). Rather than questioning whether physicians and patients will continue to demand their services following ACA reforms, embedded organizations will alleviate their uncertainty by strengthening their relationship with post-acute care providers they depend on to provide a full continuum of services (Podolny & Page, 1998). Concerns about corporate strategy needs and service offerings will be addressed by the enhanced competitiveness, legitimacy, and quality enjoyed as a result of network embeddedness and the valuable information exchange and joint problem-solving commitment it provides (Podolny & Page, 1998). Furthermore, the uncertainty and risk of forging new contractual agreements in ACOs or bundled payment systems will have been addressed by the ethical orientation guiding the exchange partner relationship, as buyers and sellers "make relationship-specific investments without contractual guarantees protecting those investments" because they trust each other to act in the interest of the network rather than self-interest (Podolny & Page, 1998, p. 60). As a result, bargaining power is no longer sought, as embedded organizations are willing to exceed "the letter of a contract" and engage in joint problem-solving efforts rather than bargaining activities (Uzzi, 1997, p. 51). With sources of uncertainty within idiosyncratic exchange relationships addressed by the benefits of network embeddedness, factors that dictate integration decisions following ACA reforms are seen in a different light by organizations.

Proposition *Following the implementation of ACOs and bundled payments, acute and post-acute care organizations exhibiting greater degrees of network embeddedness will be less likely to integrate vertically.*

CONCLUSION

A consideration of economic and sociological perspectives highlights the different directions that an organization may take in its integration activities depending on the organization's environmental uncertainty, asset specificity, or network embeddedness. As organizations vary in the degree of their environmental uncertainty and their network embeddedness, their approach to integration decision factors will also vary, resulting in a spectrum of integrative behavior. Figure 1 summarizes the two opposing theoretical perspectives' predictions for organizations in response to the environmental changes resulting from bundled payments and ACO models.

This article's predictions are solely theoretical and require both time and data to be empirically tested. As expressed by some post-acute care industry representatives, the introduction of ACOs and a bundled payment system may indeed yield anticipated outcomes, but it will also surely create unanticipated consequences that will require further attention. Perhaps this is to be expected for a sector of the healthcare industry that has already experienced considerable regulation and change. As has always been the case, in today's post-ACA healthcare industry, "there are prone to be significant winners and losers" (CPS, 2009, p. 16). Who will win and who may lose, however, remains an issue of uncertainty.

NOTES

1. First introduced in the 1980s, a bundled payment model incorporating post-acute care as a model of interest was revived following a report by the Congressional Budget Office in December 2008 proposing ways to reduce federal healthcare spending. Elliott Fisher and colleagues first proposed the concept of ACOs in 2006 as a means to encourage Medicare savings and improve quality of care through heightened accountability and performance measurement (Fisher, Staiger, Bynum, & Gottlieb, 2006).

2. Several organizational theories speak to organizations' motivations to integrate, including the popular resource dependence perspective (Mick, 1990). However, as resource dependence theory views vertical integration as a possible response to the management of organizational interdependence, emphasizing organizations' desire to enhance power and autonomy in interorganizational relationships (Scott & Davis, 2007), TCE more directly addresses organizations' decisions to draw organizational boundaries or integrate. In this sense, TCE may be considered a subtheory of the resource dependence perspective as it explains vertical integration (Mick, 1990). Given its focus, we employ a TCE perspective to predict integration behaviors. Additionally, frameworks such as resource dependence theory are largely silent on the contrasting relationship between vertical integration and network embeddedness.

FIGURE 1

Organizational
Decision Factors
for Vertical
Integration (VI) with
Post-Acute Care
(PAC) Providers

Anticipated Changes	Predicted Responses
Patients may prefer care from providers offering a full continuum of care	*TCE*: VI encouraged to enhance organizational service offerings
	Network theory: VI not required for embedded organizations maintaining strong relationships with PAC providers
Infrastructure (e.g., legal, technical, financial) may be required to discourage opportunistic behavior among accountable care organization and bundled payment partners	*TCE*: VI encouraged to reduce transaction costs of monitoring and negotiations
	Network theory: VI not required for embedded organizations operating on conditions of trust with network members and resisting opportunistic behavior
Competitors may pursue new reforms as a strategic means to enhance competitiveness, legitimacy, and quality in the marketplace	*TCE*: VI encouraged to ensure competitive advantage over other market competitors
	Network theory: VI not required for embedded organizations that enjoy enhanced competitiveness, legitimacy, and quality as a result of network information sharing and joint problem solving
Acute care and PAC providers may realize competing interests, philosophies, preferences, or treatment decisions	*TCE*: VI encouraged to align interests of PAC providers with acute care organization
	Network theory: VI not required for embedded organizations guided by ethical orientation toward network members rather than motivations driven by self-interest

REFERENCES

American Medical Rehabilitation Providers Association (AMRPA). (2009). *An option for the future of medical rehabilitation and other post acute care hospital providers: The continuing care hospital*. Retrieved from AMRPA website: http://www.amrpa.org

Banks, D., Parker, E., & Wendel, J. (2001). Strategic interaction among hospitals and nursing facilities: The efficiency effects of payment systems and vertical integration. *Health Economics, 10*(2), 119–134.

Berenson, R. (2010). Shared savings program for accountable care organizations: A bridge to nowhere? *American Journal of Managed Care, 16*(10), 721–726.

Buntin, M. B., Colla, C. H., & Escarce, J. J. (2009). Effects of payment changes on trends in post-acute care. *Health Services Research, 44*(4), 1188–1210.

Byrne, M. M., & Ashton, C. M. (1999). Incentives for vertical integration in healthcare: The effect of reimbursement systems. *Journal of Healthcare Management, 44*(1), 34–44.

Center for Post-Acute Studies (CPS). (2009). *Bundling payment for post-acute care: Building blocks and policy options.* Washington, DC: National Rehabilitation Hospital.

Centers for Medicare & Medicaid Services (CMS). (2011). Proposed rules—Medicare program; Medicare Shared Savings Program: Accountable care organizations. *Federal Register, 76*(67), 19528–19654.

Clement, J. P. (1992). Counterpoint: Issue five. In W. J. Duncan, P. M. Ginter, & L. E. Swayne (eds.), *Strategic issues in health care management: Point and counterpoint* (pp. 103–111). Boston, MA: PWS-Kent.

Congressional Budget Office (CBO). (2008). *Budget options: Volume 1: Healthcare.* Retrieved from CBO website: http://www.cbo.gov

Conrad, D. A. (1992). Point: Issue five. In W.J. Duncan, P. M. Ginter, & L. E. Swayne (eEds.), *Strategic issues in health care management: Point and counterpoint* (pp. 96–102). Boston, MA: PWS-Kent.

Craver, M. L. (2010, March). Why the health care bill may eventually curb medical costs. *The Kiplinger Letter.* Retrieved from http://www.kiplinger.com/business resource/forecast/archive/health-care-bill-may-eventually-curb-costs.html

Currie, G. A. (1996). Creating value through integrating postacute care. *Home Care Provider, 1*(6), 322–323.

Dacin, M. T., Ventresca, M. J., & Beal, B. D. (1999). The embeddedness of organizations: Dialogue and directions. *Journal of Management, 25*(3), 317–356.

Devers, K., & Berenson, R. (2009). *Can accountable care organizations improve the value of healthcare by solving the cost and quality quandaries?* Washington, DC: Urban Institute.

DeVore, S., & Champion, R. W. (2011). Driving population health through accountable care organizations. *Health Affairs, 30*(1), 41–50.

Diana, M. L. (2009). Exploring information systems outsourcing in U.S. hospital-based health care delivery systems. *Health Care Management Science, 12*(4), 434–450.

Dresevic, A., & Kalmowitz, C. F. (2011, December 10). Group practice integration in light of PPACA and Stark. *Michigan Medical Law Report*. Retrieved from http://milawyers weekly.com/wp-files/mimlr/mimlr_dec10.pdf

Fisher, E. S., Staiger, D. O., Bynum, J. P., & Gottlieb, D. J. (2006). Creating accountable care organizations: The extended medical staff. *Health Affairs, 26*(1), w44–w57.

Galewitz, P. (2009, October 25). Can "bundled" payments help slash health costs? *USA Today*. Retrieved from *USA Today* website:http://www.usatoday.com

Goldsmith, J. (2011). Accountable care organizations: The case for flexible partnerships between health plans and providers. *Health Affairs, 30*(1), 32–40.

Greis, J. S., Rawlings, R. B., & Jackson. J. B. (2009). *To bundle or not to bundle: Lawmakers explore the question* (McGuire-Woods LLP white paper). Retrieved from http://greisguide.com/wp-content/uploads/2009/06/9wp12-mka-to-bundle-or-not-to-bundle.pdf

Harrigan, K. R. (1985). Vertical integration and corporate strategy. *Academy of Management Journal, 28*(2), 397–425.

Harris, J. M., Grauman, D. M., & Hemnani, R. (2010). Solving the ACO conundrum. *Healthcare Financial Management, 64*(11), 67–74.

Jackson, J. B., Greis, J. S., & Rawlings, R. B. (2009, April 6). Exploring potential benefits and drawbacks of acute-care and post-acute care payment bundling. *McGuireWoods Legal Updates*. Retrieved from http://www.mcguirewoods.com/news-resources/item.asp?item=3855

Joskow, P. L. (2008). Vertical integration. In C. Menard & M. M. Shirley (Eds.), *Handbook of New Institutional Economics* (pp. 319–348). Heidelberg, Germany: Springer.

Keckley, P. H., & Hoffmann, M. (2010). *Accountable care organizations: A new model for sustainable innovation*. Washington, DC: Deloitte center for Health Solutions.

Lubell, J. (2009). Paying by the bundle: Docs, hospitals "at risk" under new CMS bundling demonstration project. *Modern Healthcare, 39*(14), 32, 34.

Luke, R. D., Walston, S. L., & Plummer, P. M. (2004). *Healthcare strategy: In pursuit of competitive advantage.* Chicago, IL: Health Administration Press.

Mick, S. S. (1990). Explaining vertical integration in health care: an analysis and synthesis of transaction-cost economics and strategic-management theory. In S. S. Mick (ed.), *Innovations in health care delivery: Insights for organization theory* (pp. 207–240). San Francisco, CA: Jossey-Bass.

Mick, S. S., & Conrad, D. A. (1988). The decision to integrate vertically in health care organizations. *Hospital & Health Services Administration, 33*(3), 345–360.

Moriya, A. S., Vogt, W. B., & Gaynor, M. (2010). Hospital prices and market structure in the hospital and insurance industries. *Health Economics, Policy and Law, 5*(4), 459–479.

Murer, C. G. (2009). Post-acute care bundling plan. *Rehab Management, 22*(6), 32.

Podolny, J. M., & Page, K. L. (1998). Network forms of organization. *Annual Review of Sociology, 24*(1), 57–76.

Provan, K. G. (1993). Embeddedness, interdependence, and opportunism in organizational supplier-buyer networks. *Journal of Management, 19*(4), 841–856.

Rittenhouse, D. R., Shortell, S. M., & Fisher, E. S. (2009). Primary care and accountable care: Two essential elements of delivery-system reform. *New England Journal of Medicine, 361*(24), 2301–2303.

Robinson, J. C. (1996a). Administered pricing and vertical integration in the hospital industry. *Journal of Law and Economics, 39*(1), 357–378.

Robinson, J. C. (1996b). The dynamics and limits of corporate growth in health care. *Health Affairs, 15*(2), 155–169.

Robinson, J. C. (1997). Physician-hospital integration and the economic theory of the firm. *Medical Care Research and Review, 54*(1), 3–24.

Scott, W. R., & Davis, G. F. (2007). *Organizations and organizing: Rational, natural, and open system perspectives.* Upper Saddle river, NJ: Pearson Prentice Hall.

Shortell, S. M., Casalino, L. P., & Fisher, E. S. (2010). How the Center for Medicare and Medicaid Innovation should test accountable care organizations. *Health Affairs, 29*(7), 1293–1298.

Taft Stettinius & Hollister LLP. (2010, June 15). PPACA and market demands may trigger next generation of physician hospital integration. Retrieved from Taft Stettinius & Hollister website: http://www.taftlaw.com/news/publications/

Terry, K. (2009). Payment bundling: Like it or not, it's coming. *Physicians Practice, 19*(9), 22–23.

Tocknell, M. D. (2012). M&A: Hospitals take control. Retrieved from http://www.health leadersmedia.com/intelligence/012/industry-insight-report.html

Town, R., Wholey, D., Feldman, R., & Burns, L. R. (2006). *The welfare consequences of hospital mergers* (Working Paper 12244). Cambridge, MA: National Bureau of Economic Research.

Uzzi, B. (1997). Social structure and competition in interfirm networks: The paradox of embeddedness. *Administrative Science Quarterly, 42*(1), 35–67.

Walston, S. L., Kimberly, J. R., & Burns, L. R. (1996). Owned vertical integration and health care: Promise and performance. *Health Care Management Review, 21*(1), 83–92.

Weinstock, M. (2010). are you ready for bundled payments? *Trustee, 63*(3), 28–31.

Welch, W. P. (1998). Bundled medicare payment for acute and postacute care. *Health Affairs, 17*(6), 69–81.

Williamson, O. E. (1975). *Markets and hierarchies*. New York, NY: Free Press.

Yip, J. Y., Wilber, K. H, & Myrtle, R. C. (2002). The impact of the 1997 Balanced Budget amendment's prospective payment system on patient case mix and rehabilitation utilization in skilled nursing. *The Gerontologist, 42*(5), 653–660.

Zigmond, J. (2010). Post-acute: M&A on the way. *Modern Healthcare, 40*(1), 29.

Zinn, J. S., Mor, V., Feng, Z., & Intrator, O. (2007). Doing better to do good: The impact of strategic adaptation on nursing home performance. *Health Services Research, 42*(3), 1200–1218.

Zuckerman, a. m. (2009). The next wave of mergers and acquisitions: What's your company's position? *Healthcare Financial Management, 63*(5), 60–63.

CHAPTER 7

THE SAFETY NET

One of the major policy problems addressed by the ACA is the lack of health insurance for many Americans. However, lack of insurance does not always mean individuals go without healthcare. Many services are provided by the nation's safety net—public hospitals[1], rural hospitals, and community health centers. For years, safety-net organizations have filled important roles, including providing:

◆ care to those without insurance;

◆ extensive training for physicians and other healthcare professionals;

◆ services that are culturally competent to the many unique communities throughout the nation; and

◆ services to those who live in rural communities.

Because safety-net providers receive a high percentage of their revenue from government sources, payment policies have been used to promote specific behaviors. For example, federally funded community health centers need to have independent community-based boards, and these boards must be composed mostly of consumers. Another example is the special payments made to some hospitals to provide for their uncompensated care, based on the percentage of Medicaid patients served.

Although the expansion of health insurance to almost all Americans may make the safety net less necessary in the future, the ACA contains many sections that support its continued success.

ELIGIBILITY

One of the most important strategies to increase access to health insurance is the expansion of the Medicaid program and the Children's Health Insurance Program (CHIP). This expansion is contained in Title II: "Role of Public Programs." Improved access is accomplished by mandating a maximum income level (138 percent of the federal poverty level[2]) to be used by every state for eligibility; such a policy also eliminates the many categories that Medicaid has historically used to determine eligibility. For example, single men were not covered under previous Medicaid policies.

In its review of the ACA, the Supreme Court ruled that the Medicaid expansion was optional for each state. As a result, the ACA Medicaid expansion has been controversial in many states. It is estimated that in 2014, nearly 8 million of the uninsured would have received coverage had their state opted for the expansion. States that have opted into the Medicaid expansion will experience a decrease of 48.9 percent in their uninsured population, versus an 18.1 percent decrease in opt-out states (Dickman et al. 2014). Continued pressure from providers will likely encourage states to opt in, but this may be a slow journey. The original form of Medicaid was also a state option that took many years for every state to adopt. The last state, Arizona, joined in 1983.

One of the frustrating aspects of the Medicaid system over the years has been its close ties to cash assistance programs (i.e., welfare). Because of a concern that individuals were erroneously receiving cash assistance, most states implemented complex enrollment processes for both cash benefits and Medicaid. Unfortunately, this complexity deterred many individuals from enrolling. Researchers have estimated that in 2002, more than 60 percent of all uninsured children were eligible for public coverage, a figure that climbed to 74 percent in 2005 (Sommers 2007).

The ACA addressed this problem in §2201, which provides for simplification and coordination with online health insurance exchanges. In addition, §2202 permits hospitals to make presumptive eligibility determinations for Medicaid. This solves a long-standing problem—safety-net hospitals would provide emergency services, and because the patient had little incentive to apply later for Medicaid, the hospital would not be reimbursed.

NAVIGATORS

Historically the individual health insurance market has been served by private insurance brokers. Although these professionals have provided access to health insurance to many individuals, they have not had a primary focus on the low-income population of the United States. The ACA attempts to remedy this issue through §1311, which provides the funding and authority for a new health profession—the patient navigator. Navigators conduct public education activities to raise awareness about the expanded availability of health insurance and ways to enroll. They help consumers with private insurance, premium credits, Medicaid, and CHIP. Navigators are expected to provide these services in a manner that is culturally and linguistically appropriate. The final rules for the navigator program are found at bit.ly/Reform7_1.

The Medicaid provisions in the ACA create an interesting challenge for safety-net providers. These new eligibility systems *should* decrease uncompensated care. However, the safety-net population has historically shown a reluctance to fully embrace new governmental programs, so these new policies may not be successful. In addition, the culture of complexity may not diminish if existing state government staff continue to administer the systems. Finally, individuals illegally present in the country will require services (usually in an emergency), and these will most likely be provided by the safety net.

DUAL-ELIGIBLE BENEFICIARIES

A unique aspect of the US health system is the diversity in its public payment systems. Medicare is managed by the federal government but also oversees each state-operated Medicaid program. Each state's Medicaid system is unique, and many individuals are eligible for both Medicare and Medicaid, leading to complex interactions between the payment systems. Coordination between programs is seen by many providers as problematic—particularly in the area of pharmaceuticals. For example, Medicare has Part D, which is subscribed to by the beneficiary. Medicaid provides drugs free, but has more limited sets of drugs, hence the confusion.

A new office (the Federal Coordinated Health Care Office) is established in §2602 to more effectively coordinate this care, and its goals are to ensure that dual-eligible individuals receive all benefits to which they are entitled, to eliminate regulatory conflicts between rules of the Medicare and Medicaid programs, and to eliminate cost shifting between the Medicare and Medicaid programs and among related healthcare providers. Because this problem is finally acknowledged in the ACA, coordination likely will significantly improve in the future.

HOSPITALS

The authors of the ACA anticipated the success of these simplified enrollment systems and enacted a policy for disproportionate-share hospital (DSH) payments to phase out (§1203), beginning in 2014. This additional Medicare payment has been made to hospitals that treat a disproportionate share of low-income patients. Unfortunately the authors of the bill did not anticipate that the Supreme Court would rule that the Medicaid expansion would be optional to the states. As a result safety-net hospitals in states that did not expand Medicaid could have been caught with both continued high levels of uncompensated care and reduced DSH payments. Congress has delayed this reduction until 2016, but this delay is not a long-term solution.

Chapter 6 discussed the new Center for Medicare & Medicaid Innovation. The ACA contains other interesting and creative policy ideas—the Medicaid Global Payment System demonstration project (§2705) is an example. This project will "adjust the payments made to an eligible safety net hospital system or network from a fee-for-service payment structure to a global capitated payment model."

Global payment systems significantly reduce administrative costs for hospitals and doctors. A recent study of physician practices found that "12 percent of their net patient services revenue was used to cover the costs of excessive administrative complexity" (Blanchfield et al. 2010). If this demonstration succeeds, it could lead to more global budgeting by other payers and significant administrative savings within the total healthcare system. No US hospitals have yet taken up this challenge.

RURAL HEALTHCARE

The United States has a total resident population of more than 310 million, but the population is urbanized, with 82 percent residing in cities and suburbs as of 2008 (CIA 2014). Rural healthcare—particularly small rural hospitals—has been a payment policy target for federal officials for many years. (These providers are also helped that every state—regardless of population—has two senators.) The general policy direction has been to provide enough Medicare (and in some cases Medicaid) funding to rural hospitals for them to stay fiscally healthy, even if they are providing small volumes of care. The payment tool for this goal is cost-based reimbursement, as opposed to the fixed-payment prospective payment system used for most US hospitals. The most visible policy is the Medicare cost reimbursement for critical access hospitals that have fewer than 25 beds (CMS 2014b; Rural Assistance Center 2014a).

This policy agenda is expanded in the ACA. The ACA reinstitutes reasonable cost payment for outpatient clinical lab tests performed by hospitals with fewer than 50 beds in qualified rural areas (§3122).

The Centers for Medicare & Medicaid Services (CMS) will extend the Rural Community Hospital Demonstration for five years and expand the number of participating hospitals to 30 (§3123). For this demonstration, hospitals must be located in one of the ten most sparsely populated states: Alaska, Idaho, Montana, Nebraska, Nevada, New Mexico, North Dakota, South Dakota, Utah, or Wyoming. Hospitals selected for participation in the demonstration will receive enough reimbursement to cover reasonable costs for covered inpatient services. CMS information on this project can be found at bit.ly/Reform7_2.The Medicare wage index is a complex set of rules that uses average wages of healthcare workers in an area to calibrate diagnosis-related group (DRG) payment by metropolitan statistical area and state. In 2011, the ACA (§10324) required that hospitals located in "frontier states" that are paid with the DRG system have a wage index[3] of at least 1.0 (if their index is already over 1.0 they keep this higher number). A frontier state is one in which at least 50 percent of counties have a population density of less than six persons per square mile. CMS determined that the following states are frontier states: Montana, Wyoming, North Dakota, Nevada, and South Dakota. This designation moves the DRG payment rates in these states closer to the national average.

The rural and safety-net hospital demonstrations in the ACA are rarely discussed, yet the cost-based emphasis in rural healthcare and the global payment system for safety-net hospitals might be the future models for hospital payment, as they can significantly reduce administrative costs.

COMMUNITY CLINICS

The third strand in the safety net is the growing list of community clinics. At the end of 2010, more than 1,000 federally qualified health centers (FQHCs) existed (CMS 2014c; Rural Assistance Center 2014b). Because community clinics are connected to their local neighborhoods, they have been popular with Democratic and Republican officials. This fondness continues in the ACA with significant funding increases in §5601 for FQHCs. The regulations surrounding FQHCs can be found here: bit.ly/Reform7_3.

Section 5602 improves the methodology and criteria for designating medically underserved populations and health professions shortage areas. This improvement is critical to community clinics as they recruit physicians and other health professionals. This program offers health professionals federal subsidies of up to $145,000 for their education. In return, these professionals must practice in an underserved area for some portion of their careers. If they practice in underserved areas for six years, this debt is completely forgiven (HHS 2014).

HEALTHCARE DISPARITIES

A historical mission of many safety-net providers has been to reduce the disparities in healthcare access and outcomes for some groups of Americans. Care is distributed inefficiently and unevenly across populations, and some patients receive worse care than others. In some cases, care is delivered too late or without full consideration of a patient's preferences and values. These disparities may occur for a variety of reasons, including differences in access to care, social determinants, provider biases, poor provider–patient communication, and poor health literacy. The Agency for Healthcare Research and Quality produces a periodic report on disparities, found at bit.ly/Reform7_4.

The ACA contains a number of policies to address healthcare disparities. In addition to the Medicaid expansion, access to subsidized insurance on the exchanges, improved funding for community health centers, and maternal and child health programs, the ACA also specifies two other important initiatives to address disparities. Section 10334 restructures the current federal agencies dealing with disparities. A key lead agency is the National Institute on Minority Health and Health Disparities: bit.ly/Reform7_5.

Section 4302 requires that population surveys and federally funded health and healthcare programs enhance their collection and reporting of data on race, ethnicity, sex, primary language, disability, and the status of those living in rural and frontier areas. In addition the ACA has multiple sections within the law that are aimed at increasing the diversity within the primary care, dental, mental health, and long-term care workforce.

Reading 7A provides an overview of the current actions being undertaken by American hospitals to reduce healthcare disparities.

SUMMARY

An important aspect of healthcare in the United States is the set of providers that comprise the safety net: public hospitals, rural providers, and community clinics. The ACA supports the continuation of their role through improved eligibility systems for Medicaid and CHIP and better coordination between Medicare and Medicaid.

The ACA provides substantial increases in funding for federally qualified health centers and improves rural hospital reimbursement. In addition, the law contains a new demonstration project for safety-net hospital global budgeting and a continuation of the rural demonstration project.

Two challenges remain for the safety net: the financial impact of the uneven expansion of Medicaid by the states and the needed reduction in healthcare disparities.

NOTES

1. The term *public hospital* continues to be used for large, urban hospitals that serve the safety-net mission. Most of these institutions began as local government units but have converted to some type of nonprofit status with independent governance.

2. The ACA specifies the modified adjusted gross income level for subsidies is at 133 percent of the federal poverty level. "However, §2002(a)(14)(I)(i) of ACA adds a five percentage point deduction from the FPL—one of several ways in which the AGI is 'modified.' With this five percent disregard, the Medicaid eligibility threshold is effectively 138 percent FPL" (SHADAC 2011).

3. The wage index is calculated each year by CMS. It is measured for a specific region and reflects the relative hospital wage level in the geographic area of the hospital compared to the national average hospital wage level (CMS 2014).

APPLICATIONS: DISCUSSION AND RESEARCH

1. What are the causes of individuals not enrolling in Medicaid even when eligible? What can be done? Contact a local community clinic and interview their financial staff to get their views. Also find agencies in your area that have contracted with the state or federal government to be navigators and collect their experiences with the Medicaid population (search example *Texas navigators*).

2. Is the disproportionate share program an effective policy to deal with the uninsured even after the full implementation of the ACA? If not what should replace it? Search journals such as *Health Affairs*, *Journal of the American Medical Association*, or *New England Journal of Medicine* for *DSH*, *disproportionate share*, or *safety net*.

3. What other options to the provision of rural and frontier healthcare exist beyond subsidizing hospitals in these areas? Search the Internet on *rural healthcare* and *telemedicine* to identify innovations in healthcare delivery in rural areas.

4. What specific actions can healthcare organizations take to ensure that their staff has the cultural competence to effectively treat a diverse patient base? See **Reading 7A**.

REFERENCES

Blanchfield, B. B., J. L. Heffernan, B. Osgood, R. R. Sheehan, and G. S. Meyer. 2010. "Saving Billions of Dollars—and Physicians' Time—by Streamlining Billing Practices." *Health Affairs* 29 (6): 1248.

Central Intelligence Agency (CIA). 2014. "The World Factbook." Accessed July 30. https://www.cia.gov/library/publications/the-world-factbook/index.html.

Centers for Medicare & Medicaid Services (CMS). 2014a. "Wage Index." Accessed August 6. www.cms.gov/Medicare/Medicare-Fee-for-Service-Payment/AcuteInpatientPPS/wageindex.html

———. 2011b. "Critical Access Hospital Center." Accessed August 6, 2014. www.cms.gov/Center/Provider-Type/Critical-Access-Hospitals-Center.html.

———. 2011c. "Federally Qualified Health Centers (FQHC)." Accessed July 30, 2014. www.cms.gov/center/fqhc.asp

Dickman, S., D. Himmelstein, D. McCormick, and S. Woolhandler. 2014. "Opting Out of Medicaid Expansion: The Health and Financial Impacts." *Health Affairs Blog.* Published January 30. http://healthaffairs.org/blog/2014/01/30/opting-out-of-medicaid-expansion-the-health-and-financial-impacts.

Rural Assistance Center. 2014a. "Critical Access Hospitals." Accessed August 6. www.raconline.org/topics/critical-access-hospitals.

———. 2014b. "Federally Qualified Health Centers." Accessed August 6. www.raconline.org/topics/federally-qualified-health-centers.

Sommers, B. D. 2007. "Why Millions of Children Eligible for Medicaid and SCHIP are Uninsured: Poor Retention Versus Poor Take-Up." *Health Affairs* 26 (5): w560.

State Health Access Data Assistance Center (SHADAC). 2011. "ACA Note: When 133 Equals 138—FPL Calculations in the Affordable Care Act" Accessed August 6, 2014. www.shadac.org/blog/aca-note-when-133-equals-138-fpl-calculations-in-affordable-care-act.

US Department of Health and Human Services (HHS). 2014. "National Health Service Corps." Accessed July 30. http://nhsc.hrsa.gov/.

READING 7A

EQUITY OF CARE—ELIMINATING HEALTHCARE DISPARITIES: THE CALL TO ACTION

Richard J. Umbdenstock

From *Futurescan 2014: Healthcare Trends and Implications 2014–2019* (2014), Chapter 7, 36–40. Chicago: Society for Healthcare Strategy & Market Development of the American Hospital Association and Health Administration Press, a division of the Foundation of the American College of Healthcare Executives.

Racial and ethnic minorities now make up about one-third of the US population, but by 2042 they will become the majority.

While all patients are equal, they are not the same. They may, for example, be exposed to different environments and workplace hazards, have different diets, interact differently with healthcare providers, and face different challenges in complying with medical advice. For these reasons and many others, some still unknown, patients from traditional racial and ethnic minority groups often receive a lower quality of healthcare, even when the comparisons control for income and health insurance status (IOM 2003; Mayberry, Mili, and Ofili 2000). Healthcare disparities can lead to increased medical errors, longer hospital stays, avoidable hospital admissions and readmissions, and the over- or underutilization of procedures.

THE REAL CHALLENGE

Despite our best efforts, we know that race, ethnicity, and language preference (REAL) continue to affect the likelihood that patients will receive the care they need and the outcomes they deserve (IOM 2003; Mayberry, Mili, and Ofili 2000). For example, Hispanic adults with diabetes are far less likely to receive recommended preventive services, and African-American women are more likely to die after they are diagnosed with breast cancer, than are their white counterparts (AHRQ 2009; American Cancer Society 2011). As health insurance coverage expands, each provider will be challenged to provide the best possible care to a patchwork of patient populations with different beliefs, lifestyles, family structures and support, and healthcare experiences.

Futurescan Survey Results: Equity of Care

How likely is it that the following will be seen in <u>your hospital</u> by 2019?

Very Likely (%)		Somewhat Likely (%)	Somewhat Unlikely (%)	Very Unlikely (%)

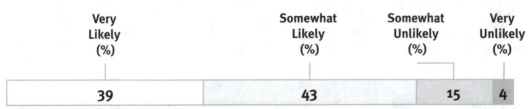

39	43	15	4

Your hospital's strategic plan will include goals for improving quality of care for culturally and linguistically diverse patient populations.

20	52	22	6

Your hospital will see a reduction of 50 percent in the disparities in quality of care among racially, culturally, and linguistically diverse patient populations.

ACHE

48	38	12	2

SHSMD

30	40	27	3

Both

43	38	16	2

The race/ethnicity diversity of your hospital board will represent your community.

ACHE

38	45	15	2

SHSMD

20	43	33	4

Both

34	44	19	3

The race/ethnicity diversity of your hospital's leadership team will represent your community.

NOTE: Percentages may not total to exactly 100% due to rounding.

(continued)

Futurescan Survey Results: Equity of Care *(continued)*

What Practitioners Predict
Strategic plans will address diverse patient populations. The majority (82 percent) of CEOs responding to the survey think it likely that goals for improving the quality of care for diverse patient populations will be part of their organization's strategic plan by 2019.

Care disparities will be reduced by half. Almost three-quarters of survey respondents believe that disparities of care among racially, culturally and linguistically diverse patient populations will be reduced by half in their organizations by 2019.

Governing boards and leadership will reflect the community. A majority of those answering the survey (nearly 86 percent of ACHE respondents and 70 percent of SHSMD respondents) predict that by 2019 the racial/ethnic diversity of their board will reflect their community. Similarly, 83 percent of ACHE respondents and more than 63 percent of SHSMD respondents predict that the racial/ethnic diversity of the hospital's leadership team will represent their community by that time.

Planning for equitable care involves developing ongoing relationships with community organizations that can support providers' efforts to build cultural competency in delivering that care. Providers must anticipate community needs to ensure access for those with limited or no English proficiency, for example, or to develop patient education materials that consider differences in both language and culture.

The use and types of measures of clinical quality and patient experience have increased significantly in recent years, and they are driving improvements across the board. But overall, national quality measures cannot be readily broken down by REAL. Recently, the Institute for Diversity in Health Management surveyed hospitals and found that although 81 percent of hospitals collect REAL data, only 18 percent have used those data for quality interventions (AHA and Institute for Diversity in Health Management 2012). Hospitals that collect accurate REAL data can begin to correctly identify their patient population. These data can also be used to break down quality outcomes by race and ethnicity and reveal if certain patient populations have lower-quality outcomes. Only at this level of data granularity can a hospital begin to implement quality interventions to reduce or eliminate disparities.

CALL TO ACTION

The need to address the problem of healthcare disparities led to the National Call to Action to Eliminate Health Care Disparities. In 2011, the American Hospital Association (AHA) stood in partnership with America's Essential Hospitals (formerly the National Association of Public Hospitals and Health Systems), the American College of Healthcare Executives, the Association of American Medical Colleges, and the Catholic Health Association of the United States to urge hospitals to speed up action to eliminate healthcare disparities. This was a bold but necessary step. To seek the field's support for action during a time of great change in healthcare was to acknowledge the urgency of improving equity of care.

The Call to Action focuses on three core areas that we believe will lay the foundation for all hospitals to reduce healthcare disparities:

1. increased collection of REAL data;

2. broader cultural competency training; and

3. diversity in governance and leadership.

Call to Action partners have set up the Equity of Care website (www.equityofcare. org) to help hospitals, healthcare systems, clinicians, and others improve the quality of care for each and every patient by sharing resources and best practices. We believe that most healthcare providers are moving in the right direction and that many are taking important steps to make care more equitable. But given the speed of change in our communities, we feel that this process must be accelerated and that information sharing is an important way to facilitate equitable care.

Call to Action partners recently set goals for each core area. By 2020, we hope to

1. increase collection and use of REAL data to 75 percent;

2. increase cultural competency training to 100 percent; and

3. increase governance and leadership team diversity to 20 and 17 percent, respectively, or to a composition reflective of the hospital's community.

For the field to achieve these goals and to sustain progress and momentum, hospitals need to make equity of care a priority and look beyond the immediate future.

FUTURESCAN SURVEY RESULTS

What are hospitals doing to promote equity of care? The *Futurescan* survey provides us with a view into hospitals' strategic thinking over the next five years. The majority (82 percent) of CEOs responding to the survey think it likely that goals for improving the quality of care for diverse patient populations will be part of their organization's strategic plan by 2019. This is a key step for equity of care. We know that for real, meaningful change to occur, it must come from a hospital's leadership team. We also know that embedding key goals into a hospital's strategic process raises the issue to a level where results are seen. It becomes part of the work the hospital does and something to be believed in and integrated into its culture.

Understanding that disparities in healthcare are a problem is the first step toward achieving equity of care. Finding ways as an organization to reduce those disparities comes next. Again, we can look to the survey for an indication of what the future holds. Almost three-quarters of survey respondents believe that disparities of care among racially, culturally, and linguistically diverse patient populations will be reduced by half in their organizations by 2019.

Eliminating healthcare disparities is the ultimate point of the Call to Action and the goal of those who support equitable care. We do not have all the answers yet, but through the Call to Action and the Equity of Care platform, we are sharing resources and guides to help the field navigate toward high-quality care for all. To realize the goal of eliminating healthcare disparities, hospital leaders must believe that results can be achieved. The survey data highlight that this belief and commitment exist.

A hospital strives to reflect its community. As the demographic makeup of communities changes, hospital boards and leadership teams must change accordingly to reflect their community and align the hospital's work with the needs of a new population of patients. Call to Action goals around diversity address this movement and need for action.

A majority of those answering the survey (nearly 86 percent of ACHE respondents and 70 percent of SHSMD respondents) predict that by 2019 the racial/ethnic diversity of their hospital's board will reflect that of their community. Similarly, 83 percent of ACHE respondents and more than 63 percent of SHSMD respondents predict that the racial/ethnic makeup of the hospital's leadership team will represent their community.

The governing board is crucial because it establishes the overarching direction of the hospital or healthcare system. A board whose makeup reflects that of its community has a far better chance of understanding its community's unique needs. This insight helps a hospital's leadership team strategically shift the approach to care, specifically in the area of equity.

IMPLICATIONS FOR HOSPITAL LEADERS

What does achieving equity in care mean for hospitals and healthcare systems? It results in better care and better outcomes, higher patient satisfaction, and a deeper and more meaningful connection to the community. Equity of care also has a strong business imperative; a study by the Joint Center for Political and Economic Studies found that eliminating healthcare disparities for minorities would have reduced direct medical care expenditures by $229.4 billion between 2003 and 2006 (LaVeist, Gaskin, and Richard 2009). As healthcare transitions to a value-based system of care, hospitals must ensure that their outcomes improve.

Hospitals can act immediately to address equity of care by developing consistent processes to collect and use REAL data. For example, they can ask patients to self-report their information and train staff, using scripts, to appropriately discuss patients' cultural and language preferences during the registration process. Hospitals should generate data reports stratified by REAL group to examine disparities. REAL data can be used to develop targeted interventions to improve quality of care (e.g., scorecards, equity dashboards) and can help create the case for building access to services in underserved communities.

In the area of cultural competency, hospitals should educate all clinical staff during orientation about how to address the unique cultural and linguistic factors affecting the care of diverse patients and communities and require all employees to attend diversity training. Hospitals should also provide culturally and linguistically competent services (e.g., interpreters, diverse community health educators) and features (e.g., a bilingual workforce, multilingual signage). In the area of diversity, a hospital should actively work to diversify its board and leadership team to include a voice and perspective that reflect its community. Accountability through the use of regular reporting on the racial and ethnic makeup of the leadership team will support actionable approaches. Diversification strategies include the creation of a community-based diversity advisory committee, engagement of the broader public through community-based activities and programs, and use of search firms.

The mission of the AHA and its members is to advance the health of individuals and communities. We are accountable to the community and committed to health improvement. We cannot succeed unless we eliminate healthcare disparities. As a partner in the Call to Action, we will keep the drumbeat steady and work closely with our members to foster success in the realm of equitable care. Equity in care is more than the right thing to do; it's the smart thing to do—for patients, for communities, and for hospitals.

REFERENCES

Agency for Healthcare Research and Quality (AHRQ). 2009. *National Healthcare Disparities Report, 2008*. AHRQ Publication No. 09-0002. www.ahrq.gov/research/findings/nhqrdr/nhdr08/nhdr08.pdf.

American Cancer Society. 2011. *Breast Cancer Facts & Figures, 2011–2012*. www.cancer.org/acs/groups/content/@epidemiologysurveilance/documents/document/acspc-030975.pdf.

American Hospital Association (AHA) and Institute for Diversity in Health Management. 2012. *Diversity and Disparities: A Benchmark Study of U.S. Hospitals*. Published June. www.hpoe.org/Reports-HPOE/diversity_disparities_chartbook.pdf.

Institute of Medicine (IOM). 2003. *Unequal Treatment: Confronting Racial and Ethnic Disparities in Health Care*. Washington, DC: National Academies Press.

LaVeist, T.A., D.J. Gaskin, and P. Richard. 2009. *The Economic Burden of Health Inequalities in the United States*. Joint Center for Political and Economic Studies. Published September. www.jointcenter.org/hpi/sites/all/files/Burden_Of_Health_FINAL_0.pdf.

Mayberry, R.M., F. Mili, and E. Ofili. 2000. "Racial and Ethnic Differences in Access to Medical Care." *Medical Care Research and Review* 57 (Suppl 1): 108–45.

CHAPTER 8

THE PERFECT MARKET: HEALTH INSURANCE REFORM

The current version of the US Pledge of Allegiance reads, "I pledge allegiance to the flag of the United States of America, and to the Republic for which it stands, one nation, under God, indivisible, with *Liberty and Justice for all.*" "Liberty and Justice for all" summarizes the conflicting values in the US government that have been present since its founding. *Liberty:* we are on our own to succeed or fail; therefore, keep the government off my back. *Justice for all:* we are all in this together; government is a tool to advance the common good.

The final theory of the ACA is based in liberty and the force of the free market to optimize healthcare costs and value. Chapter 2 provides an overview of the markets theory as applied to healthcare, and this chapter explores some of the market-based policies in the ACA that will shape US healthcare in the future.

Throughout the debate surrounding the ACA, the title of the legislation vacillated between "health reform" and "health insurance reform." The final product does make substantial changes to the health insurance system, but it also makes significant changes to the structure and functioning of the healthcare delivery system, as outlined in previous chapters.

However, four key policies in the new health insurance system will also have a major effect on the operation of the total system. They are key elements in the markets theory of the ACA and are based on best practices in the health insurance industry. The policies are universal coverage, health insurance exchanges, standard benefits, and increased government regulation to maintain a fair playing field.

UNIVERSAL COVERAGE

Many problems prompted the reform of the healthcare system. However, the strongest force was the increasing number of uninsured people with resultant untreated illnesses and financial disasters. Hence, the most prominent feature of the ACA is its multiple mechanisms to increase the rate of health insurance.

The problem of the lack of insurance is illustrated by a study of individuals with three chronic conditions: diabetes mellitus, hypertension, and elevated cholesterol (Wilper et al. 2009). Insurance status was related to the rates at which people with these chronic conditions were undiagnosed or inadequately treated. For all three conditions, people without insurance were undiagnosed at higher rates. The same was true when uncontrolled, or *inadequately treated*, conditions were examined. For diabetes mellitus, however, the difference between the rates of uncontrolled disease for those with insurance and those without insurance was small. Wilper and colleagues conclude in their study, "Gaining insurance and a diagnosis might not guarantee optimal treatment of chronic conditions, unless these achievements are coupled with other system improvements such as expanded access to primary and preventive care, reducing financial barriers to care, and a focus on chronic disease management in lieu of the current episodic care model."

However, the first important step on the road to an improved system is the expansion of coverage, a principal goal of the ACA. Eibner, Hussey, and Girosi (2010) have developed simulation models that predict 94.6 percent of US workers will be covered by comprehensive health insurance once the ACA is fully implemented. This estimate assumes that all states will enact the Medicaid expansion (27 states have expanded Medicaid as of 2014).

Universal coverage promotes a stable and competitive market and eliminates the need for many of the worst practices of the prior health insurance system—for example, rating or exclusions for preexisting conditions. In addition, universal coverage provides prevention, early treatment, and chronic disease management—all of which have been demonstrated to improve quality and decrease costs (see Chapters 3 and 4).

Another benefit of universal and portable coverage is its support of innovation and enterprise. If an inventor has a preexisting condition, she may choose to remain with her current employer to keep her health insurance. However, after the implementation of the ACA, this "job lock" is eliminated, and the inventor can start her own company and still retain affordable health insurance. A study by the Urban Institute found that "the number of self-employed people in the United States will be about 1.5 million higher following the universal availability of non-group coverage, the financial assistance available for it, and other related market reforms" (Blumberg, Corlette, and Lucia 2013). The sections of the ACA that drive this expanded coverage are contained in Title I: "Quality, Affordable Health Care for all Americans," and Title II: "Role of Public Programs" (see Chapter 6).

HEALTH INSURANCE EXCHANGES

The most visible portion of the ACA has been the health insurance exchange websites operated by both the state and federal governments (§1311). The roll out of these marketplaces was problematic, and the details of these shortcomings were well reported in the press. However, it is important to remember a few characteristics of the health exchange model that are critical for the future:

◆   The consumer can choose from a broad array of products.

◆   The exchange promotes price and quality competition.

◆   The financial responsibility of the employer (or government) and the individual is clearly delineated.

Some issues in the ACA exchanges are worth exploration, as they will likely impact both public and private exchange development into the future.

RISK MANAGEMENT

The science of risk adjustment and pooling has become more sophisticated, which will protect most insurance companies from adverse selection and create price competition much more on true operational costs. These cost pressures will radiate throughout all aspects of the providers' systems. Health plans are buffered from large financial losses and gains through three mechanisms:

1. Reinsurance: Provides funding to health plans that incur high claims costs for enrollees (§1341)

2. Risk corridors: Limit plan losses and gains caused by inaccurate rate setting (§1342)

3. Risk adjustment: Transfers funds from plans with lower-risk enrollees to plans with higher-risk enrollees (§1343)

SUBSIDIES

The largest single expenditure in the ACA is the funding of the subsidies for those individuals and small employers purchasing health insurance on the exchanges. An income-based subsidy is available to individuals and families up to 400 percent of the poverty level (§1401). Subsidies are also available to companies with fewer than 25 employees that have average employee wages of less than $50,000 per year (§1421). Funds for the subsidies in the exchanges come from reduced Medicare payment to providers and a variety of new taxes, as discussed in Chapter 2.

NARROW NETWORKS

Because underwriting of individuals is now prohibited, an increasingly prevalent response to price competition in the exchanges has been to narrow the network of providers. A 2013 national study by the McKinsey Center for US Health System Reform found that narrow network insurance products had a 26 percent lower one-year price increase (2013 to 2014) than did broad networks, which include most providers (McKinsey 2013).

The narrow network issue has attracted considerable concern from providers. In response, the Centers for Medicare & Medicaid Services (CMS) issued draft regulations on network sufficiency for the 2015 enrollment year (CMS 2014). Specifically they address whether an issuer meets the reasonable access standard. CMS will focus most closely on those areas that have historically raised network adequacy concerns, including the following:

◆   Hospital systems

◆   Mental health providers

◆   Oncology providers

◆   Primary care providers

Network adequacy will be an ongoing issue as health plans struggle to maintain competitive rates.

MEDICAID EXPANSION

The ACA Medicaid expansion has been controversial in many states. It is estimated that nearly 8 million of the uninsured would have received coverage had their state opted for the expansion in 2014. States that have opted into the Medicaid expansion will experience a decrease of 48.9 percent in their uninsured population, versus an 18.1 percent decrease in opt-out states (Dickman et al. 2014); continued pressure from providers will likely encourage states to opt in, but this may be a slow journey.

SURPRISES FROM THE ACA EXCHANGES

As part of the political compromise to exclude the "public option" from the ACA exchanges, the expansion of healthcare co-ops was encouraged with legislation and funding (§1322). The public option would have been a government-run health insurance agency that would compete with private health plans on the exchanges. Although co-ops were expected to be a minor player, many have been surprisingly successful, with more than 300,000 individual nationwide signing up in 2014. Co-ops in Maine and Kentucky have achieved market shares of 80 percent and 61 percent, respectively (Hancock 2014).

Regional cost differences are also now apparent. In approximately half of the states, a 27-year-old will pay between $195 and $250 a month for the second-lowest-cost silver plan. In five states, he will pay more than $320 a month. The most expensive silver premiums for a 27-year-old are along the Eastern Seaboard; at the higher end is Vermont, at $413 a month (PWC 2014). Because these data are visible, a region with low healthcare costs may begin to use this attribute for economic development and attracting business relocations.

PURCHASING ACROSS STATE LINES

One controversial policy is the ability of individuals to purchase health insurance across state lines. The argument for this policy is to provide a much broader choice of insurance options to consumers. However, opponents have argued that this would damage the ability of states to regulate the type of insurance a state's residents could purchase.

Section 1333 of the ACA permits states to form "health care choice" interstate compacts and allow insurers to sell policies in any state participating in the compact. Two or more states may enter into compacts under which one or more insurance plans may be offered in such states, subject to the laws and regulations of the state in which it was written. This law takes full effect in 2016. It is not yet evident if this policy will be useful to states or will prove attractive to consumers.

PRIVATE EXCHANGES, PRIVATE INSURANCE MARKET

The private healthcare market has also been making significant changes independent of the ACA. Private exchanges are growing as they operate with the three fundamental characteristics described previously: broad choice, price and quality competition, and clear lines of financial responsibility. While this market segment has remained small, with fewer than 1 million enrollees in 2012, employers are expressing strong interest. Recent employer surveys indicate that more than one in four employers is considering moving to a private exchange in the next three to five years (Accenture 2013).

A leading example of a private exchange is Aon Corporation's, which serves 18 companies, including Walgreens, Sears Holding Corporation, and Darden Restaurants, Inc. More than 20 insurers participated in Aon's exchange in 2014, and most employers have access to five carriers, which each have five plans, giving each worker a choice of 25 options.

An important aspect of private exchanges is they provide defined contribution plans, which can insulate employers from healthcare inflation in the future. The exchange model then becomes very attractive for both employers (defined contribution) and employees (broader choice).

The private exchange model is a strategic option for many employers, as it controls costs and fits into a human resources mission to attract and maintain talented employees. Therefore large employers will not likely eliminate health insurance as a benefit and pay the ACA fine ($2,000 per employee per year), as some had predicted during the ACA debate.

Healthcare exchanges are discussed in depth in **Reading 8A**. Regulations on the operations of the ACA exchanges can be found at http://bit.ly/Reform8_1.

MEDICARE EXCHANGES

The Medicare program has two interesting examples of marketplace competition that predate the ACA. Medicare beneficiaries can access the CMS website and choose both Medicare Advantage plans and Medicare drug coverage (Part D) plans. These websites are comprehensive and exhibit the same characteristics of broad choice and competition that are present in the private and ACA exchanges.

The Medicare Advantage exchange can be found here: http://bit.ly/Reform8_2. The Medicare drug benefit exchange is here: http://bit.ly/Reform8_3.

STANDARD BENEFITS

To be effective, the exchanges must ensure that each participating health plan has comparable products. The ACA accomplishes this through two mechanisms: standard benefits and a standard method to calculate premiums. Standardization promotes fair market competition and is a key to the success of the markets theory of the ACA.

Benefit design in health insurance has always been controversial, with extended debates on coverage for mental health and substance abuse, disease-specific plans, and plans with such high deductibles as to be equivalent to no insurance. The benefit design question is left to the US Department of Health and Human Services (HHS) (§1302) but must include "at least the following general categories and the items and services covered within the categories:

- ambulatory patient services;
- emergency services;
- hospitalization;
- maternity and newborn care;
- mental health and substance use disorder services, including behavioral health treatment;
- prescription drugs;
- rehabilitative and habilitative services and devices;
- laboratory services;

◆ preventive and wellness services and chronic disease management; and

◆ pediatric services, including oral and vision care."

The details of the essential benefit design are set either by states or by the federal government. Twenty-five states have chosen to do so, and the remaining states have left this task to the federal government. The details of these benefits can be found here: http://bit.ly/Reform8_4.

Consumers can choose varying levels of coinsurance and copays for the insurance policy they select. The policy with the lowest monthly premium is the bronze level; this provides a level of coverage that is designed to provide benefits that are equivalent to 60 percent of the full actuarial value of the benefits. Other levels include silver (70 percent), gold (80 percent), and platinum (90 percent).

The markets theory of the ACA predicts that these two standardizations will promote price competition by health plans and a general reduction in the growth of healthcare costs.

INCREASED GOVERNMENT REGULATION

The exchanges should promote aggressive competition between health plans, which in some markets does not currently exist. In fact, critics have asserted that in some geographic areas health plans practice shadow pricing, where all competitors' prices in the area rise at approximately the same rate.

In a study from 2001 to 2003, Chollet and Liu (2005) examined 52 insurers in three contiguous jurisdictions: Maryland, Virginia, and the District of Columbia. They found that "monopolistic pricing was observed among the largest insurers and could be measured against the pricing behavior of mid-sized insurers in the market. In addition, shadow pricing by the smallest insurers in the market was observed, even controlling for potential diseconomies of scale associated with small size."

Shadow pricing has not yet been observed in the exchanges, but if it occurs legislators may look to increased regulation of rates.

MEDICAL LOSS RATIOS

The ACA mandates that insurance sold in the United States have medical loss ratios (MLRs) of 85 percent for large employers and 80 percent for small employers (§1001). The MLR is the percentage of the revenue a health plan receives that is spent on healthcare services. The regulations surrounding this section are complex, and HHS has worked closely with the National Association of Insurance Commissioners to develop them.

The effects of MLR rules may be unpredictable. Some smaller insurance companies that are focused on the individual market may be unable to meet these rules and may cease to exist. Some services that were provided directly by health plans (e.g., disease management) may be subcontracted back to providers to meet the MLR. Even though the MLR penalties are part of the ACA, it is unlikely that any health plans can succeed in the future in a price-competitive health exchange with high overhead costs.

RATE INCREASES

One of the intense issues preceding the enactment of the ACA was the large rate increases for individuals in some markets. The ACA addressed this issue in §1003, "Ensuring that Consumers Get Value for Their Dollars." This section provides for a review of rate increases each year by the states and the federal government and possible exclusion of health plans whose rate increases are too large. Some states already have rate approval authority, and the coordination of these policies will require intricate regulations.

ADMINISTRATIVE SIMPLIFICATION

The high administrative costs of the US health system are addressed in §1104. This section provides a mechanism to create a single set of operating rules for each financial transaction between health plans and providers. It builds on the regulations contained in the Health Insurance Portability and Accountability Act of 1996. In addition to standards for electronic transactions, the section includes improvements to unravel much of the complexity of the current system, such as

- ◆ determining an individual's eligibility and financial responsibility for specific services prior to or at the point of care;

- ◆ requiring minimal augmentation of electronic systems by paper or other communications; and

- ◆ providing for timely acknowledgment, response, and status reporting that supports a transparent claims and denial management process.

This work coincides with the expansion of health information technology into medical practices. With any luck, this new clinical automation will coincide with the adoption of the new standardized operating rules, and much of today's complex paper systems will be eliminated.

A True Marketplace?

Although the exchanges are designed to support the markets theory in the ACA, innovation will be difficult for health plans. The standard benefit set will restrict some creativity in benefit design, and the MLR would not be required in a functioning market.

However, the large numbers of people who will buy their insurance through exchanges will provide new opportunities to create national products—in insurance and in provider systems. If all of these exchanges models continue to be successful, a unique American model of health access and competition will have been created.

SUMMARY

The third major theory of the ACA is that a competitive marketplace will deliver value in costs and quality. The new state-based health insurance exchanges are the most visible portion of the ACA that supports this theory.

Estimates predict that when the ACA is fully implemented, 94.6 percent of Americans will have health insurance as a result of the exchanges and the mandate to have health insurance once Medicaid is expanded in all states. The new market for health insurance in the exchanges is made competitive by standardized healthcare benefits and four levels of deductibles and coinsurance. The ACA and private exchanges will support the creation of other new and innovative private forms of health insurance.

The ACA adds new rules for the health insurance market, including mandatory medical loss ratios and a rate increase review process. The ACA has increased efforts to reduce costs in the health insurance system through administrative simplification of claims processing.

APPLICATIONS: DISCUSSION AND RESEARCH

1. The majority of states chose not to develop their own exchange but to take the federal-default plan. Was this the right decision? Discuss the advantages and disadvantages of state-based versus federal-default exchanges (Morrisey 2013; see **Reading 8A**).

2. You are an insurance broker. What do the ACA and the exchanges mean for you (Morrisey 2013; see **Reading 8A**)?

3. Under what circumstances would you expect a market facilitator exchange to lead to enhanced insurer competition? How would an active purchaser be expected to lead to greater competition (Morrisey 2013; see **Reading 8A**)?

4. The early estimates of premiums in the exchanges suggest that premiums will increase in the vast majority of states over what they would have been in the absence of the ACA. What factors lead to this result (Morrisey 2013; see **Reading 8A**)?

5. What are the advantages and risks of narrow networks?

6. What are the advantages of purchasing a health plan from another state? What might make this less attractive? (Review the National Center for State Legislatures analysis regarding this topic at http://bit.ly/Reform8_5.)

7. What benefits should be added to the essential benefits? Why?

NOTE

Portions of the chapter previously appeared in "Health Insurance Update," *Healthcare Executive* (29) 4: 50–52.

REFERENCES

Accenture. 2013. "Are You Ready? Private Health Insurance Exchanges Are Looming." Accessed August 11, 2014. www.accenture.com/sitecollectiondocuments/pdf/accenture-are-you-ready-private-health-insurance-exchanges-are-looming.pdf.

Blumberg, L. J., S. Corlette, and K. Lucia. 2013. "The Affordable Care Act: Improving Incentives for Entrepreneurship and Self Employment." Accessed July 31, 2014. www.rwjf.org/content/dam/farm/reports/issue_briefs/2013/rwjf406367.

Chollet, D., and S. Liu. 2005. "The Elephants in Your Back Yard: Monopolistic Pricing in Health Insurance Markets." *Abstracts AcademyHealth Meeting* 22: Abstract no. 3486.

Centers for Medicare & Medicaid Services (CMS). 2014. "2015 Letter to Issuers in Federally-Facilitated Marketplaces." Accessed August 4. www.cms.gov/CCIIO/Resources/Regulations-and-Guidance/Downloads/2015-final-issuer-letter-3-14-2014.pdf.

Dickman, S., D. Himmelstein, D. McCormick, and S. Woolhandler. 2014. "Opting Out of Medicaid Expansion: The Health and Financial Impacts." *Health Affairs Blog*. Published January 30. http://healthaffairs.org/blog/2014/01/30/opting-out-of-medicaid-expansion-the-health-and-financial-impacts.

Eibner, C., P. S. Hussey, and F. Girosi. 2010. "The Effects of the Affordable Care Act on Workers' Health Insurance Coverage." *New England Journal of Medicine* 363 (15): 1393–95.

Hancock, J. 2014. "Co-Ops Report Early Enrollment Successes and Expansion Plans." *Kaiser Health News*. Published February 27. http://capsules.kaiserhealthnews.org/index. php/2014/02/co-ops-report-early-enrollment-successes-and-expansion-plans.

McKinsey Center for US Health System Reform. 2013. "Hospital Networks: Configurations on the Exchanges and Their Impact on Premiums." Published December 14. www. mckinsey.com/~/media/mckinsey/dotcom/client_service/healthcare%20systems%20 and%20services/pdfs/hospital_networks_configurations_on_the_exchanges_and_ their_impact_on_premiums.ashx.

PricewaterhouseCoopers (PWC). 2014. "ACA State Exchange Premiums." Accessed July 31. www.pwc.com/us/en/health-industries/health-research-institute/aca-state-exchanges. jhtml.

Wilper, A. P., S. Woolhandler, K. E. Lasser, D. McCormick, D. H. Bor, and D. U. Himmelstein. 2009. "Hypertension, Diabetes, and Elevated Cholesterol Among Insured and Uninsured US Adults." *Health Affairs* 28 (6): w1151.

READING 8A

HEALTH INSURANCE EXCHANGES

Michael A. Morrisey

From *Health Insurance*, 2nd ed. (2013), Chapter 22, 393–416. Chicago: Health Administration Press.

The Patient Protection and Affordable Care Act (ACA) calls for the establishment of health insurance exchanges, now officially called *marketplaces*. These virtual marketplaces are intended to be the vehicles through which individuals and small businesses can compare a number of health insurance plans and buy coverage. They are also intended as the mechanism whereby eligibility for individual subsidies is determined and the subsidy applied to the selected coverage. Finally, the exchanges are intended to serve as the point of entry for coverage in Medicaid (both existing and expanded) and to the state's Children's Health Insurance Program.

In this chapter we will outline the organizational, functional, and financial options that the states have in establishing an exchange. As part of this outline, we will discuss the essential health benefits and the "medals levels" of coverage that the exchanges will offer. This will lead us into brief discussions of the exchanges' obligations in determining qualified health plans, organizing premium payment systems, and providing outreach and assistance to potential purchasers. Because more than half the states have declined to establish their own exchanges, we will discuss the implications for exchanges run by the federal government and the partnership models that seven states have indicated they will establish. Finally, the chapter includes some microsimulation analyses that explore the enrollment and premium implications of implementing the exchanges.

STATE VERSUS FEDERAL EXCHANGES

Each state had until early 2013 to submit blueprints to the federal government for state-run exchanges. If states did not adopt either a state-run model or a state–federal partnership model, the legislation required the federal government to operate a default exchange in the state. Exhibit 22.1 shows the distribution of the choices made by the states. A total of 17 states and the District of Columbia have chosen a state-based model, seven chose a partnership approach, and the remaining 26 elected to take the federal default

State-Based Exchanges	Partnership Exchanges	Default Federal Exchanges	
California	Arkansas	Alabama	New Jersey
Colorado	Delaware	Alaska	North Carolina
Connecticut	Illinois	Arizona	North Dakota
District of Columbia	Iowa	Florida	Ohio
Hawaii	Michigan	Georgia	Oklahoma
Idaho	New Hampshire	Kansas	Pennsylvania
Kentucky	West Virginia	Indiana	South Carolina
Maryland		Louisiana	South Dakota
Massachusetts		Maine	Tennessee
Minnesota		Mississippi	Texas
Nevada		Missouri	Virginia
New Mexico		Montana	Wisconsin
New York		Nebraska	Wyoming
Oregon			
Rhode Island			
Utah			
Vermont			
Washington			

EXHIBIT 22.1
State Decisions on Creating Health Insurance Exchanges

SOURCE: Data from KFF (2013a).

option. Even with these decisions, the states have the flexibility to change their approach over time. Illinois, for example, a partnership state, has indicated that it plans to run a state-based exchange in 2015 (KFF 2013a). Other states have taken more nuanced positions; Utah has proposed a state-based exchange for small employers but a federal default for individuals.

It is perhaps not surprising that the majority of states chose to accept the federal default. While federal startup money was available to establish the exchanges in the states and to fund their operation in the first year, the exchanges were required to be financially self-sufficient in their second year of operation (i.e., in 2015). Thus, the states would be responsible for the costs of running the exchanges after only one year. In addition, the regulations providing details on the operation of the exchanges were not complete even in the second quarter of 2013, even though the exchanges were required to begin their open enrollment period October 1. As a result, there was also concern that any public blame for deficiencies in a state-based exchange would fall on state officials. These financial and political concerns, together with the ability to convert to a state-based model in the future, undoubtedly played a significant role in the states' decisions.

ROLE AND STRUCTURE OF THE EXCHANGES

Perhaps the key decision that the states have had to face in creating a state-based exchange is what sort of exchange they want. The states have three options:

1. *Market facilitator.* With this model, the state's exchange accepts all health plans that meet the federal minimum requirements for qualified health plans. As such, the exchange serves as an impartial source of information and provides a structure in which people and businesses can compare plans and plan options. In some sense, this approach is analogous to the Internet-based insurance websites. In principle, a consumer would provide the exchange with some basic demographic information, and the market facilitator exchange would provide an easily readable comparison of the plans available, their premiums, and a quality rating for each. This approach seeks to maximize the number of plan choices available. As a market facilitator, the exchange would be expected to provide some meaningful guidance to purchasers about the definition of terms and the implications of choosing one type of plan over another.

2. *Selective contractor.* In this model, the state-based exchange provides additional constraints on health plans that otherwise meet the minimum federal requirements, selecting some plans while rejecting others. The state might require that the plans offered meet some quality threshold, for example. It might require that networks of providers in plans be sufficiently deep or geographically broad. It may impose limits on the nature of the deductibles or copays that may be assessed in each of the tiers of coverage; it may impose additional limits on underwriting. It may only accept plans with premiums at or below some level.

3. *Active purchaser.* In this model, the exchanges functions much as an employer would. The exchange would select which plans with which sets of benefits, copays, and deductibles it wishes to offer and then negotiate premiums with insurers. Individuals and small employers would then purchase coverage from the exchanges, but only for the plans that have been selected by the exchange.

The top panel of Exhibit 22.2 shows the distribution of initial decisions about the approaches taken by the 17 states and the District of Columbia adopting state-based

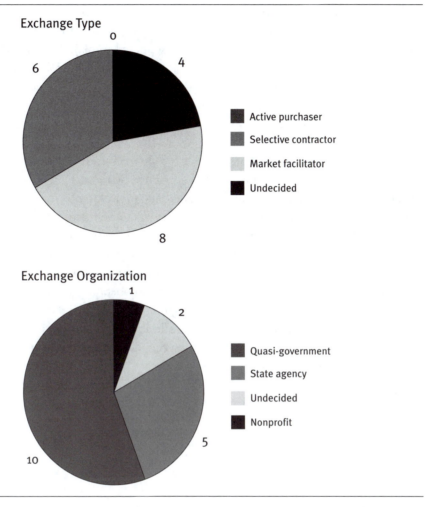

EXHIBIT 22.2
Characteristics
of State-Based
Exchanges, 2013

SOURCE: Data from KFF (2013a).

exchanges. The majority intend to be market facilitators. The states that adopt the federal default or the partnership are also required to be market facilitators. Four states, as of early 2013, were still undecided.

GOVERNANCE

The states have several options for organizing and governing their exchanges. The states can establish a new state agency or assign the responsibilities to an existing agency, such as the department of insurance, the state Medicaid agency, or the agency that runs the state employees' health plans. There are advantages and disadvantages to using a state agency. On the plus side, as government entities, oversight is clearly established and access to sensitive or confidential data related to enrollment and income, among other elements, is maintained in-house. However, state agencies may lack the flexibility and speed necessary to hire and adequately staff an expanded or new organization. Procurement and financial rules may inhibit the role that an exchange is supposed to play. There are also potential conflicts of interest and lack of expertise. Can a department of insurance, for example, which is typically charged with regulating insurers, also provide outreach and marketing for plans within an exchange? Can a Medicaid agency dealing with a major Medicaid expansion also provide adequate attention to interactions with private insurers seeking to participate in an exchange?

A quasi-governmental agency is a second alternative. These entities are established by the legislature and governed by a board appointed by the state. They can be chartered with the power to interact with the Medicaid agency, for example, in the use of Medicaid data for the determination of eligibility and the state revenue department to determine income levels for eligibility for exchange subsidies. However, they are also sufficiently independent from state personnel and financial procedural requirements that would allow them flexibility in establishing an exchange. The challenge with this approach is the creation of a management structure, accountability, and operating procedures.

Finally, a state may choose to create a nonprofit organization to run its exchange(s). Such an organization would provide even more flexibility in organizing an exchange. However, it may not be appropriate for determining eligibility for government programs, granting exemptions to rules, and in assessing penalties.

The bottom panel of Exhibit 22.2 shows that states have taken all of these approaches, with the quasi-government agency being the most popular. Obviously, if a state takes the federal default option, no governance issues need to be decided. However, as we discuss later in the chapter, the states may play several roles in both the partnership and default models.

THE NUMBER OF EXCHANGES AND RISK POOLS

The ACA calls for the creation of two exchanges: an individual exchange and a Small Business Health Options Program, or SHOP exchange. The states have the options to combine the administration of the two exchanges into a single entity and/or to combine the two risk pools into a single pool.

The expectation is that the state-based plans will combine the administration into a single entity because there are likely to be substantial economies of scale in running the exchanges.

However, the states will likely establish distinct risk pools for each segment. The key issue in this decision is adverse selection. The concern is that small employers with low claims experience will seek to remain outside the exchanges and be charged premiums that more closely reflect their actual claims experience. In contrast, small firms with higher claims experience have an incentive to purchase coverage through the exchanges, where their higher claims experience will blend in with other purchasers and keeping their premiums lower than would otherwise be the case. By keeping the individual and small-group risk pools separate, the view is that the individual market, to some extent, will be shielded from the premium-increasing aspects of this phenomenon.

Adverse selection may be enhanced if small employer plans become self-insured in large numbers. Virtually all large firms that offer insurance offer one or more self-insured plans. A small employer may do so as well by purchasing stop-loss coverage. The small employer would pay all claims costs until some threshold, say, 125 percent of expected claims. Then the stop-loss feature would be activated and the firm would pay no additional claims that year. Thus, a small employer with a healthy workforce would have low claims experience that was not averaged among others through the exchange. Moreover, because exchange plans must meet guaranteed issue provisions, a small employer could switch to an exchange plan at a later date if its claims experience is worse than anticipated.

FUNCTIONS OF THE EXCHANGES

The exchanges have five core functions to perform:

1. *Eligibility determination.* The exchange must be able to determine eligibility for Medicaid, CHIP, and individual subsidies for purchasing coverage through an exchange. To do this the exchange needs virtually real-time access to data on household income, citizenship, and residence, and whether the individual has access to affordable coverage through her employer. (*Affordable* means the out-of-pocket premium contribution is no more than 9.5 percent of household income.) Moreover, coverage is not assured for 12 months, so the exchanges must be able to deal with changing individual circumstances. In doing this it is almost a given that the exchanges will interface with the state Medicaid program (and possibly CHIP). The federal government is developing a data hub that will make the relevant federal data available in a timely fashion. In the summer of 2013, the federal government determined that the data hub would not be ready by the October 1, 2013, open enrollment period, and people would be on their honor to report correct information.[1]

2. *Enrollment.* The exchanges must be able to enroll people in Medicaid and CHIP as well as enroll individuals and small employers in their selected private exchange plans. They must also be able to disenroll individuals and businesses for reasons such as nonpayment of premiums or changes in plan choice. In the individual market these duties are straightforward.

However, they are much more complicated in the small group exchange, depending on how the state organizes small-employer options. The exchange could function much as a small employer currently does: The small employer chooses one plan for all of his employees. Alternatively, an employer may be allowed to choose the carrier, say Blue Cross or Aetna, and the employees may choose plans from any of those offered by the carrier. A third approach would have the employer choose a plan tier, say *silver*, and the employees may choose any plan offered by any carrier in that tier. Finally, the exchange could allow employees to choose any plan from any carrier offered through the exchange. In this case the employer plays no role in carrier or plan selection. In the summer of 2013 the federal government also determined that its SHOP exchange would not be fully functional. Instead of the full set of options across all plans and tiers, in the first year the SHOP exchange would only be able to let an employer choose a single plan for all of its workers—much as small employers typically have done heretofore.

3. *Plan management.* The exchanges must certify qualified health plans. This means the plans must provide the essential health benefits specified in the ACA and any other terms or limits on coverage as specified by final rules from the Department of Health and Human Services and from the state's own requirements. (See the earlier discussion about the exchanges as selective contractors or active purchasers.) The exchanges are also responsible for assigning a quality ranking to each plan offered in the exchange and for reviewing and (in some cases) approving rates. They are responsible for reviewing marketing, network adequacy, accreditation, and quality improvement programs. In addition, the exchanges, working with the state department of insurance, will provide general oversight of the health plans.

4. *Consumer assistance.* The exchanges must provide a single application process that an individual can access online, by phone, or in person. They are required to conduct outreach and education. Evidence from Massachusetts suggests that people need considerable assistance in enrolling in an exchange health plan (Sinaiko et al. 2012). This is not surprising, given that most people have either obtained health insurance through an employer or have been enrolled in a public program. The exchange concept requires a deeper understanding of insurance and insurance terms than has been necessary previously. As part of this requirement, the exchanges are to retain *navigators*. These people or organizations are either exchange employees or contracted groups, such as chambers of commerce or community centers, that will assist people in working through the process of enrolling and in understanding their options. It is important to note that the exchanges must also help individuals and small employers compare coverage and premiums. As part of this effort, the

exchanges must have premium calculators that will allow people to determine their premiums, net of any subsidy across various plan options. Premium calculators may go further and incorporate likely health services utilization, deductibles, and copays into the computation.

5. *Financial management.* Obviously, the exchanges are responsible for accounting, auditing, and reporting. However, they can also collect premiums directly or serve simply as a pass-through of premiums from purchasers to insurers. An issue of paramount significance to the states is that each state-based exchange is to be self-sufficient by January 2015. An exchange could attain self-sufficiency in a variety of ways. The simplest, but perhaps least desirable, is to simply fund the exchange out of the state's general tax collections. More likely models include imposing a fee on all policies sold through the exchange, or imposing a fee on all individual and small-group policies, whether offered through the exchange or not.

States that accepted the federal default exchange can still perform some functions of the exchanges, if they choose. The state may determine Medicaid and CHIP eligibility and/or may perform some reinsurance activities (discussed later in this chapter). States that are establishing a state partnership exchange may undertake either or both of these functions and can also undertake the plan management and/or consumer assistance roles outlined previously. See Goodell (2013) and Carey (2011a) for more detailed discussions of the functions of the exchanges.

ESSENTIAL HEALTH BENEFITS

The ACA was relatively silent on the nature of the coverage that is to be provided through the exchanges. It listed ten essential benefits that each plan must provide (see sidebar). However, the legislation required the secretary of the Department of Health and Human Services to develop regulations defining the essential benefits in more detail. The secretary allowed the states to use one of four general benchmark health plans to define the benefits in their states. The four options are:

1. One of the three largest small-group plans in the state, by enrollment;

2. One of the three largest state employee health plans, by enrollment;

3. One of the three largest federal employee health benefit plan options, by enrollment; or

4. The largest HMO plan offered in the state's commercial market, by enrollment.

The 10 Essential Health Benefits Required by the ACA

1. Ambulatory patient services
2. Emergency services
3. Hospitalization
4. Maternity and newborn care
5. Mental health and substance abuse services
6. Prescription drugs
7. Rehabilitative services and devices
8. Laboratory services
9. Preventive and wellness services and chronic disease management
10. Pediatric services, including oral and vision care

This is not to imply that the deductibles, copays, coinsurance, or limits on units of service in the benchmark plan are made part of the essential benefits. Rather, the services covered in the benchmark plan selected would be the services required to be offered by plans in the state's exchange(s). All states that have chosen to default to the federal exchange are required to use the largest small-group plan in their state as the benchmark. Most state-based or partnership exchanges (18) have chosen to do the same. Four will use the coverage offered by the state's largest HMO as a model, and three will use a state employee benefit plan. The National Conference of State Legislatures (2013) has an excellent website (www. ncsl.org/issues-research/health/state-ins-mandates-and-aca-essential-benefits.aspx) with links to each state's benchmark and a comparison of the options that were open to the state.

The exchanges will offer four tiers of coverage, "the medals levels," plus a catastrophic plan. Each tier of benefits is to cover all of the services included in the essential benefit package. The differences between the plans come in two dimensions. First, plans in each tier cover an increasing share of the actuarial cost of the essential benefit package. As shown in Exhibit 22.3, silver plans must cover 70 percent of the cost of the covered services. Gold and platinum plans cover larger percentages and will have higher premiums. Bronze plans cover a smaller share.

Second, the plans within a tier will differ by how the consumer satisfies his or her share of the actuarial cost. One approach may be a plan that offers a relatively large deductible, but has low copays once the deductible is satisfied. Another plan in the same tier may have a modest deductible, but copays for some services and a coinsurance rate for others. The only requirement in the legislation is that the cost sharing for each plan in tier is actuarially expected to cover the remaining share of the costs of care. Thus, in the silver tier the out-of-pocket cost sharing for each plan will cover 30 percent of the costs of service.

Insurers are not required to offer plans in every tier. They are required, however, to offer one silver and one gold plan in every exchange in which they participate.

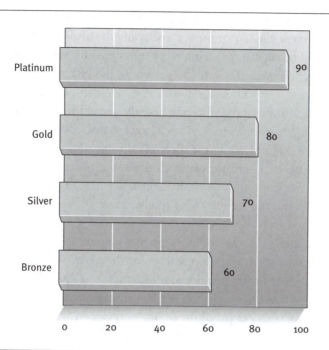

EXHIBIT 22.3
Percentage of the
Actuarial Cost
of the Essential
Benefits Covered
by Exchange Plan
Tiers

The catastrophic plan is somewhat different than the others. It is only available in the individual exchange, and it may only be sold to people under age 30 and to those who would otherwise be exempt from buying coverage because the premiums would be greater than 8 percent of their income. These plans don't have to meet actuarial cost percentages, but the size of the deductible and out-of-pocket maximum must meet the current requirements for a health savings account (HSA) plan. (In 2013 these values were $1,250 and $6,250, respectively.)

SUBSIDIES WITHIN THE EXCHANGES

In general, anyone may purchase coverage in the individual exchange and, as we note later, the expectation is that many people who currently buy nongroup coverage will do so. The ACA provides for an advanceable, refundable tax credit as a subsidy for lower-income people, many of whom currently do not have insurance. It also provides subsidies for the out-of-pocket cost of healthcare services.

TAX CREDITS

The tax credit is designed to cover the cost of the second-least costly silver plan offered in the area. However, regardless of the cost of that plan, the tax credit may be no greater than a specified percentage of the person's income, as defined by the legislation. Tax credits are provided from 100 to 400 percent of the federal poverty level (FPL). The poverty level depends on the number of people in the household and is adjusted every year. Exhibit 22.4 shows the income levels eligible for the tax credits and the income range for a family of two in 2013 that would be eligible for each level of subsidy. Thus, some living in a two-person family with income between 100 and 138 percent of the FPL would have annual income between $15,510 and $21,404. As Exhibit 22.4 shows, that person would have to pay no more than 2 percent of her income to purchase the second-lowest-cost silver plan in her area. People with higher incomes have to pay a larger share of their income for the coverage.

Suppose the second-lowest-cost silver plan in the area costs $5,000. Exhibit 22.4 shows the maximum tax credit people at the midpoint of each income level would be eligible to receive. Someone with an annual income of $18,457 (the midpoint of the 100 to 138 percent FPL income range) would receive a maximum subsidy of $4,631 toward the purchase of the silver plan. He would have to pay $369 of his own money for the coverage. The size of the subsidy declines at higher income levels. Notice that in the 300 to 400 percent income level, $5,000 premium for the silver plan is less than 9.5 percent of the income of someone with the midpoint income (i.e., $5,000 is less than 0.095 times $54,285). It is important to note that an individual may buy a plan from any tier, but the size of the subsidy remains pegged to the second-least expensive silver plan.

An advanceable, refundable tax credit is one that can be obtained prior to submitting one's tax forms and can be obtained even if one doesn't owe any taxes. A tax credit is typically obtained when one completes one's annual income tax forms. A credit of, say, $4,000 would mean that one's tax liability is reduced by $4,000. If one had no tax liability one could not use the tax credit. A refundable credit means that one would get the credit even if no taxes were owed. Thus, one could get a refund based on the credit. This sort of subsidy may not help someone who is eligible for a credit to buy insurance, but cannot get the subsidy until she files her tax forms in the following year. As a consequence, the ACA tax credit is advanceable. What that means is that the exchange will make an estimate of the

Exhibit 22.4 Individual Exchange Subsidies			
Income Level	**2013 Federal Poverty Level (FPL) Income Range for a Family of Two**	**Maximum Percentage of Income to Be Paid for Insurance**	**Maximum Subsidy for a $5,000 Silver Plan at the Midpoint of the FPL**
100 to 138% FPL	$15,510–$21,404	2.00	$4,631
138 to 150% FPL	$21,404–$23,265	3.00 to 4.00	$4,219
150 to 200% FPL	$23,265–$31,020	4.00 to 6.30	$3,602
200 to 250% FPL	$31,020–$38,775	6.30 to 8.05	$2,496
150 to 300% FPL	$38,775–$46,530	8.05 to 9.50	$1,255
300 to 400% FPL	$46,530–$62,040	9.50	No subsidy

size of the tax credit one can receive and then apply it to the premium of the plan selected. When one completes the tax forms the following year the actual credit is determined, and one may owe more taxes or receive a somewhat larger credit than originally estimated.

COST-SHARING SUBSIDIES

These subsidies reduce the liability that lower-income people face when using health services. If one were to purchase a silver plan, the out-of-pocket liability would be 30 percent. For lower-income people the out-of-pocket liability is reduced. For those with incomes between 100 and 150 percent of the FPL, the out-of-pocket liability is 6 percent. For those 150 to 200 percent of the FPL, the out-of-pocket liability is 13 percent. For those with incomes of 200 to 250 percent of the FPL, the out-of-pocket liability for services is 27 percent. Thus, the deductibles, copays, and coinsurance that would be required are to be commensurately reduced.

SMALL-EMPLOYER SUBSIDIES

Small employers with fewer than 50 full-time employees are not required to offer health insurance to their workers. However, those with 25 or fewer employees are eligible for a tax credit of up to 50 percent of the "employer's contribution" toward the insurance premium. However, this subsidy is only available if the firm's contribution is at least 50 percent of the full premium and the average annual wage is less than $50,000. The size of the subsidy is reduced as firm size and average wage levels increase. The subsidy is only available for two years.

EXCHANGES WITH NO STATE MEDICAID EXPANSION

The Supreme Court declared in June 2012 that the ACA overreached when it required the states to expand their Medicaid program or lose all the federal matching funds for

---

Default Exchanges and the Availability of Individual Subsidies

There is some contention as to the authority of the federal default exchanges to provide subsidies to those with incomes below 400 percent of the FPL. Goodell (2013) notes that opponents of the legislation argue that the language of the legislation only provides for state-based exchanges to make premium tax credits available. She also notes that the IRS has issued regulations stating that the credits are available through all exchanges. This point is currently being litigated.

their existing Medicaid program. As a result each state is free to decide whether or not to expand coverage.

Here we want to briefly highlight the implications for the exchanges if a state decides not to expand its Medicaid program. The Medicaid expansion is intended to cover individuals between the ages of 19 and 64 inclusive who had incomes below 138 percent of the FPL. If a state does not expand its program, these people are not eligible for Medicaid. They may purchase coverage through an exchange. However, only those with incomes above 100 of the FPL will be eligible for the individual subsidies. Thus, the exchanges in states that didn't expand will not see all or most of those who would have been Medicaid-eligible enrolled in their exchange. At this writing, some states are in discussions with the federal government over using potential Medicaid expansion money to subsidize the purchase of coverage through their state exchange for people who would have been eligible for Medicaid coverage had the state expanded its Medicaid program, but such alternative models have yet to be approved.

RISK ADJUSTMENT

Plans offered through the exchanges (as well as those offered outside the exchanges) are limited in the measures they may use in setting premiums. The ACA allows the use of age, with a maximum premium differential of 1 to 3 between the lowest and highest premium; geographic area; family composition; and tobacco use, in a band of 1 to 1.5. Plans may not use gender or preexisting health conditions. This last prohibition also implies that the plans may not use any measures of health status.

Nonetheless, it is likely that plans will not get a balanced distribution of enrollees. Some may get more higher-cost women and others more lower-cost men. Some may have physician and hospital networks that are located in lower-cost neighborhoods. Some may have a panel of specialist physicians that attracts a disproportionate number of enrollees with chronic conditions. Thus, adverse selection will continue to be a significant problem and will destabilize the market because those plans that enroll higher-cost subscribers will not be able to differentially charge premiums that reflect their subscriber mix.

ACA deals with this by requiring the exchanges to risk adjust the payments that are made to individual health plans (Weiner et al. 2012). It does so in three ways.

1. *Transitional reinsurance.* Over the period 2014 through 2016, states must establish a reinsurance program for the individual market. This program will collect payments from insurers in the individual, small-group, and administrative services–only markets and make payments to the insurers in the individual market to cover the costs of high-risk individuals. The fee in 2014 is $5.25 per covered individual per month. Essentially, the exchange will set a threshold or *attachment point* defining high-cost claims. Then the

exchange will use the money from the fees collected to compensate plans for some proportion of the costs of their high-cost claims.

2. *Risk-corridor program.* This program is also in effect from 2014 through 2016. The concern is that plans may experience large gains or losses over the first years of the exchange. Each health plan will be given a target amount for medical expenses, equal to their total premiums less allowable administrative costs. If their actual costs are more than 3 percent above or below this target, they will either receive or make a payment.

3. *Risk adjustment.* The ACA calls for a diagnosis-based risk adjustment mechanism that is to begin in 2014. It will include all populations covered by insurers in the individual and small-group markets, both inside and outside the exchanges. An insurer that has a disproportionately sicker population will receive a risk adjustment payment paid for by assessments on those insurers with disproportionately less-sick enrollment. While a model has not been released at this writing, it is anticipated that the methodology will closely resemble the CMS Hierarchical Condition Categories. Obviously, such conditions as pregnancy would have to be built into the system that was designed for the Medicare population.

Financing State Exchanges

The federal government bears the cost of running state-based exchanges in 2014. However, by 2015 the exchanges are to be self-sufficient. States could choose to fund an exchange in many ways. They could use general fund tax dollars or they could raise the state cigarette tax rate, as examples. More likely the states will impose a fee either on the plans sold through each exchange or on all individual and small-group plans sold in the state regardless of whether they are sold through an exchange or not. Federal default exchanges will charge a 3.5 percent fee on all plans sold in an exchange (Goodell 2013).

The size of the fees necessary to fund an exchange depends upon the costs of the activities undertaken by an exchange, the number of people to be covered, and whether the fee applies only inside the exchanges.

The State of Alabama decided to let the federal government run its exchanges. Nonetheless, it did undertake a number of analyses to gauge the costs of running a state-based model. The following estimates are drawn from Bob Carey's (2011a) analysis.

(continued)

(continued from previous page)

Alabama was estimated to have approximately 500,000 people who would potentially be eligible to participate in an individual exchange. Another 600,000 were estimated to be eligible for a state SHOP exchange. Not everyone eligible to enroll will do so, of course. Carey presented a range of estimates; his "moderate" estimate was that 60 percent of those eligible for the individual exchange and 5 percent of those eligible for the SHOP exchange would participate.[2]

The following table shows the cost estimates of running an administratively combined Alabama exchange for moderate combined enrollment of 330,000 in 2015.

EXHIBIT 22.5
Estimated Administrative Costs of Alabama Exchange— Moderate Enrollment of 330,000 People, 2015

Budget Category	Estimated Annual Cost
Eligibility determination	
Cost per enrollee	$17.50
Total cost	$5,775,000
Health plan enrollment	
Annual per enrollee	$96.00
Total cost	$31,680,000
Outreach and marketing	$4,000,000
Exchange staff	$2,750,000
Facilities	$300,000
Total	
Aggregate	$44,505,000
Per enrollee per month	$11.24

SOURCE: Data from Carey (2011a).

Eligibility determination includes such activities as determining eligibility for Medicaid and for tax credits, notifying applicants, adjudicating appeals, and responding to inquiries. Health plan enrollment costs relate to maintaining the infrastructure for comparing plans, maintaining the web portal and the decision support systems, and other duties. Outreach includes the navigator program as well as direct marketing about the exchange and its ability to assist consumers in obtaining care. Staff is estimated to

(continued)

(continued from previous page)

include 25 to 30 people. The aggregate annual cost was estimated at $44.5 million, or $11.24 per enrollee. For comparison, Massachusetts retains 3.0 percent of monthly premiums, or about $12.00 per enrollee.

Thus, if a fee were to be assessed only on those who purchase coverage through the individual or SHOP exchange, under these estimates the fee would be $11.24 per month in addition to the premium for coverage. In contrast, if a fee was assessed on all those who purchase coverage in the individual and small-group markets, regardless of whether they buy coverage through the exchange, the per enrollee per month cost would be $3.21.

Obviously, assessing a fee on all participants regardless of whether they buy through an exchange is controversial. Small employer groups, particularly, argue that they would be made to pay for the operation of an exchange that the estimates suggest they wouldn't use. The proponents argue that any reduction in premiums that arise from increased insurer competition would benefit all those who buy coverage whether or not they use an exchange.

ESTIMATED ENROLLMENT IN THE EXCHANGES

Parente and Feldman (2013) have the most extensive simulation of the likely effects of the ACA on enrollment in the individual and group markets. They are unable to provide estimates of the exchanges, per se, as that would require assumptions about the proportion of people getting coverage in and outside of an exchange. However, they can look at everyone below age 65. Exhibit 22.6 presents their baseline estimates; these estimates do not take into account the Supreme Court decision making the Medicaid expansion voluntary. Overall, the number of uninsured decreases by 38 percent between 2012 and 2014, from 54.8 to 34.1 million. This is because of large increases in both the number of privately insured and in those covered by Medicaid.

The individual market will see an increase of more than 12 million people between 2012 and 2014 in the Parente and Feldman simulation. Their model uses Medical Expenditure Panel Survey (MEPS) data among other elements. They viewed the least restrictive PPOs, those with low deductibles and no copays, as the equivalent of platinum plans. Gold plans were mid-restrictive PPOs, and silver plans were considered PPOs with narrower panels of providers, higher deductibles, and larger copays. Bronze and catastrophic plans were considered to be high-deductible health plans. From this perspective, individual enrollment in silver, gold, and platinum plans increases by 55 percent with the first year implementation of the ACA. Bronze and catastrophic plans increase enrollment by an estimated 27 percent.

The group market considered here includes both small and large groups. The anticipated shifts are more complicated. First, there is a decrease in enrollment of approximately 12 million from restrictive PPOs. These are the plans with limited provider networks and

EXHIBIT 22.6
Estimates of Under
Age 65 Insurance
Enrollment
Before and After
Implementation
of ACA, in Millions

	2012	2014	Change
Total Coverage			
Privately insured	205.7	226.9	21.2
Medicaid	34.9	52.0	17.1
Uninsured	54.8	34.1	−20.7
Individual Market			
Platinum, gold, or silver	13.1	20.3	7.2
Bronze or catastrophic	19.5	24.7	5.2
Total individual	32.6	45.0	12.4
Group Market			
PPO – least restrictive	22.4	18.5	−3.9
PPO – mid-restrictive	2.8	3.4	0.6
PPO – most restrictive	81.9	69.8	−12.1
HMO	5.9	5.9	0.0
HRA	18.1	17.7	−0.4
HSA-funded	2.0	3.9	1.9
ESI to self-pay PPO	0.1	3.5	3.4
ESI to other/exchange	19.6	30.4	10.8
Refused coverage	5.9	5.5	−0.4

SOURCE: Data from Parente and Feldman (2013).

high deductibles and/or copays. These folks largely move to "ESHI to other/exchange," which see increased enrollment of 10.8 million. Many of these are the people who currently have insurance coverage through a small employer who is not required to offer coverage. Recall that employers with fewer than 50 employees are not required to offer coverage. If these firms have a large proportion of workers with low income, they and their workers can be money ahead by dropping coverage, raising wages, and taking coverage through an individual exchange where many of them would be eligible for a subsidy. The group of switchers in Exhibit 22.6 also includes some with spousal coverage who will switch plans.

Second, there is an anticipated reduction of nearly 4 million in enrollment in the most generous plans, the "PPO–least restrictive." Some people in these plans shift to less costly options. Third, there are also anticipated to be approximately 3.4 million people who buy coverage from a qualified exchange plan and the employer pays a penalty. These are the "ESHI to self-pay PPO" in the exhibit.

The estimates change if the states do not expand their Medicaid programs. The challenge, of course, is predicting which states, if any, choose not to expand their programs. However, for our consideration of the exchanges the key issue is what happens to private insurance coverage. Parente and Feldman (2013) consider the case when six states opt out: Florida, Louisiana, Mississippi, Nebraska, South Carolina, and Texas. Exhibit 22.7 displays their simulation results. Their work suggests that initially enrollment in private plans will increase by about 3.3 million people. Many of these people have incomes between 100 and 138 percent of the FPL and will have subsidies through the exchanges. Others will remain in employer plans. However, over time, health insurance premiums increase and the number of insured declines under both scenarios. After 2018, Parente and Feldman expect that the higher premium costs of private coverage will lead many people to drop private coverage. As Exhibit 22.7 shows, the drop-off is larger when some states don't expand Medicaid.

ESTIMATED PREMIUM COSTS IN THE EXCHANGES

Ideally, we would like to know, with some precision, what the premium purchased by an individual of defined characteristics would be just prior to the implementation of the ACA, just after, and say, three years after that. That is, as a 26-year-old male, how much is my nongroup insurance premium today, and how much would coverage cost me if purchased through an exchange? Those sorts of computations, if they exist, do not appear to be publicly available. There are good reasons for this. Such computations require a number of assumptions and decisions. Do we want to compare identical coverage before and after?

EXHIBIT 22.7

Estimates of Private Coverage with and Without Full Medicaid Expansion

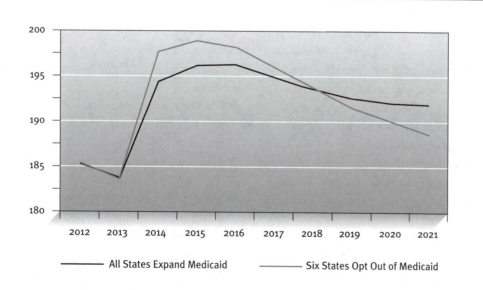

SOURCE: Data from Parente and Feldman (2013).

Do we want the premium differences to reflect changes in coverage that are required? The amount of premium change will depend, in part, on the regulatory environment in place in a given state. Do we want a national average comparison, or one that is state specific? Are we interested in gold coverage . . . or silver? And so on, and so on.

We do have some actuarial work that begins to address these questions. The Society of Actuaries (SOA 2013) released a report that estimates the average premium consequences of the ACA on the nongroup market. Exhibit 22.8 provides the SOA's overall estimates both nationally and for selected states. In 2017, three years after implementation, the SOA estimates that, on average, the per-member per-month premiums for coverage purchased through an exchange will be 31.5 percent higher under the ACA than they would have been otherwise. There is considerable variation in both the pre-ACA premium levels and the forecast premium increases. States like Ohio and Wisconsin have premium increases estimated to be 80 percent. In contrast, New York and Massachusetts are forecast to see declines in average premiums on the order of 13 percent.

The states with the largest increases in premiums also appear to have the lowest pre-ACA premiums. If insurers in these states are allowed to medically underwrite, for example, the *average* premium will encompass more healthier and fewer sicker subscribers. Thus, when the ACA eliminates the use of these underwriting practices, greater numbers of sicker individuals are brought into the risk pool, resulting in higher average premiums.

In contrast, the states with the smallest increases and with actual declines in average premiums are much more likely to have regulated underwriting rules. New York, Massachusetts, and Vermont were among the states that eliminated medical underwriting. Thus, it is not surprising that we see in Exhibit 22.7 that these states have high pre-ACA *average* premiums. Eliminating medical underwriting would lead to higher average premiums at baseline. Healthier individuals would have seen higher premiums and disproportionately chosen not to enroll. Sicker individuals, averaged into a common risk pool, would have found lower premiums, and they disproportionately would have joined. The consequence of this earlier action is that the insurance mandate in the ACA, requiring most people to have coverage, means that disproportionately healthier people are joining the risk pool in these states. This would reduce the average premium.

The SOA report also provides some insight into how premiums may vary across personal characteristics once the ACA is implemented. As we know, the ACA prohibits the use of gender in setting premiums and differences by age may only extend to a 1-to-3 range. Exhibit 22.9 provides some selected cost ratios for men and women at different ages for a standard benefit package. It shows, for example, that in a population of insured men and women (drawn from the MEPS), a 30-year-old male has expected claims experience of 62.25 percent of average; a 30-year-old woman has expected claims experience of 117.80 percent of average. Indeed, women have claims experience that is higher than men until age 55, after which women have lower expected claims.

The ACA says that women and men may not be treated differently. Thus, with equal numbers of 30-year-old men and women, their combined expected claims experience would be 91.53 of average. Thus, with no other changes, a 30-year-old man's premium

State	Pre-ACA	Post-ACA	Percent Change
Ohio	$223	$403	80.9%
Wisconsin	$258	$464	80.0
Indiana	$272	$455	67.6
Maryland	$284	$473	66.6
Idaho	$211	$343	62.2
California	$260	$420	61.6
Alabama	$263	$422	60.3
Missouri	$238	$378	58.8
District of Columbia	$348	$528	51.9
Illinois	$304	$459	50.8
National Average	$314	$413	31.4%
Washington	$314	$357	13.7
North Carolina	$361	$409	13.5
Iowa	$350	$384	9.7
North Dakota	$326	$353	8.4
Maine	$468	$487	4.1
New Jersey	$481	$474	−1.4
Rhode Island	$587	$548	−6.6
Vermont	$587	$514	−12.5
Massachusetts	$519	$453	−12.8
New York	$619	$533	−13.9

EXHIBIT 22.8

Average Forecast Premium Increases in the Non-Group Market—National Average and States with Largest and Smallest Increases, 2017

NOTE: Premiums are per member per month. The analysis assumes that all states expand their Medicaid programs. If none do so, the estimated national increase in premium was 28.9 percent.

SOURCE: Data from SOA (2013).

would be expected to increase by 70.5 percent, and a 30-year-old woman's would decrease by 29.3 percent. Other things equal, men below age 55 should expect that their insurance premiums will increase relative to what they paid prior to the ACA; women should expect, for the most part, that their premiums decline.

	Age	Male	Female	Combined	"Smoothed" Age Groups	3-to-1 Rating Band
EXHIBIT 22.9 Gender and Age Rating for Single Coverage	20	0.4303	0.8518	0.6411		
	25	0.4662	1.3368	0.9015	<25	0.6355
	30	0.5368	1.2937	0.9153		
	35	0.6225	1.1780	0.9003	25–34	0.7517
	40	0.7450	1.2852	1.0151		
	45	0.9105	1.1092	1.0099	35–44	1.0635
	50	1.1522	1.2747	1.2135		
	55	1.4966	1.4966	1.4966		
	60	1.9568	1.8045	1.8807	55+	1.9144
	65	2.8144	2.3277	2.5711		

SOURCE: Data by gender from Figure B-4, rating bands from Figure B-5 (SOA 2013). Combined values computed based on equal numbers of men and women in each age strata.

The SOA also provided some insight into the effects of the 3-to-1 rating band that is allowed for premium differentials based on age. The plans offered through the exchanges may charge different premiums based upon age. However, the oldest subscriber may not be charged a premium that is more than three times the premium for the youngest subscriber for the same coverage. From Exhibit 22.9 we can see that the range of premiums for 65-year-old males is more than six times the premium for a 20-year-old. For both genders combined it was more than four times greater. The SOA reports that their simulation suggests that a 3-to-1 premium range would have people under age 25 with a premium that was 63.55 percent of the average, while those aged 55 and older would pay premiums of 191.44 percent of average. Thus, the required narrowing of the allowable age band has the effect of still leaving men younger than 55 worse in terms of premiums than they were prior to the ACA, and those over age 60 are made better off. For women, post-ACA premiums are lower for those younger than 45, but worse off for those aged 60 and above. All of this, of course, ignores the effects of health status on premiums.

NOTES

1. The potential for fraud is limited, however, in that people do have to report their income and any ACA insurance subsidy they receive on their federal income tax forms in the next year.

2. The 5 percent estimate is probably too high. As Carey notes, as of July 2011, fewer than 2,500 employees were covered by the Massachusetts Health Connector (that state's small-group exchange). This represented only 0.5 percent of the small-group market.

Summary

◆ Twenty-six states have opted for the federal-default exchange, in which the federal government runs the exchanges in their state.

◆ These states and the majority of the state-based exchanges will be market facilitators. They will offer all qualified health plans on their exchanges.

◆ The majority of state-based exchanges will be quasi-governmental entities with their boards appointed by the state government.

◆ An exchange has five core functions: determining eligibility for Medicaid and for tax subsidies, enrollment, plan management, consumer assistance, and financial management.

◆ The ten essential health benefits defined in the ACA are operationalized at the state level by the selection of a benchmark plan, typically the plan in the small-group market with the largest enrollment.

◆ Most people who would have been eligible for Medicaid coverage through the ACA Medicaid expansion will not be eligible for a tax subsidy to buy coverage through an exchange, if their state decides not to expand Medicaid.

◆ The exchanges must implement risk adjustment methodology to account for the adverse selection across health plans.

◆ Exchanges must be self-sufficient by 2015.

For the Interested Reader

Goodell, S. 2013. "Federally Facilitated Exchanges." Health Policy Brief. Published January 31. www.healthaffairs.org/healthpolicybriefs/brief.php?brief_id=84.

Parente, S. T., and R. Feldman. 2013. "Microsimulation of Private Health Insurance and Medicaid Take-Up Following the US Supreme Court Decision Upholding the Affordable Care Act." *Health Services Research* 48 (2, Part II): 826–49.

Weiner, J. P., E. Trish, and K. Lemke. 2012. "Adjusting for Risk Selection in State Health Insurance Exchanges Will Be Critically Important and Feasible, but Not Easy." *Health Affairs* 31 (2): 306–15.

References

Carey, R. L. 2011a. "Financial Sustainability of the Alabama Exchange." National Governors Association. Accessed May 23, 2013. http://statepolicyoptions.nga.org/policy_article/financial-sustainability-alabama-exchange.

Goodell, S. 2013. "Federally Facilitated Exchanges." *Health Policy Brief*. Published January 31. www.healthaffairs.org/healthpolicybriefs/brief.php?brief_id=84.

Kaiser Family Foundation (KFF). 2013a. "Establishing Health Insurance Marketplaces: An Overview of State Efforts." Published May 2. http://kff.org/health-reform/issue-brief/establishing-health-insurance-exchanges-an-overview-of/.

LoSasso, A. T., and I. Z. Lurie. 2009. "Community Rating and the Market for Private Non-Group Health Insurance." *Journal of Public Economics* 93 (1–2): 264–79.

National Conference of State Legislatures (NCSL). 2013. "State Health Insurance Mandates and the PPACA Essential Benefits Provisions." Accessed June 20. www.ncsl.org/issues-research/health/state-ins-mandates-and-aca-essential-benefits.aspx.

Parente, S. T., and R. Feldman. 2013. "Microsimulation of Private Health Insurance and Medicaid Take-Up Following the U.S. Supreme Court Decision Upholding the Affordable Care Act." *Health Services Research* 48 (2, Part II): 826–49.

Sinaiko, A. D., D. Ross-Degnan, S. B. Soumerai, T. Lieu, and A. Galbraith. 2012. "The Experience of Massachusetts Shows That Consumers Will Need Help in Navigating Insurance Exchanges." *Health Affairs* 32 (1): 78–86.

Society of Actuaries (SOA). 2013. "Cost of the Future Newly Insured Under the Affordable Care Act (ACA)." Accessed May 29, 2013. www.soa.org/files/research/projects/research-cost-aca-report.pdf.

Weiner, J. P., E. Trish, C. Abrams, and K. Lemke. 2012. "Adjusting for Risk Selection in State Health Insurance Exchanges Will Be Critically Important and Feasible, but Not Easy." *Health Affairs* 31 (2): 306–15.

CHAPTER 9

HEALTH POLICY AND ADVOCACY

The Affordable Care Act (ACA) was enacted in 2010, and as time passes it will be modified—the health policy journey continues. Looking at the process of policymaking is useful for understanding how these changes may unfold over the coming years.

HEALTH POLICY PROCESS

Policymaking has been part of the world since government has existed. As a result, scholars have studied this process for many years and developed a variety of theories to explain it.

Longest **(Reading 9A)** has articulated a useful model, which includes the five major activities in health policymaking:

1. *Agenda setting:* Who decides which issues need attention, and how do they bring these issues into the public debate?

2. *Policy formulation:* How does legislation get drafted, passed, and signed into law?

3. *Rules:* How does the government write the detailed rules?

4. *Implementation:* How are new policies implemented by healthcare organizations?

5. *Modification:* All policies are improved over time—how does this occur?

All of these steps must be considered in the context of the healthcare system stakeholders (e.g., federal officials, states, provider organizations, consumer advocacy groups).

Reading 9A provides a detailed examination of both systems and markets views of healthcare policymaking.

THE STATES

Although most of the ACA involves actions by the federal government, the states also play a key role in its implementation. Historically states have served as laboratories for testing new policy initiatives. For example, the federal healthcare exchanges are based on a similar successful model pioneered in Massachusetts.

Examples of states' activities related to the ACA are:

◆ Connecting state Medicaid systems to either the state or federal exchanges

◆ Expanding the eligibility limits of Medicaid to 133 percent of the federal poverty level, a state option

◆ Operating healthcare exchanges as a state option

◆ Helping to operate navigator programs to encourage enrollment

◆ Establishing the details of the essential benefits set

◆ Continuing to administer scope of practice laws that influence the delivery of primary care

◆ Enact "any willing provider" statues to reduce or eliminate narrow networks (predominately targeted at pharmacies)

◆ Establishing state compacts that allow insurance to be sold across state lines

Although state policymaking is similar in some aspects to the federal system, it also has key differences. **Reading 9B** provides an overview and case studies related to state-level health policymaking.

HEALTH POLICY AND ADVOCACY

This is an invitation for you, the reader, to get into the game. Active participation, innovation, and creativity built the US government, and your expertise is needed. The thoughtful healthcare leader has three opportunities to become involved: through associations, through innovations and demonstrations, and as a policy expert.

HEALTHCARE ASSOCIATIONS AND LOBBYING

The easiest path for involvement in health policy is through the numerous healthcare associations. These associations may represent organizations (e.g., American Hospital Association) or individual professionals (e.g., American Medical Association). Much of the US healthcare system is affected by governmental policy; most associations have a legislative affairs committee. By joining these committees, leaders have an opportunity to shape and influence policy. Start with state associations, as these are more accessible and much of the ACA will be implemented through state legislation and regulation.

Within these committees, members can fill two roles. One role is to create policy positions (e.g., "we need to increase the supply of nurse practitioners") and the other is to direct advocacy—otherwise known as lobbying.

Because of the intensity of the arena, lobbying is not for the faint of heart or those with thin skins. However, it can be deeply rewarding and can have a significant and wide-reaching effect on your community.

Healthcare professionals who want to be become effective lobbyists should do the following:

◆ Develop a 30-second elevator speech about your proposal. Successful pitches can lead to appointments with elected officials for more in-depth briefings. Here is an example:

Hello, Senator Berglin, I am Dan McLaughlin, the CEO of Vincent Valley Health System, and we have an interesting proposal for our state that could reduce obesity in children by 25 percent through a cooperative program with schools and hospitals. Can I come to your office and provide you with more details?

◆ Know the topic. Once you have your meeting scheduled, be able to present your proposal in depth or briefly. Know who knows the topic in more depth so you can refer the official's staff to them if she wants to explore the topic further.

◆ Know the legislative process. Never ask a legislator to do something that is prohibited by the rules (e.g., introduce a bill into the wrong committee). Engage a professional lobbyist to provide you with this information.

◆ Know the opposition. Surprisingly, the most innocent policy proposal will have opposition (in some cases bureaucrats protecting budgets or turf). Your elected official may agree to carry your legislative proposal; your duty is to provide her with information on the opposition and its arguments.

◆ Be respectful. Almost all elected officials strive to do the best for their constituencies and the country. They are almost never thanked and frequently take abuse from the general public. A thank you for their service will be highly appreciated.

INNOVATIONS IN CARE DELIVERY

The Center for Medicare & Medicaid Innovation (CMI) is designed to experiment with new delivery and payment systems. If your organization has developed an innovation, consider applying to CMI to execute a pilot. If your innovation is a success, it may be the basis for ACA version 2.

POLICY EXPERTISE

The third option to influence policy is to become an expert for an elected official. Most legislators choose one of two paths while in office. The first path is to focus on leadership, which requires an emphasis on party relationships, fundraising, media appearances, and the like. The second path is to focus on policy and become an expert in some subject. These legislators tend to craft the details of legislation and rely on experts to assist them. You can be their expert.

One of the most famous examples of this approach was chronicled in the book *The Dance of Legislation* by Eric Redman (2001). In 1971, Dr. Abe Berman of Seattle, Washington, became passionate about physician shortages in underserved areas of the country. He met regularly with US Senator Warren Magnuson and his staff to press the issue. Eventually Magnuson authored legislation to address this problem and did what was necessary to get it passed and signed by President Nixon. The legislation continues today as the National Health Service Corps, which is expanded in the ACA, Title V.

SUMMARY

As Longest (**Reading 9A**) explains,

Health policies, like those in other domains, are made within the context of the political marketplace, where demanders for and suppliers of policies interact. The federal and state governments have important health policy roles, and their policymaking processes are quite similar.

The demanders of policies include those who view public policies as a mechanism for meeting their health-related objectives or other objectives, such as economic advantage. Although individuals alone can demand public policies, the far more effective demand emanates from organizations and especially from organized interest groups. The suppliers of health policy include elected and appointed members of all three branches of government and the civil servants who staff the government.

The interests of the various demanders and suppliers in this market cannot be completely coincident—often, they are in open conflict—and the decisions and activities of any participant always affect and are affected by the activities of other participants. Public policymaking in the health domain is a human process, a fact with great significance for the outcomes and consequences of the process and one that argues for ethical behavior by all involved in the process.

The policymaking process itself is a highly complex, interactive, and cyclical process that incorporates formulation, implementation, and modification phases. These phases are discussed in detail in subsequent chapters.

Those who wish to actively engage in health policy have three options: engage in policy development and lobbying through a professional association, develop a project to be implemented by the CMI, or develop a specific area of policy expertise and assist other health policy professionals in their policy advocacy.

APPLICATIONS: DISCUSSION AND RESEARCH

1. Discuss the roles of states in health policy (Longest 2010; **Reading 9A**).

2. Who are demanders and suppliers of health policies? What motivates each in the political marketplace (Longest 2010; **Reading 9A**)?

3. Compare and contrast the pluralist and elitist perspectives on interest groups in the political marketplace (Longest 2010; **Reading 9A**).

4. Define power and influence. What are the sources of power in political markets (Longest 2010; **Reading 9A**)?

5. Draw a schematic model of the public policymaking process (Longest 2010; **Reading 9A**).

6. Describe the general features of the model drawn in question 5 (Longest 2010; **Reading 9A**).

7. Describe, and provide an example of, the policymaking process at the US local level.

8. What are the health policy–related activities of private health research institutes? Of private health foundations?

9. What kinds of public health information and initiatives are contributed by private industry?

10. List three characteristics of health policy development in the US state government, local government, and private sectors.

REFERENCE

Redman, E. 2001. *The Dance of Legislation*. Seattle: University of Washington Press.

READING 9A

THE CONTEXT AND PROCESS OF HEALTH POLICYMAKING

Beaufort B. Longest, Jr.
From *Health Policymaking in the United States*, 5th ed. (2010), Chapter 2, 33–74. Chicago: Health Administration Press.

Whether health policies take the form of laws, rules or regulations, operational decisions, or judicial decisions, all policies are decisions made through a complex process. With certain variations, policies at the federal, state, and local levels of government are made through similar processes. Furthermore, the structure of the decision-making process is the same for all policy domains, whether health, education, defense, taxes, welfare, or another area.

The domain of health policy is broad, because health is a function of multiple determinants: the physical environment in which people live and work, their behaviors and biology, social factors, and the health services to which they have access. The health domain also overlaps with other policy domains. For example, it is impossible to consider health policy apart from its relationship to tax policy. Health policy cannot be separated from the fact that government finances, essentially through taxes, many of the services or programs health policy establishes. At a minimum, any dollars spent as a result of public health policies have alternative uses in other domains.

Another example of overlapping policy domains is the 1996 Personal Responsibility and Work Opportunity Reconciliation Act (P.L. 104-193), also known as the Welfare Reform Act, which had significant health implications. In addition to the obvious effect of changes to the nation's welfare policy regarding such health determinants as the social and economic environments affected people face, this law fundamentally affected eligibility for Medicaid. Since the establishment of the Medicaid program in 1965, families receiving Aid to Families with Dependent Children (AFDC) have been automatically enrolled in the Medicaid program. The Welfare Reform Act, however, replaced AFDC with the Temporary Assistance to Needy Families (TANF) block grant. Under the provisions of the TANF block grant, states were given broad flexibility to design income support and work programs for low-income families with children and were required to impose federally mandated restrictions, such as time limits, on federally funded assistance.

The Welfare Reform Act provided for children and parents who would have qualified for Medicaid based on their AFDC eligibility to continue to be eligible for Medicaid. But in the absence of AFDC, states found it necessary to use different mechanisms to identify and enroll former AFDC recipients in their Medicaid programs. This example is typical of the overlap between policies in different domains. A former European Commissioner for Health and Consumer Protection describes this relationship as follows: "To achieve good health, we need to look at the grass root problems—poverty, social exclusion, healthcare access. We need to understand how different socio-economic and environmental factors affect health. And then we need to make all these factors work together for good health. Good health must become the driving force behind all policy-making" (Byrne 2004, 7).

The main purposes of this chapter are to provide a description of the political context within which health policymaking takes place and to present a model of the public policymaking process. The political context is discussed first, beginning with the fact that health policymaking is both a federal and a state responsibility. Subsequently, we describe features of the political marketplace and present a model of the policymaking process.

THE CONTEXT OF HEALTH POLICYMAKING: FEDERAL AND STATE GOVERNMENTS MAKE HEALTH POLICY

Health policy is a joint federal-state responsibility. Although much of this book is devoted specifically to policymaking at the federal level, almost all of the content applies equally at the state level. The two levels have somewhat different health policy responsibilities, but their organization, structure, and policymaking process are similar. As Weissert and Weissert (2006, 250–51) point out, each state has a constitution and a bill of rights. These documents set forth the structure and function of the state government and of the local governments within their boundaries. Each state has three branches of government, and the duties of each branch are essentially the same as those in the federal government. The legislative branch passes laws and oversees the executive branch, which implements the laws. The judiciary branch determines the constitutionality of laws and adjudicates violations of them at both levels.

An unsettled debate over the appropriate distribution of health policy responsibilities between federal and state governments dates from the nation's founding. Over the years, the balance has occasionally shifted, with the federal government dominating health policy for most of the period since the mid-1960s. Recent changes in states' responsibilities for operating the Medicaid program and the failure in the early 1990s of federally led attempts at comprehensive health reform have reinforced the states' traditional health policy roles, and some states have undertaken new, broader roles.

Current information about state health policy can be found at the Kaiser Family Foundation website (www.kff.org) in the section on State Health Policy. State-level data on demographics, health, and health policy, including health coverage, access, financing, and state legislation and budgets, are available at www.statehealthfacts.org.

STATES' ROLES IN HEALTH POLICY

The states' role in protecting and ensuring the public's health is their fundamental responsibility in the pursuit of health. However, states' health policy roles have expanded (Leichter 2008; King 2005). The key health policy responsibilities of states are briefly summarized in the following sections, beginning with the states' continuing role as guardians of the public's health.

States as Guardians of the Public's Health

States were granted constitutional authority to establish laws that protect the public's health and welfare. This responsibility engages states in protecting the environment; ensuring safe practices in workplaces and food service establishments; mounting programs to prevent injuries and promote healthy behaviors; and providing health services such as public health nursing and communicable disease control, family planning and prenatal care, and nutritional counseling. Since the attacks of September 11, 2001, state and regional public health departments have become vital participants in protecting the public from the health consequences of terrorist attacks.

States as Purchasers of Healthcare Services

Typically, the state government is the largest purchaser of healthcare services in a state (King 2005). States assume significant responsibility for funding their Medicaid programs. Although the costs of these programs are shared with the federal government, this program typically consumes 17–20 percent of state budgets (Kaiser Commission on Medicaid and the Uninsured 2009; National Governors Association and National Association of State Budget Officers 2009). Medicaid is among the highest policy—let alone health policy—priorities for the states. In addition to their Medicaid funding roles, the states also typically pay the costs of providing health insurance benefits to state employees and their dependents and, in many states, for other public-sector workers, such as teachers. The states also purchase services under the Children's Health Insurance Program (CHIP), and many have established state-only programs to assist the uninsured. Examples include Pennsylvania's AdultBasic plan, which expands coverage to more of the state's uninsured adults, and Oregon's Family Health Insurance Program, aimed at low-income working citizens and their dependents. States will likely continue to play increasingly important funding roles as part of their health policy responsibilities.

States as Regulators

States have legal authority to regulate almost every aspect of the healthcare system and many aspects of the overall pursuit of health. The states license and regulate health professionals through the provisions of their practice acts, and they license and monitor health-related organizations. States also establish and monitor compliance with environmental quality standards.

A particularly important aspect of the role of states in health-related regulation is their responsibility for the health insurance industry as it operates within their boundaries. States control the content, marketing, and price of health insurance products and health plans because the 1945 McCarran-Ferguson Act (P.L. 79-15) left most insurance regulation to the states. However, recent changes in federal law illustrate the tenuous line between federal and state regulation of this industry and portend continued vagueness in this relationship.

For example, the 1974 Employee Retirement Income Security Act (P.L. 93-406), commonly known as ERISA, preempts the states' regulation of pensions and self-insured employer health plans. The 1985 Consolidated Omnibus Budget Reconciliation Act (P.L. 99-272), also known as COBRA 1985, gives people leaving a job in any state the right to retain their existing employer-provided health insurance for up to 18 months by paying the premiums directly, plus a small surcharge. The 1996 Health Insurance Portability and Accountability Act (P.L. 104-191), also known as HIPAA, guarantees access to health insurance to employees who work for companies that offer health insurance benefits if and when they change jobs or become unemployed. The legislation also guarantees renewability of health insurance coverage so long as premiums are paid.

States as Safety Net Providers

States provide safety nets—although these are often porous—through their support for community-based providers, hospitals that provide charity care, local health departments and clinics that serve low-income people, and other programs that ensure access to appropriate healthcare services (King 2005).

An especially important category of community-based providers are the federally qualified health centers (FQHCs). These can be community health centers, migrant health centers, healthcare for the homeless programs, and other service providers. FQHCs receive much of their funding from federal grants but also depend in part on Medicaid and Medicare patients to subsidize care for their uninsured patients.

States as Educators

States subsidize medical education, often but not exclusively in state-supported medical schools. They also subsidize graduate medical education (GME) through Medicaid payments to teaching hospitals, state appropriations, and scholarship and loan programs. Most states provide incentives such as student loan repayments to students who help the state achieve its goals—for example, by choosing nursing or family practice or serving in low-income or rural areas.

More broadly, states provide funding and expertise for large-scale campaigns to improve population health through such educational programs as informing parents about immunization benefits and requirements or encouraging the general public to use seat belts and motorcycle helmets. They also provide funding to schools to support efforts to encourage healthy lifestyles by addressing such topics as nutrition, sex education, and drug and alcohol abuse among students.

States as Laboratories

In the health policy domain, the popular view considers states laboratories in which experimentation with such policy ideas as comprehensive approaches to health reform take place. According to this view, states try various solutions to problems, and the results demonstrate the usefulness of these solutions for other states and, in some instances, for federal policymakers.

Other views of this role are less positive. For example, Davidson (1997, 894), speaking of the states' efforts at comprehensive reform of their healthcare systems, notes, "On the one hand, we have fifty individual political markets which, implicitly, act or fail to act for their own reasons; on the other hand, we have the phenomenon of many, if not most, states taking up the same thorny topic in the same period." In other words, a variety of states, each pursuing solutions to the same problem in idiosyncratic ways under unique sets of reasons in the same time frames, are unlikely to treat each other as laboratories or to benefit much from the others' experiences. Oliver and Paul-Shaheen (1997, 721) support this view. They concluded from their study of six states that enacted major health reform legislation that the wide variation among their approaches to reform "casts doubt on the proposition that states can invent plans and programs for other states and the federal government to adopt for themselves."

Whether or not the states are particularly good laboratories for other states or for the federal government, their roles in health policy innovation are expanding. In the absence of federal solutions, some states have found at least partial solutions to some of the health policy challenges they face.

THE CONTEXT OF HEALTH POLICYMAKING: THE POLITICAL MARKETPLACE

The political marketplace for health policies has characteristics in common with a traditional economic market. Many different products and services, including those used in the

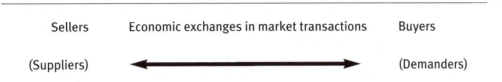

Sellers	Economic exchanges in market transactions	Buyers
(Suppliers)	⟵————————————⟶	(Demanders)

EXHIBIT 2.1
Relationships in the Political Marketplace

pursuit of health, are bought and sold in the context of economic markets. Willing buyers and sellers enter into economic exchanges in which each party attains something of value. One party demands, and the other supplies. By dealing with each other through market transactions, individuals and organizations buy needed resources and sell their outputs. These relationships are summarized in Exhibit 2.1.

NEGOTIATION IN MARKETS

Because people are calculative regarding the relative rewards and costs of market exchanges, they negotiate. Negotiation, or bargaining, involves two or more parties attempting to settle what each shall give and take (or perform and receive) in an economic transaction. The next section shows a parallel between this feature of economic markets and the operation of political markets. In the negotiations that take place in an economic market, the parties seek a mutually acceptable outcome in a situation where their preferences are usually negatively related (e.g., buyers prefer lower prices, while sellers prefer higher prices). Indeed, if the preferences for outcomes are positively related, an agreement can be reached almost automatically.

More typically, at least two types of issues must be resolved through the negotiations. One type involves the division of resources—the so-called tangibles of the negotiation, such as who will receive how much money and what products or services. Another type centers on the resolution of the psychological dynamics and the satisfaction of personal motivations of the negotiating parties. These issues are the intangibles of the negotiation and can include such notions as appearing to win or lose, to compete effectively, and to cooperate fairly.

Negotiations in economic exchanges usually follow one of two strategic approaches: cooperative (win/win) or competitive (win/lose) strategies. The better negotiating strategy in a particular situation is a function of the interaction of several variables (Watkins 2006). Greenberger and colleagues (1988) contrast the optimal conditions for cooperative negotiating strategies with the optimal conditions for competitive strategies as follows.

Cooperative negotiating strategies work best when

◆ the tangible goal of both negotiators is to attain a specific settlement that is fair and reasonable;

◆ sufficient resources are available in the environment for both negotiators to attain their tangible goal, more resources can be attained, or the situation can be redefined so that both negotiators can "win";

◆ each negotiator thinks it is possible for both to attain their goals through the negotiation process; or

◆ the intangible goals of both negotiators are to establish a cooperative relationship and to work together toward a settlement that maximizes their joint outcomes.

Competitive negotiating strategies work best when

◆ the tangible goal of both negotiators is to attain a specific settlement or to get as much as they possibly can;

◆ the available resources are not sufficient for both negotiators to attain their goals, or their desire to get as much as possible makes it impossible for one or both to actually attain their goals;

◆ both negotiators think it is impossible for both to attain their goals simultaneously; or

◆ the intangible goal of each negotiator is to beat the other.

THE OPERATION OF POLITICAL MARKETS

Health policies—indeed, all public policies—are made in the context of political markets, which in many ways operate like traditional economic markets. However, there are notable differences. The most fundamental is that buyers or demanders in economic markets express their preferences by spending their own money. That is, they reap the benefits of their choices, and they directly bear the costs of those choices. In political markets, on the other hand, the link between who receives benefits and who bears costs is less direct. Feldstein (2006), for example, observes that public policies that impose costs on future generations are routinely established. The nature of the political marketplace dictates that many decisions made by contemporary policymakers are influenced by the preferences of current voters, perhaps to the detriment of future generations. Such allocative policies as Medicare and Social Security are examples of this phenomenon. In the case of Social Security, outlays are projected to exceed revenues in the future; it is currently projected that this could occur first in 2019 (Congressional Budget Office 2008b).

The CBO (2008b) suggests that there are only four approaches to closing that gap, each of which has substantial drawbacks:

1. The benefits that are scheduled to be paid to future recipients under current law could be reduced, lowering Social Security's contribution to their income.

2. The taxes that fund Social Security could be raised to draw additional resources from the economy to the program.

3. The resources consumed by other federal programs could be reduced to cover the gap between Social Security's outlays and revenues.

4. The federal government's borrowing could be increased, which would be another way to draw more resources from the economy to Social Security. That borrowing would need to be repaid by future generations, however, either through increased taxes or reduced federal spending.

Of course, Social Security is not the only source of pressure on the federal budget. The financial crisis that engulfed the United States and most of the world beginning in late 2008 is causing an unprecedented increase in the federal deficit as government seeks a resolution. In addition, the aging of the U.S. population—which is the main cause of the projected increase in Social Security spending—will raise costs for other entitlement programs. In particular, the CBO projects that Medicare and Medicaid expenditures will grow even faster than Social Security outlays because of rising healthcare costs. Unless taxation reaches much higher levels in the United States, current spending policies are likely to prove financially unsustainable over the long term. The resulting burden of federal debt will have a corrosive and potentially contractionary effect on the economy.

Feldstein (2006) also points out that decision makers in political markets use different criteria from those used in traditional economic markets. In both markets, thoughtful decision makers take benefits and costs into account. In political markets, however, decision makers may use different time frames. Because legislators stand for periodic reelection, they typically favor policies that provide immediate benefits to their constituencies, and they tend to weigh only, or certainly more highly, immediate costs. Unlike most decision makers in economic markets, who consider costs and benefits over the long run, decision makers in political markets are more likely to base decisions on immediate costs and benefits. An obvious consequence of this is policies with immediate benefits but burdensome future costs.

In political markets, suppliers and demanders stand to reap benefits or incur costs because of the authoritative decisions called policies. Policies are therefore valued commodities in the political marketplace. These relationships are shown in Exhibit 2.2.

Given that demanders and suppliers will enter into exchanges involving policies, it is helpful to know who the demanders and suppliers are and what motivates their decisions and actions in political markets.

EXHIBIT 2.2
The Operation of
Political Markets

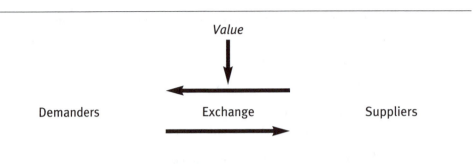

Usually involves negotiation

Structurally and operationally, a political market is much like an economic market.

DEMANDERS AND SUPPLIERS OF HEALTH POLICIES

As we noted, political markets operate similarly to economic markets. In both markets, something of value is exchanged between suppliers and demanders. Considering political markets in this way permits us to view public policies as a means of satisfying certain demanders' wants and needs in much the same way that products and services produced and sold in economic markets serve to satisfy demanders (or, in an economic context, consumers). In commercial markets, demanders seek products and services that satisfy them. In political markets, demanders seek public policies that satisfy their preferences. Policymakers are in a position to supply the public policies that demanders seek.

THE DEMANDERS OF HEALTH POLICIES

Broadly, the demanders of health policies can include (1) anyone who considers such policies relevant to the pursuit of their own health or that of others about whom they care and (2) anyone who considers such policies a means to some other desired end, such as economic advantage. These desires motivate participation in political markets, just as desires motivate participation in economic markets.

For individuals, however, effective participation in the political marketplace presents certain problems and limitations. To participate effectively, individuals must acquire substantial policy-relevant information, which can require considerable time and money. Beyond this, individual participants or demanders often must be prepared to expend additional time and money in support of achieving desired policies. Any particular health policy might have significant, or even noticeable, benefits for only a few individuals. Consequently, individual demander participation is limited in the political markets for policies.

Organizations, such as large health systems, health insurance companies, and technology suppliers, have a significant advantage over individuals in the political marketplace. They may have the necessary resources to garner needed policy-relevant information and to support their efforts to achieve desired policies. In addition, an organization's health policy interests may be concentrated. A change in Medicare policy that results in an increased deductible of $100 per year for certain individuals is one thing; a policy change that results in several million dollars of revenue for a health services organization is quite another. Organizations tend to be more effective demanders of health policy than individuals, in part because the stakes for them tend to be higher.

The most effective demanders of policies, however, are well-organized interest groups. These are groups of people or organizations with similar policy goals that enter the political process to try to achieve those goals. By combining and concentrating the resources of their members, interest groups can have a much greater impact than individuals or organizations alone.

In effect, interest groups provide their members—whether individuals or organizations—with greater opportunities to participate effectively in the political marketplace (McGarity and Wagner 2008; Cigler and Loomis 2007). This is what the American Medical Association (AMA; www.ama-assn.org) does for individual physicians, what the American Association of Retired Persons (AARP; www.aarp.org) does for older individuals, and what PhRMA does for its member companies. Because of their power in political markets, interest groups, as demanders of health policy, are described more fully in the next section.

INTEREST GROUPS IN THE POLITICAL MARKETPLACE

Interest groups (also called advocacy groups, lobby groups, pressure groups, or special interest groups) arise in democratic societies because the opportunities to achieve particular outcomes are enhanced through collective action in the political marketplace, specifically through influencing the public policymaking process. They are ubiquitous in the United States, in the health policy domain as in any other. However, as Exhibit 2.3 shows, the relative influence of interest groups in political markets varies by state.

The First Amendment to the U.S. Constitution guarantees the American people the right "peaceably to assemble, and to petition the Government for a redress of grievances." However, constitutional guarantees notwithstanding, political theorists from the nation's beginning to the present day have disagreed about whether interest groups play positive or negative roles in American political life (Ornstein and Elder 1978; Moe 1980; Cigler and Loomis 2007; Peters 2003; Edwards, Wattenberg, and Lineberry 2009).

James Madison, writing in the *Federalist Papers* in 1787, discusses the relationship of groups, which he called "factions," to democratic government. In *Federalist* Number 10,

EXHIBIT 2.3

Comparing Interest
Group Strength
Across the States

Dominant (4)	Dominant/ Complementary (26)	Complementary (15)	Complementary/ Subordinate (5)	Subordinate (0)
Alabama	Alaska	Colorado	Kentucky	
Florida	Arizona	Connecticut	Michigan	
Hawaii	Arkansas	Indiana	Minnesota	
Nevada	California	Maine	South Dakota	
	Delaware	Massachusetts	Vermont	
	Georgia	Montana		
	Idaho	New		
	Illinois	Hampshire		
	Iowa	New Jersey		
	Kansas	New York		
	Louisiana	North Carolina		
	Maryland	North Dakota		
	Mississippi	Pennsylvania		
	Missouri	Rhode Island		
	Nebraska	Washington		
	New Mexico	Wisconsin		
	Ohio			
	Oklahoma			
	Oregon			
	South Carolina			
	Tennessee			
	Texas			
	Utah			
	Virginia			
	West Virgina			
	Wyoming			

NOTE: This classification of interest group strength across the states is a composite of the judgments of experienced political observers in each state. Interest groups have an overwhelming influence in dominant states. In dominant/complementary states, interest group influence is strong but limited by the influence of other political actors such as party organizations, governmental institutions, or the electorate. In complementary states, interest group influence strikes a balance with other political actors. In complementary/subordinate states, interest group influence is secondary to the influence of other political actors. To be placed in the subordinate category, interest group influence in a state would have to be weak or inconsequential—a situation not apparent in any of the states.
SOURCE: Adapted from A. J. Nownes, C. S. Thomas, and R. J. Hrebenar (2008).

he defines a faction as "a number of citizens, whether amounting to a majority or a minority of the whole, who are united and actuated by some common impulse of passion, or of interest, adverse to the rights of citizens, or to the permanent and aggregate interests of the community." Madison felt strongly that factions, or interest groups, were inherently bad. He also believed, however, that the formation of such groups was a natural outgrowth of human nature (he writes in *Federalist* Number 10 that "the latent causes of faction are sown into the nature of man") and that government should not seek to check this activity.

Madison felt that what he called the "mischiefs of faction" could and should be contained by setting the "ambition" of one faction against the selfish preferences and behaviors of others. So began the uncertainty about and ambiguity toward the role of interest groups in public policymaking in the United States. One point about which there is neither uncertainty nor ambiguity, however, is that interest groups play an active role in the public policymaking process. Reflecting widely divergent views on the manner in which interest groups play their role in this process, two distinct perspectives on ways in which groups influence policymaking have emerged: the pluralist and the elitist models.

The Pluralist Perspective

People who hold the pluralist perspective on the role of interest groups in policymaking believe that because so many interest groups are operating, everyone's interests can be represented by one or more of them. Adherents to the pluralist model usually maintain that interest groups play an essentially positive role in public policymaking. They argue that various interest groups compete with and counterbalance each other in the political marketplace. Pluralists do not question that some groups are stronger than others. However, they contend that as groups seek their preferred outcomes, power is widely dispersed among competing groups, with each group winning some of the time and losing some of the time.

Pluralist theory about how the policymaking process works includes several interconnected arguments that, taken together, constitute what has come to be called a group theory of politics (Truman 1992). The central tenets of the group theory include the following:

- Interest groups provide essential links between people and their government.

- Interest groups compete among themselves for outcomes, with the interests of some groups counterbalanced by the interests of others.

- No group is likely to become too dominant in the competition; as groups become powerful, other countervailing interests organize or existing groups intensify their efforts. An important mechanism for maintaining balance among the groups is their ability to rely on various sources of power. Groups representing concentrated economic interests may have money, but consumer groups may have more members.

- The competition among interest groups is basically fair. Although there are exceptions, groups typically play by the rules of the game.

Some observers have concluded that the pluralist approach is out of control. There are more than 11,000 associations of national scope today and another 16,000 state or regional associations in such domains as business, education, religion, science, and health—all actively pursuing a variety of policy interests on behalf of their members (Concept Marketing Group, Inc. 2009). The problem, according to the critics of pluralism, is not merely the large number of groups but also the fact that government seems to consider the demands and preferences of all interest groups to be legitimate. There is little debate that government does attempt to satisfy the preferences of many interests, sometimes in conflicting ways.

Critics of the pluralist approach to the role of interest groups in the public policy-making process strongly agree on two points:

1. Interest groups have become too influential in the policymaking process. Satisfying their multiple and often conflicting demands seems to drive government rather than government being driven by a desire to base policy decisions on considerations of what is best for the nation as a whole—that is, on the public interest.

2. Seeking to satisfy the multiple and often conflicting demands of various interest groups leads to confusion, contradiction, and even paralysis in the policymaking process. Rather than making a difficult choice between satisfying X or Y, government seems frequently to pretend that there is no need to make the choice and seeks to satisfy both X and Y.

In addition to those who criticize the pluralist approach as dysfunctional and out of control are those who believe that the perspective itself is misguided, or even wrong. Instead of everyone having a chance to influence the policymaking process through one group or another, some people believe that such influence actually resides only in the hands of an elite few.

The Elitist Perspective

Whereas pluralists point with pride to the remarkable number of organized groups actively and aggressively participating in the American process of public policymaking, elitists point out how most groups are fairly powerless and ineffectual. The elitist perspective on the role of interest groups, which is the opposite of the pluralist viewpoint, grows out of a power elite model of American society.

This model is based on the idea that real political power in the United States is concentrated in the hands of the small proportion of the population that controls the nation's key institutions and organizations and much of its wealth. In the elitist perspective, these so-called "big interests" look out for themselves in part by disproportionately influencing, if not controlling, the public policymaking process. It is debatable whether this model accurately reflects the American political marketplace, but it does represent the opinions of a growing majority of Americans concerning which members of the society have the most influence.

The elitist theory holds that a power elite, often referred to as "the establishment," acts as a gatekeeper to the public policymaking process. Unless the power elite considers an issue important, the issue does not get much attention in policymaking circles. Furthermore, the theory holds, once an issue is on the policy agenda, public policies made in response reflect the values, ideologies, and preferences of this governing elite (Dye 2008). Thus, the power elite dominates public policymaking through its superior position in society. Its powerful roles in the nation's economic and social systems allows the elite to shape the formulation of policies and control their implementation. It has been argued that the nation's social and economic systems depend on the power elite's consensus regarding the system's fundamental values, and the only policy alternatives that receive serious consideration are those that fall within the shared consensus (Dye 2002).

The central tenets of the power elite theory stand in stark contrast to the pluralist perspective. These tenets are as follows (Dye and Zeigler 2009; Edwards, Wattenberg, and Lineberry 2009):

◆ Real political power resides in a very small number of groups; the large number of interest groups is practically meaningless because the power differentials among them are so great. Other groups may win minor policy victories, but the power elite always prevails on significant policy issues.

◆ Members of the power elite share a consensus or near consensus on the basic values that should guide public policymaking: private property rights, the preeminence of markets and private enterprise as the best way to organize the economy, limited government, and the importance of individual liberty and individualism.

◆ Members of the power elite have a strong preference for incremental changes in public policies. Incrementalism in policymaking permits time for the economic and social systems to adjust to changes without feeling threatened, with minimal economic dislocation or disruption and with minimal alteration in the social system's status quo.

◆ Elites protect their power bases. Some limited movement of non-elites into elite positions is permitted to maintain social stability, but only after non-elites clearly accept the elites' consensus values.

Which Perspective Is Correct?

Those who hold the power elitist perspective challenge those who hold the pluralist perspective by pointing to the highly concentrated and interlocked power centers in American society. Studies of the concentration of power do find that many of the top leadership positions in the United States—on corporate, foundation, and university governing boards, for example—are held by people who occupy more than one such position (Domhoff 2009).

Those who prefer the pluralist perspective, however, are equally quick to cite numerous examples in which those who traditionally have been grossly underrepresented in the inner circles of the power elite have succeeded in their collective efforts to significantly influence the public policymaking process. African Americans, women, and consumers in general provide examples of the ability of groups once ignored by policymakers to organize as effective interest groups and redirect the course of the public policymaking process.

Neither the pluralist nor the elitist perspective alone fully explains how the interests of individuals or organizations relate to the public policymaking process. The results of that process affect the interests of all individuals and all organizations to varying degrees. Many, if not all, individuals and organizations with interests can influence the policymaking process, although, again, not to equal degrees. The elitist and pluralist approaches each have something to contribute to an understanding of the roles interest groups play in the marketplace for public policies. Whether such groups work proactively, by seeking to stimulate new policies that serve the interests of their members, or reactively, by seeking to block policy changes that they do not believe serve their members' best interests, they are intrinsic to the public policymaking process. Interest groups provide their members with a way to link their policy preferences into a more powerful, collective voice that greatly increases the likelihood of a significant influence on policymaking.

THE SUPPLIERS OF HEALTH POLICIES

Because policies are made in the executive, legislative, and judicial branches of government, the list of potential policymakers is lengthy. Members of each branch of government supply policies in the political market, although each branch plays its role differently.

Legislators as Suppliers

One important group of public policy suppliers is elected legislators, whether members of the U.S. Congress, state legislatures, or city councils. Few aspects of the political marketplace are as interesting, or as widely observed and studied, as the decision-making behaviors of legislators and the motives and incentives behind those behaviors. To a large extent, this intense interest in the motivations of policy suppliers reflects the desire of policy demanders to exert influence over the suppliers.

Although neither extreme fully reflects the motivations of legislators, the end points on a continuum of behaviors that policymakers might exhibit can be represented by those who seek to maximize the public interest on one end and by those who seek to maximize self-interest on the other end. A legislator at the public interest extreme would always seek policies that maximize the public interest, although the true public interest might not always be easy to identify. A legislator whose motivations lie at the self-interest extreme would always behave in a manner that maximizes self-interest, whether that interest is reelection, money, prestige, power, or whatever appeals to the self-serving person.

In the political marketplace, legislators can be found all along the continuum between extreme public-interest and extreme self-interest motivations. Although some people incorrectly ascribe dominant self-interest motives to all legislators, the actions and decisions of most legislators reflect a complex mixture of the two motivations, with exclusively self-interested or public-interested motives only rarely dominating decisions.

Motives aside, legislators at all levels of government are key policy suppliers, especially of policies in the form of laws. For example, only Congress can enact new or amend existing public laws. In political markets, legislators constantly calculate the benefits and costs of their policymaking decisions and consider who will reap these benefits and bear these costs. Factoring in the interests they choose to serve, they make their decisions accordingly. Their calculations are complicated by the fact that the costs and benefits of a particular decision often affect many people in different ways.

In effect, policies typically create winners and losers. The gains some people enjoy come at the financial expense of others, or at least at the expense of having someone's problems ignored or someone's preferred solutions postponed. Most of the time, most legislators seek to maximize their own net political gains through their policy-related decisions, because reelection is an abiding objective.

In view of the reality that most policies create winners and losers, legislators may find that their best strategy is to permit the winners their victory, but not by a huge margin, and in so doing cushion the impact on the losers. For example, suppose a legislator is considering a policy that would increase health services for an underserved population at the expense of higher taxes on others. Options include various policies with the following outcomes: (1) few services at relatively low cost, (2) more services at higher cost, and (3) many services at very high cost. Facing such a decision, and applying the concept of net political gain, policymakers might opt for the provision of a meaningful level of services, but one far below what could have been provided and at a cost below what would have been required for a higher level of services. The "winners" receive more services, but the expense for the "losers," who have to pay for the new services, is not as great as it might have been. Through such calculations and determinations legislators routinely seek to maximize their net political gains.

Executives and Bureaucrats as Suppliers

At all levels of government, members of the executive branch are important policy suppliers, although their role differs from that of legislators. Presidents, governors, mayors, and other senior public-sector executives offer policies in the form of legislative proposals and seek to have legislators enact their preferred policies. Chief executives and those in charge of government departments and agencies are directly responsible for policies in the form of rules or regulations used to guide the implementation of laws and operational protocols and procedures for the policies they implement. Career bureaucrats who participate in these activities and thus become suppliers of policies in the political marketplace join elected and appointed executives and managers in their rulemaking and operational duties.

Elected and appointed officials of the executive branch are often affected by the same self-interest/public-interest dichotomy that affects legislators; reelection concerns in particular often influence their decisions. Like legislators, elected and appointed members of executive branches are apt to calculate the net political gains of their policy-related decisions and actions. As a result, their motivations and behaviors in the political marketplace can be similar to those of legislators. However, the behaviors of members of the executive branch of a government and members of its legislative branch show some important differences.

The most fundamental difference derives from the fact that the executive branch generally bears greater responsibility than the legislative branch for the state of the economy, and it is widely perceived to bear even more responsibility than it actually does. Presidents, governors, and mayors, along with their top appointees, are held accountable for economic conditions much more explicitly than are Congress, state legislatures, or city councils. Although legislators do not escape this responsibility altogether, the public typically lays most of the responsibility at the feet of the executive branch. This can be seen in the financial crises facing the United States and much of the world beginning in 2008. The executive branch, especially the president, is expected to spur development of legislation to rescue the nation from this circumstance. When people do blame the legislative branch, they tend to hold the entire Congress or the state or city legislature collectively responsible rather than to blame individual legislators.

The concentration of responsibility for the economy in the executive branch influences the decision making that takes place there. Because of the close connection between government's budget and the state of the economy, the budget implications of policy decisions are carefully weighed in the executive branch. Not infrequently, the legislative and executive branches will hold different positions on health policies because members in the two branches give different weight to the budget implications of the policies they are considering.

Career bureaucrats, or civil servants, in the executive branch also participate in policymaking in the legislative branch when they collect, analyze, and transmit information about policy options and initiate policy proposals in their areas of expertise. However, the motivations and behaviors of career bureaucrats tend to differ from those of legislators and those of members of executive branches.

The behaviors and motivations of career bureaucrats in the public sector are often analogous to those of employees in the private sector. Workers in both settings typically seek to satisfy certain personal needs and desires through their work. This can obviously be categorized as self-serving in both cases. But government employees are no more likely to be totally motivated by self-interests than are private sector workers. Most workers in both sectors are motivated by blends of self-interest and interest in what is good for the larger society.

However, most career bureaucrats watch a constantly changing mix of elected and senior government officials—with an equally dynamic set of policy preferences—parade past, while they remain as the most permanent human feature of government. It should surprise no one that career bureaucrats develop a strong sense of identification with their home department or agency or that they become protective of it. This protectiveness is most visible in the relationships between government agencies or departments and those with legislative oversight of them, including authorization, appropriation, and performance review responsibilities. Many career bureaucrats equate the well-being of their agencies, in terms of their size, budgets, and prestige, with the public interest. Obviously, this is not always the case.

The Judiciary as Supplier

The judicial branch of government is also a supplier of policies. For example, whenever a court interprets an ambiguous law, establishes judicial procedure, or interprets the U.S. Constitution, it makes a policy. These activities are conceptually no different from those involved when legislators enact public laws or when members of the executive branch establish rules and regulations to guide implementation of laws or make operational decisions regarding their implementation. All of these activities are policymaking, because they lead to authoritative decisions made within government for the purpose of influencing or directing the actions, behaviors, and decisions of others.

Policymaking in the judicial branch, however, differs from that in the legislative and executive branches, not only in focus but also in operation. The responsibilities of courts require them to focus narrowly on the issues involved in specific cases or situations. This stands in stark contrast to the wide-open political arena in which most other public policymaking occurs.

The courts are involved in numerous and diverse aspects of health policy, reflecting the entire range of health determinants (i.e., physical environment, behavior and genetics, social factors, and health services). For example, in a 1980 opinion in what is called the benzene case, the U.S. Supreme Court invalidated an Occupational Safety and Health Administration (OSHA; www.osha.gov) rule limiting benzene to no more than one part per million in the air in workplaces. In the court's view, OSHA had not found a significant risk to workers' health before issuing the rule.

In a 1905 landmark ruling in *Jacobson v. Massachusetts*, the U.S. Supreme Court upheld compulsory vaccination as an appropriate use of state police power to protect the health, welfare, and safety of a state's citizens. Police powers granted to the states by the U.S. Constitution provide the legal basis for state authority in the field of public health. This case involved a compulsory vaccination regulation of the Cambridge, Massachusetts, Board of Health. Defendant Jacobson refused to be vaccinated and contended that the requirement invaded his liberty. The Court held, however, that

> the liberty secured by the Constitution to every person...does not import an absolute right in each person to be at all times and in all circumstances wholly freed from restraint...it was the duty of the constituted authorities primarily to keep in view the welfare, comfort and safety of the many, and not permit the interests of the many to be subordinated to the wishes or convenience of the few.

Furthermore, the Court stated that

> it is equally true that in every well-ordered society charged with the duty of conserving the safety of its members the rights of the individual in respect of his liberty may at times, under the pressure of great dangers, be subjected to such restraint, to be enforced by reasonable regulations, as the safety of the general public may demand... .

The heart of the judiciary's ability to supply policies lies in its role in interpreting the law. The courts can exercise the powers of nullification, interpretation, and application to the rules and regulations established by the executive branch in carrying out its implementation responsibilities. This includes the power to declare federal and state laws unconstitutional—that is, to declare laws enacted by the legislative branch to be null and void. This role of the courts is clearly illustrated in a ruling by the 9th U.S. Circuit Court of Appeals that overturned Arizona legislation requiring abortion clinics in that state to submit to warrantless searches and to make patient files available to state regulators. These onerous state regulations had been established following the death of a patient having a clinic abortion. The appeals court based its ruling on an interpretation that the regulations violated constitutional restrictions on searches and seizures and that requiring the clinics to submit patient files to state regulators on demand violated the patients' privacy rights (Kravets 2004).

Another example of the interpretative role of the courts in health policymaking is the ruling by the U.S. Supreme Court in April 1995 that ERISA (P.L. 93-406) does not preclude states from setting hospital rates. The case that resulted in this ruling arose out of New York's practice of adding a surcharge to certain hospital bills to help pay for health services for some of the state's low-income citizens. The state's practice was challenged by a group of commercial insurers and HMOs and by New York City (Green 1995). A number of health-related interest groups filed a joint *amicus curiae* (friend of the court) brief in which they asserted that Congress, in enacting ERISA, never intended for it to be used to challenge state health reform plans and initiatives. The Supreme Court's ruling is generally seen as supportive of state efforts to broaden access to health services for their poorer residents through various reforms and initiatives.

Health policymaking within the judicial branch is far more prevalent in state courts and lower federal courts than in the U.S. Supreme Court. A state-level example of courts making important health policy can be seen in Pennsylvania cases involving the tax-exempt status of healthcare organizations. In one 1995 case, for example, the Indiana County, Pennsylvania, Court of Common Pleas rebuffed the leaders of Indiana Hospital in their appeal to have the hospital's tax-exempt status restored after the exemption had been revoked by the county in 1993. In making its ruling, the court held that the hospital failed to adequately meet one of the state's tests through which an organization qualifies for tax exemption. Among other criteria, at the time of this case, the state required a tax-exempt organization "to donate or render gratuitously a substantial portion of its services."

In making its ruling, the Indiana County court took note of the fact that Indiana Hospital's uncompensated charity care in fiscal year 1994 had amounted to approximately 2 percent of its total expected compensation and contrasted this with an earlier case resulting from the revocation of the tax-exempt status of a nursing home in the state. The state supreme court decision in the St. Margaret Seneca Place nursing home case (*St. Margaret Seneca Place v. Board of Property Assessment Appeals and Review, County of Allegheny, PA*) had been that the nursing home did meet the state's test because it demonstrated that it bore more than one-third of the cost of care for half of its patients.

The variation in these and several other Pennsylvania cases in the courts' interpretation of the state's partial test for tax-exempt status (i.e., the requirement that a tax-exempt organization is "to donate or render gratuitously a substantial portion of its services") led to enactment in 1997 of clarifying legislation on this and other points regarding the determination of tax-exempt status. Late in that year, the governor of Pennsylvania signed into law House Bill 55, known as the Institutions of Purely Public Charity Act, or Act 55. This act permits an institution to meet the charitable purpose test and qualify for tax exemption if it has a charitable mission, is free of private profit motive, is designated a 501(c)(3) by the federal government, and is organized for any of the following reasons:

◆ relief of poverty

◆ advancement and provision of education, including secondary education

◆ advancement of religion

◆ prevention and treatment of disease or injury, including mental retardation and mental illness

◆   government or municipal purposes

◆   accomplishment of a purpose that is recognized as important and beneficial to
     the public and that advances social, moral, or physical objectives

The act specifically clarified, quite liberally, how an institution could meet the requirement for donating or rendering gratuitously a substantial portion of its services. Act 55 established 3 percent of an institution's total operating expenses as the necessary contribution of charitable goods or services. In this instance, court decisions were policies themselves, and the impact of the decisions eventually led to a significant change in Pennsylvania's public laws.

It is generally acknowledged that, because the pursuit of health in the United States is so heavily influenced by laws and regulations, the courts are a major factor in the development and implementation of health policies (Rosenblatt 2008; Gostin 2008). The courts include not only the federal court system but also the court systems of the states and the territories. Each of these systems has developed in idiosyncratic ways, and each has a constitution to guide it, specific legislation to contend with, and its own history of judicial decisions. A great deal of information on the structure and operation of the U.S. legal system can be found in the outline of the legal system provided by the U.S. Department of State (2004).

Although the federal and state courts play significant roles as policy suppliers, their behaviors, motivations, and roles differ significantly from those of participants in the legislative and executive branches. In their wisdom, the drafters of the U.S. Constitution created the three branches, and Article III ensured the judicial branch's independence, at least mostly so, from the other branches.

An independent judiciary facilitates adherence to the rules all participants in the policymaking process must follow. Federal judges are appointed rather than elected, and the appointments are for life. Consequently, federal judges are not subject to the same self-interest concerns related to reelection that many other policymakers face. This enhances their ability to act in the public interest, although judges, like all policymakers, vary in their personal commitments to this objective (Cass 2008).

INTERPLAY AMONG DEMANDERS AND SUPPLIERS IN THE POLITICAL MARKETPLACE

In the political marketplace, demanders and suppliers of policies seek to further their objectives. These objectives can be based on self-interest and involve some health or economic advantage, or they can be based on what is best for the public, or at least some subset of society, such as the elderly, poor, or medically underserved. In either case, the outcome depends on the relative abilities of some participants in the marketplace to influence the actions, behaviors, and decisions of other participants.

POWER AND INFLUENCE IN POLITICAL MARKETS

Influence in political markets, just as in private economic markets, is defined as "actions that, either directly or indirectly, cause a change in the behavior and/or attitudes of another individual or group" (Shortell and Kaluzny 2006, 533). But to have influence, one must also have power. More power means more potential to influence others. Therefore, an understanding of influence requires an understanding of power.

Those who wish to exert influence in the political marketplace must first acquire power from the sources available to them (Alexander et al. 2006). The classic categories for sources of interpersonal power include legitimate, reward, coercive, expert, and referent (French and Raven 1959). These bases of interpersonal power apply to individuals, organizations, and interest groups in political markets.

Legitimate power, for example, derives from one's relative position in a social system, organization, or group; this form of power is also called *formal power* or authority. It exists because assigning or ascribing certain powers to individuals, organizations, or groups better enables them to fulfill their duties or perform their work effectively. Elected officials, appointed executives, judges, health professionals, corporation executives, union leaders, and many other individual participants in the political marketplace, possess legitimate power that accompanies their social or organizational positions. Suppliers and demanders of policies possess legitimate power. That is, they can exert influence in the policymaking process because they are recognized as legitimate in the process.

Reward power is based on the ability of one person, organization, or group to reward others for their decisions and actions. Reward power stems in part from legitimate power. It comes from many sources and takes many forms. Within organizations, it includes the obvious: control over pay increases, promotions, work and vacation schedules, recognition of accomplishments, and such status symbols or perks as club memberships and office size and location. In economic markets, the buying power of consumers is a form of reward power. In political markets, reward power is more likely to take the form of favors that can be provided or exchanged, specific influence with particular individuals or groups, and whatever influence can be stored for later use. *Coercive power* is the opposite of reward power and is based on the capacity to withhold or to prevent someone from obtaining desired rewards.

Expert power tends to reside in individuals but can also reside in a group or organization. It derives from possessing expertise valued within the political marketplace, such as expertise in solving problems or performing crucial tasks. People with expert power often occupy formal positions of authority, transferring some of the expert power to the organization or group. People who can exercise their expert power in the policymaking arena may also be trusted advisers or associates of other participants in the political marketplace.

Referent power derives from the influence that results from the ability of some people, organizations, and interest groups to engender admiration, loyalty, and emulation from others. In the marketplace for policies, this form of power, when it pertains to individuals, is called *charismatic power*. Charismatic power usually belongs to a select few people who typically have strong convictions about the correctness of their preferences, have great self-confidence in their own abilities, and are widely perceived to be legitimate agents of change. It is rare for a person, organization, or interest group to gain sufficient power to heavily influence policymaking simply from referent or charismatic power, even in political markets where charisma is highly valued. But it can certainly give the other sources of power in the political marketplace a boost.

The bases of power in the political marketplace are interdependent. They can and do complement and conflict with each other. For example, people, organizations, or groups that are in a position to use reward power and who do so wisely can strengthen their referent power. Conversely, those who abuse coercive power might quickly weaken or lose their referent power. Effective participants in the marketplace for policies—those individuals, organizations, and groups that succeed at translating their power into influence—tend to be fully aware of the sources of their power and to act accordingly. They seem to understand intuitively the costs and benefits of using each kind of power and can draw on them appropriately in different situations and with various people they wish to influence.

POWER AND INFLUENCE OF INTEREST GROUPS: BREAKING THE IRON TRIANGLES

Some interest groups, including several in the health domain, are extraordinarily powerful and influential in demanding public policies. To fully appreciate their power and the influence it permits, it is necessary to understand *iron triangles*, a model of the relationships that sometimes exist among participating individuals, organizations, and groups in the political marketplace.

Any policy domain attracts a set of participating individuals, organizations, and groups. Each participant has some stake in policies affecting the domain and thus seeks to influence policymaking. Some of the participants, or stakeholders, in a domain demand policies; others supply policies. Collectively, these stakeholders form a *policy community*.

Traditionally, the policy community formed around a particular policy domain (such as health) has included any legislative committees with jurisdiction in the domain, the executive branch agencies responsible for implementing public laws in the domain, and the private-sector interest groups involved in the domain. The first two categories are suppliers of the policies demanded by the third category. This triad of organized interests has been called an iron triangle because when all three sides are in accord, the resulting stability allows the triad to withstand attempts to make undesired changes.

A policy community that could be appropriately characterized as a strong and stable iron triangle dominated the health policy domain until the early 1960s, when battle lines began to be drawn over the eventual shape of the Medicare program. This triangle featured a few powerful interest groups with concordant views that, for the most part, had sympathetic partners in the legislative committees and in the relevant implementing agencies of government.

During this period, the private-sector interest group members of the iron triangle that dominated health policy, notably AMA and the American Hospital Association (AHA; www.aha.org), joined later by the American College of Physicians (ACP; www. acponline.org) and the American College of Surgeons (ACS; www.facs.org), generally held a consistent view of the appropriate policies in this domain. Their shared view of optimal health policy was that government should protect the interests of health services providers and not intervene in the financing or delivery of health services (Peterson 1993). Under the conditions and expectations extant in these largely straightforward relationships, it was relatively simple for the suppliers and demanders of policies to satisfy each other. This triangle was unbreakable into the second half of the twentieth century.

The dynamics of the situation began to change dramatically with the policy battles over Medicare, and they worsened with the addition of Medicaid to the debate. Fundamental differences emerged among the participants in the health policy community in terms of their views of optimal health policy. Today, there is rarely a solid block of concordant private sector interests driving health policy decisions. For example, differences over questions of optimal policy shattered the accord between AMA and AHA. Splintering within the memberships of these groups caused even more damage. For example, the medical profession no longer speaks through the single voice of AMA; organizations such as ACP and the American Academy of Family Physicians (AAFP; www.aafp.org) can and sometimes do support different policy choices. Similarly, AHA is now joined in policy debates by organizations with diverse preferences representing the specific interests of teaching hospitals, public hospitals, for-profit hospitals, and other hospital subsets. These changes have eroded the solidarity among private-sector interest groups and the public-sector members of the health policy community.

Rather than an iron triangle, the contemporary health policy community is far more heterogeneous in its membership and much more loosely structured. At most, this community can be thought of as a group of members whose commonality stems from the attention they pay to issues in the health policy domain. There is an important difference, however, between shared attentiveness to health policy issues and shared positions on optimal health policy or related issues. The loss of concordance among the members of the old iron triangle has somewhat diminished the power of certain interest groups. Nevertheless, they remain highly influential, and other interest groups have also been able to assume influential roles in health policymaking.

Ethics in the Political Marketplace

Ethics in policymaking is essential to any discussion of the political marketplace. Humans control political markets. Thus, various mixes of altruism and egoism influence what takes place. Human control of the public policymaking process means that its operation, outcomes, and consequences are directly affected by the ethics of those who participate in the process. Ethical considerations help shape and guide the development of new policies by contributing to definitions of problems and the structure of policy solutions.

Having considered the context within which health policies are made, especially the structure and operations of political markets, and having identified the demanders and suppliers who interact in these markets and the important operational and ethical aspects of these interactions, it is now possible to consider the intricate process through which public policies are made. The consideration begins in this chapter at the conceptual level; applied discussions of the component parts of the policymaking process follow in subsequent chapters.

A CONCEPTUAL MODEL OF THE PUBLIC POLICYMAKING PROCESS

The most useful way to conceptualize a process as complex and intricate as the one through which public policies are made is through a schematic model. Although such models, like the one presented here, tend to be oversimplifications, they can accurately reflect the component parts of the process and their interrelationships. Exhibit 2.4 is a model of the public policymaking process in the United States. Several key features of the policymaking process as reflected in this model are helpful in understanding the policymaking process.

POLICYMAKING IS A CYCLICAL PROCESS

As Exhibit 2.4 illustrates, the policymaking process is a continuous cycle in which all decisions are subject to modification. Public policymaking is a process within which numerous decisions are reached and then revisited as circumstances change.

POLICYMAKING IS INFLUENCED BY EXTERNAL FACTORS

Another important feature of the public policymaking process shown in Exhibit 2.4 is the influence of factors external to the process itself. The policymaking process is an *open system*, one in which the process interacts with and is affected by events and circumstances in its external environment. This important phenomenon is shown in the model by the effect of the preferences of individuals, organizations, and interest groups that are affected by policies—along with biological, cultural, demographic, ecological, economic, ethical, legal, psychological, social, and technological inputs—on the policymaking process.

Legal inputs, which include decisions made in the courts, are themselves policies. In addition, however, decisions made within the legal system influence other decisions made within the policymaking process. Legal inputs help shape all other policy decisions, including by reversing them when they are unconstitutional.

EXHIBIT 2.4
Model of the Public Policymaking Process in the United States

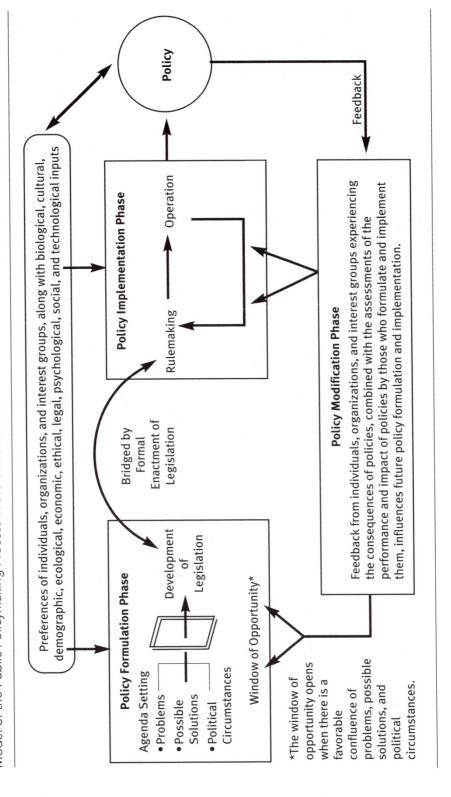

Technology provides another example of the effect of external factors on the policymaking process. The United States is the world's major producer and consumer of health-related technology. As the policymaking model shows, technological inputs flow into the policymaking process. Along with other effects, the costs of new technologies must be factored into public and private insurance programs (Congressional Budget Office 2008a). As Elmendorf (2009) noted, "given the central role of medical technology in cost growth, reducing or slowing spending over the long term would probably require decreasing the pace of adopting new treatments and procedures or limiting the breadth of their application."

THE COMPONENTS OF THE POLICYMAKING PROCESS ARE INTERACTIVE AND INTERDEPENDENT

While the model emphasizes the various distinct component parts or phases of the policymaking process, it also shows that they are highly interactive and interdependent. The public policymaking process modeled in Exhibit 2.4 includes the following three interconnected phases:

1. policy formulation, which incorporates activities associated with setting the policy agenda and, subsequently, with the development of legislation

2. policy implementation, which incorporates activities associated with rulemaking that help guide the implementation of policies and the actual operationalization of policies

3. policy modification, which allows for all prior decisions made within the process to be revisited and perhaps changed

Once enacted as laws, policies remain to be implemented. The formulation phase (making the decisions that lead to public laws) and the implementation phase (taking actions and making additional decisions necessary to implement public laws) are bridged by the formal enactment of legislation, which shifts the cycle from the formulation to the implementation phase.

Implementation responsibility rests mostly with the executive branch, which includes DHHS and the Department of Justice (DOJ; www.usdoj.gov), and independent federal agencies, such as the Environmental Protection Agency (EPA; www.epa.gov) and the Consumer Product Safety Commission (CPSC; www.cpsc.gov). These and many other departments and agencies in the executive branch exist primarily to implement the policies formulated in the legislative branch.

Some of the decisions made in the course of policy implementation become policies themselves. Rules and regulations promulgated to implement a law and operational protocols and procedures developed to support a law's implementation are policies as surely as is the law itself. Similarly, judicial decisions regarding the applicability of laws to specific situations or regarding the appropriateness of the actions of implementing organizations are public policies. Policies are established within the formulation and the implementation phases of the overall process.

The policy modification phase exists because perfection cannot be achieved in the other phases and because policies are established and exist in a dynamic world. Suitable policies made today may become inadequate with future biological, cultural, demographic, ecological, economic, ethical, legal, psychological, social, and technological changes. Pressure to change established policies may come from new priorities or the perceived needs of individuals, organizations, and interest groups affected by the policies.

Policy modification, which is shown as a feedback loop in Exhibit 2.4, may entail only minor adjustments in the implementation phase or modest amendments to existing public laws. In some instances, however, the consequences of implementing certain policies can feed all the way back to the agenda-setting stage. For example, formulating policies to contain the costs of providing health services—a key challenge facing policymakers today—is to a large extent an outgrowth of previous policies that expanded access and increased the supply of human resources and advanced technologies to be used in providing health services.

POLICYMAKING IS A HIGHLY POLITICAL PROCESS

One feature of the public policymaking process that the model presented in Exhibit 2.4 cannot adequately represent—but one that is crucial to understanding the policymaking process—is the political nature of the process in operation. While many people believe—and still others naïvely hope—that public policymaking is a predominantly rational decision-making process, this is not the case.

The process would no doubt be simpler and better if it were driven exclusively by fully informed consideration of the best ways for policy to support the nation's pursuit of health, by open and comprehensive debate about potential policies, and by rational selection from among policy choices strictly on the basis of ability to contribute to the pursuit of health. Those who are familiar with the policymaking process, however, know that a wide range of other factors and considerations influence the process. The preferences and influence of interest groups, political bargaining and vote trading, and ideological biases are among the most important of these factors. This is not to say that rationality plays no part in health policymaking. On a good day, it will gain a place among the flurry of political considerations, but "it must be a very good and rare day indeed when policymakers take their cues mainly from scientific knowledge about the state of the world they hope to change or protect" (Brown 1991, 20).

The highly political nature of the policymaking process in the United States accounts for competing theories about how this process plays out. At the opposite ends of a continuum sit strictly public-interest and strictly self-interest theories of how policymakers behave. Policies made entirely in the public interest would be the result of all participants acting according to what they believe to be the public's interest. Alternatively, policies made entirely through a process driven by self-interests would reflect the interplay of the various self-interests of the diverse participants. Policies resulting from these two hypothetical extremes would indeed be very different.

In reality, however, health policies always reflect a mix of public-interest and self-interest influences. The balance between the public and self-interests being served is important to the ultimate shape of health policies. For example, the present coexistence of the extremes of excess (the exorbitant incomes of some physicians and health plan managers, esoteric technologies, and various overcapacities in the healthcare system) and deprivation (lack of insurance for millions of people and inadequate access to basic health services for millions more) resulting from or permitted by some of the nation's existing health policies suggests that the balance has been tipped too often toward the service of self-interests.

This aside, public policymaking in the U.S. health domain is a remarkably complex process, although clearly an imperfect one. In general, policymaking is a highly political process. It is continual and cyclical in its operation, it is heavily influenced by factors external to the process, and the component phases and activities within the phases of the process are highly interactive and interdependent.

SUMMARY

Health policies, like those in other domains, are made within the context of the political marketplace, where demanders for and suppliers of policies interact. The federal and state governments have important health policy roles, and their policymaking processes are quite similar.

The demanders of policies include those who view public policies as a mechanism for meeting their health-related objectives or other objectives, such as economic advantage. Although individuals alone can demand public policies, the far more effective demand emanates from organizations and especially from organized interest groups. The suppliers of health policy include elected and appointed members of all three branches of government and the civil servants who staff the government.

The interests of the various demanders and suppliers in this market cannot be completely coincident—often, they are in open conflict—and the decisions and activities of any participant always affect and are affected by the activities of other participants. Public policymaking in the health domain is a human process, a fact with great significance for the outcomes and consequences of the process and one that argues for ethical behavior by all involved in the process.

The policymaking process itself is a highly complex, interactive, and cyclical process that incorporates formulation, implementation, and modification phases.

REFERENCES

Alexander, J. A., T. G. Rundall, T. J. Hoff, and L. L. Morlock. 2006. "Power and Politics." In *Health Care Management: Organization Design and Behavior*, 5th ed., edited by S. M. Shortell and A. D. Kaluzny, 276–310. Clifton Park, NY: Thomson Delmar Learning.

Brown, L. D. 1991. "Knowledge and Power: Health Services Research as a Political Resource." In *Health Services Research: Key to Health Policy*, edited by E. Ginzberg, 20–45. Cambridge, MA: Harvard University Press.

Byrne, D. 2004. *Enabling Good Health for All: A Reflection Process for a New EU Health Strategy.* [Online report; retrieved 9/3/09.] ec.europa.eu/health/ph_overview/Documents/pub_good_health_en.pdf.

Cass, R. S. 2008. "Judicial Partisanship Awards." *Washington Independent*, July 31. [Online material; retrieved 2/8/09.] washingtonindependent.com/350/judicial-partisanship-awards.

Cigler, A. J., and B. A. Loomis (eds.). 2007. *Interest Group Politics*, 7th ed. Washington, DC: CQ Press.

Concept Marketing Group, Inc. 2009. *Directory of Associations*. Scottsdale, AZ: Concept Marketing Group, Inc.

Congressional Budget Office. 2008a. "Accounting for Sources of Projected Growth in Federal Spending on Medicare and Medicaid." [Online brief; retrieved 2/10/09.] www.cbo.gov/ftpdocs/93xx/doc9316/05-29-SourcesHealthCostGrowth_Brief.pdf.

———. 2008b. "Updated Long-Term Projections for Social Security." [Online report; retrieved 2/6/09.] www.cbo.gov/ftpdocs/96xx/doc9649/08-20-SocialSecurity Update.pdf.

Davidson, S. M. 1997. "Politics Matters! Health Care Policy and the Federal System." *Journal of Health Politics, Policy and Law* 22 (3): 879–96.

Domhoff, G. W. 2009. *Who Rules America? Challenges to Corporate and Class Dominance*, 6th ed. Hightstown, NJ: McGraw-Hill Companies.

Dye, T. R. 2008. *Understanding Public Policy*, 12th ed. White Plains, NY: Pearson Longman.

Dye, T. R. 2002. *Who's Running America? The Bush Restoration*, 7th ed. White Plains, NY: Pearson Longman.

Dye, T. R., and H. Zeigler. 2009. *The Irony of Democracy: An Uncommon Introduction to American Politics*, 14th ed. Belmont, CA: Wadsworth Cengage Learning.

Edwards, G. C., M. P. Wattenberg, and R. L. Lineberry. 2009. *Government in America: People, Politics, and Policy*, Brief Study Edition, 10th ed. White Plains, NY: Pearson Longman.

Elmendorf, D. E. 2009. Testimony Before the United States Senate Committee on the Budget, February 10. [Online information; retrieved 2/10/09.] www.cbo.gov/ftpdocs/99xx/doc9982/02-10-HealthVolumes_Testimony.pdf.

Feldstein, P. J. 2006. *The Politics of Health Legislation: An Economic Perspective*, 3rd ed. Chicago: Health Administration Press.

French, J. R. P., and B. H. Raven. 1959. "The Basis of Social Power." In *Studies of Social Power*, edited by D. Cartwright, 150–67. Ann Arbor, MI: Institute for Social Research.

Gostin, L. O. 2008. *Public Health Law: Power, Duty, Restraint*, 2nd ed. Berkeley, CA: University of California Press.

Green, J. 1995. "High-Court Ruling Protects Hospital-Bill Surcharges." *AHA News* 31 (18): 1.

Kaiser Commission on Medicaid and the Uninsured. 2009. *The Role of Medicaid in State Economies: A Look at the Research*. [Online information; retrieved 9/25/09.] http://www.kff.org/medicaid/upload/7075_02.pdf.

King, M. P. 2005. *State Roles in Health: A Snapshot for State Legislators*. Denver, CO: National Conference of State Legislatures.

Kravets, D. 2004. "Arizona Abortion Regulation Invades Privacy, Appeals Court Says." Associated Press, June 19.

Leichter, H. M. 2008. "State Governments: E Pluribus Multa." In *Health Politics and Policy*, 4th ed., edited by J. A. Morone, T. J. Litman, and L. S. Robins, 173–95. Clifton Park, NY: Delmar Cengage Learning.

Madison, J. 1787. "The Same Subject Continued: The Union as a Safeguard Against Domestic Faction and Insurrection." *Federalist Papers* 10.

McGarity, T. O., and W. E. Wagner. 2008. *Bending Science: How Special Interests Corrupt Public Health Research*. Cambridge, MA: Harvard University Press.

Moe, T. 1980. *The Organization of Interests*. Chicago: University of Chicago Press.

National Governors Association and National Association of State Budget Officers. 2009. *The Fiscal Survey of States*. Washington, DC: National Association of State Budget Officers. [Online information; retrieved 9/25/09.] http://www.nasbo.org/ Publications/ PDFs/FSSpring2009.pdf

Nownes, A. J., C. S. Thomas, and R. J. Hrebenar. 2008. "Interest Groups in the States." In *Politics in the American States*, 9th edition, edited by V. Gray and R. L. Hanson, 98–126. Washington, DC: CQ Press.

Oliver, T. R., and P. Paul-Shaheen. 1997. "Translating Ideas into Actions: Entrepreneurial Leadership in State Health Care Reforms." *Journal of Health Politics, Policy and Law* 22 (3): 721–88.

Ornstein, N. J., and S. Elder. 1978. *Interest Groups, Lobbying and Policymaking*. Washington, DC: Congressional Quarterly Press.

Peters, B. G. 2003. *American Public Policy: Promise and Performance*, 6th ed. Chappaqua, NY: Chatham House.

Peterson, M. A. 1993. "Political Influence in the 1990s: From Iron Triangles to Policy Networks." *Journal of Health Politics, Policy and Law* 18 (2): 395–438.

Rosenblatt, R. 2008. "The Courts." In *Health Politics and Policy*, 4th ed., edited by J. A. Morone, T. J. Litman, and L. S. Robins, 127–52. Clifton Park, NY: Delmar Cengage Learning.

Shortell, S. M., and A. D. Kaluzny. 2006. *Health Care Management: Organization Design and Behavior*, 5th ed. Clifton Park, NY: Thomson Delmar Learning.

Truman, D. B. 1992. *The Governmental Process*, 2nd ed. Berkeley, CA: University of California, Institute of Governmental Studies.

U.S. Department of State. 2004. *Outline of the U.S. Legal System*. [Online booklet; retrieved 2/8/09.] www.america.gov/media/pdf/books/legalotln.pdf#popup.

Watkins, M. 2006. *Shaping the Game: The New Leader's Guide to Effective Negotiating*. Boston: Harvard Business School Publishing.

Weissert, C. S., and W. G. Weissert. 2006. *Governing Health: The Politics of Health Policy*, 3rd ed. Baltimore, MD: Johns Hopkins University Press.

READING 9B

HEALTH POLICYMAKING AT THE STATE AND LOCAL LEVELS AND IN THE PRIVATE SECTOR

Leiyu Shi
From *Introduction to Health Policy* (2013), Chapter 3, 53–73. Chicago: Health Administration Press.

A policy is a temporary creed liable to be changed, but while it holds good it has got to be pursued with apostolic zeal.

— Mohandas Gandhi

LEARNING OBJECTIVES

Studying this chapter will help you to

◆ describe features of the US state-level policymaking process and political system and provide examples of state healthcare legislation,

◆ discuss features of the US local government policymaking process and local political system and provide examples of local healthcare legislation,

◆ address the health policy–related activities of private health research institutes and foundations,

◆   understand the implications for the US healthcare system of policies created and practices followed by private industry, and

◆   appreciate the attributes of health policy development at the US state and local levels and in the private sector.

Case Study
Massachusetts Healthcare Reform

In 2006, Massachusetts enacted landmark legislation to provide health insurance coverage to nearly all state residents (Kaiser Family Foundation 2012). The legislation led to the creation of the Commonwealth Care health insurance program to provide subsidized coverage for individuals whose income is below 300 percent of the federal poverty level. It also developed a health insurance exchange for individuals and small businesses to purchase insurance at more affordable rates than could be obtained on the open market. The state's Medicaid program was expanded and merged with the Children's Health Insurance Program to form MassHealth. Children whose family's income is up to 300 percent of the federal poverty level are covered by this program.

As part of that legislation, Massachusetts mandated that residents purchase health insurance coverage or be charged a penalty of up to $912. In addition, employers with 11 or more employees were required to contribute to health insurance coverage for their employees or pay an annual fair-share contribution of up to $295 per employee.

As of 2012, Massachusetts percentage of residents without insurance had declined to 6.3 percent, in comparison to the 2006 level of 10.9 percent uninsured. Additionally, uninsurance in Massachusetts is about one-third that of the rest of the United States (18.4 percent). Employer health coverage remains the most common type of insurance, but the MassHealth public insurance plan and Commonwealth Care (which provides subsidies for families and individuals to purchase private coverage) have grown substantially (Kaiser Family Foundation 2012).

Community health centers and safety net hospitals play a dominant role in caring for those Massachusetts residents who now have health insurance as a result of the state healthcare reform legislation. In addition, they continue to provide care for those who remain uninsured.

(continued)

> *(continued from previous page)*
>
> Massachusetts' experience with healthcare reform legislation provides a real-world case study demonstrating the potential to significantly reduce the number of uninsured through an individual mandate combined with affordable health coverage options.

Although US health policies are developed primarily at the federal level, state and local governments and industries in the private sector (nonfederal arenas) also engage in health policymaking. This chapter focuses on health policymaking in these arenas. First, state-level health policymaking is presented; that discussion is followed by sections covering local government and private-sector health-related policy influencers. The attributes of health policymaking in these sectors are also summarized.

STATE GOVERNMENTAL STRUCTURE

The federal and state sectors share a common government structure composed of the legislative, executive, and judiciary branches. However, each state has its own constitution and bill of rights, which together define the structure and function of the state government and of the local governments within the state's boundary (Longest 2010). Following is a brief discussion of the typical state political system.

POLITICAL SYSTEM

State governments are modeled after the US federal government in that each is composed of an executive, legislative, and judicial branch (Exhibit 3.1). States are bound by the US (federal) Constitution to maintain a republican form of government, although they are not specifically required to adhere to the three-branch system. The executive branch of the state government is headed by the governor and other state executives, such as the attorney general, the lieutenant governor, the secretary of state, auditors, and commissioners. All states' governors are directly elected by the people, as are most other positions in their executive branch. The exact structure of the executive branch varies from state to state.

The state legislative branch is the main lawmaking body of the government; it also approves the state's budget and fulfills other functions of government. As in the federal government, the state legislature consists of a house of representatives—known in some states as the assembly or house of delegates—and a senate chamber. (Nebraska has only one chamber in its legislature.) In most states, senators are elected by the state's voters to four-year terms, and members of the house are elected to two-year terms.

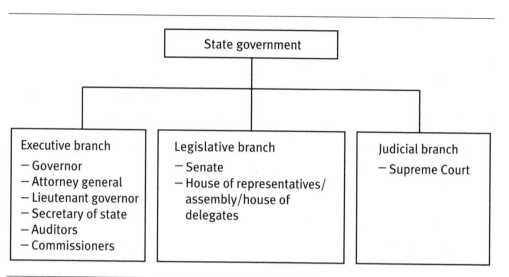

Exhibit 3.1
The US State
Political System

A state's judiciary is generally headed by its version of the Supreme Court (with some exceptions; for example, New York's Supreme Court is the trial-level court, whereas the state's highest court is referred to as the Court of Appeals). This court hears appeal cases from lower-level state courts; no trials are held in state supreme courts. Decisions made by a state's supreme court are binding unless they do not adhere to the US Constitution, in which case, decisions may be appealed in the US Supreme Court.

The exact structure of the courts and the rules governing judicial appointments and elections are determined on a state-by-state basis, either through state legislation or by the state's constitution.

POLICYMAKING PROCESS AT THE STATE LEVEL

The policymaking process at the state level can vary substantially from state to state. In general, however, states apply the same legislative system as does the federal government (see, e.g., Alabama State Legislature 2011; Maryland General Assembly 2006; Oregon State Legislature 2011; State Legislature of Alaska 2011; West Virginia Legislature 2011). The idea for a new law can come from an elected representative, a group of elected representatives, the governor, or any other concerned citizen or interest group. The proposed law is drafted into a bill, which is then sponsored by an elected member of either the state's senate chamber or its lower chamber (house of representatives, general assembly, etc.). Although a bill must be introduced into the legislature by a representative or senator, both legislators and interest groups draft significant amounts of legislation.

Bills can be introduced in either chamber of the legislature, where they are reviewed by committees. Many states require that the bill also be accompanied by a financial projection showing the budgetary impact of the potential law. The bill goes through three readings before being voted on by the elected representatives. Often, amendments are made after each reading, and the merits of the bill are debated among the members.

Once it passes one chamber, the bill proceeds to three readings in the other chamber. The same process of debates and amendments is followed. After both houses have agreed on and passed a final version of the bill, it goes to the governor to be signed into law. In many states, the governor has the ability to veto a bill that is passed by both chambers. In other states, such as Oregon, the governor's veto can be overridden by a favorable vote of two-thirds or more of the members in both houses.

EXAMPLES OF STATE HEALTHCARE LEGISLATION

The power and responsibility of states to establish laws that protect the public's health and welfare derive from the US Constitution. The focus of healthcare legislation can range from promoting health, including environmental protection, occupational health, safe food services, and injury prevention, to providing health services, such as public health nursing, communicable disease control, family planning and prenatal care, and nutritional counseling. (See Exhibit 3.2 for examples of state health policies, and review the Learning Point box titled "Illustrations of States' Involvement in Health Policy Development" for a description of health policy activity in Oregon and Connecticut.)

EXHIBIT 3.2
Examples of States'
Responsibilities
Through Health
Policy

- Serve as a major payer of healthcare services—an average of 22.3 percent of all state expenditures were Medicaid-related in 2010 (Miller 2012)

- Fund the Children's Health Insurance Program, health insurance benefits for state employees and other public-sector workers, and stand-alone state programs that provide health services to the uninsured

- Regulate the state's healthcare system (e.g., licensing and monitoring health professionals and health-related organizations, regulating states' private health insurance industry)

- Establish and monitor compliance with quality standards for environmental protection

- Provide safety net facilities through support of local health departments and community-based healthcare organizations and through programs that provide charity care to low-income populations

- Provide subsidies for graduate medical education and support large-scale educational campaigns

Learning Point
Illustrations of States' Involvement
in Health Policy Development

Oregon

Known as a leader in state healthcare reform (Oregon.gov 2011; Oregon Health Authority 2011; Health Care for All Oregon 2011), in 2009, Oregon's Legislative Assembly passed House Bill 2009, which established the Oregon Health Authority. The legislation created an insurance exchange—a federal subsidy–eligible set of standardized healthcare plans regulated by the state from which individuals may purchase health insurance—through the Oregon Health Authority for individuals and small businesses that do not have group health insurance.

The law also expanded the Oregon Health Plan, the state's Medicaid program, to cover low-income working families, and it allocated $5 billion in additional funds to the Medicaid plan over the following ten years. Other provisions contained in House Bill 2009 called for expanding the use of electronic health records through the Oregon Health Authority, establishing quality standards for hospitals and healthcare providers, and mandating that health insurance companies disclose their administrative costs and executive salaries to maintain transparency and accountability. As with the federal reforms included in the Affordable Care Act (ACA) of 2010, lifetime maximum limits on health benefits will be eliminated, insurers will be prohibited from dropping health coverage to those already enrolled in a plan, and children who are unmarried will be able to stay on their parents' health insurance plan until age 26.

The ACA is expected to provide some financial support for the reforms contained in Oregon's House Bill 2009. Once all the health reforms are implemented, an estimated 90 percent or more of Oregon residents will have health insurance coverage, with the aim to ensure coverage for all Oregon residents by 2015.

Connecticut

Connecticut, another of the first states to embrace national healthcare reform efforts (Johnson 2009; House Democrats of Connecticut 2011a, 2011b; State of Connecticut 2011), created Sustinet through legislation passed in May 2009 by the Connecticut General Assembly. Sustinet is a public healthcare plan to provide coverage for 98 percent of Connecticut residents by 2014. Governor M. Jodie Rell initially vetoed the law,

(continued)

(continued from previous page)

but her veto was overridden by more than 67 percent majorities in both the state's House of Representatives and Senate.

Sustinet functions as an insurance pool. State employees, retirees, the uninsured and underinsured, residents receiving public assistance, and small business employers were the first groups to be eligible for the plan. In June 2011, the state legislature voted to extend Sustinet coverage to nonprofit organization and local government employees. Large employers will soon have an opportunity to buy into the Sustinet plan on behalf of their employees.

Sustinet's focus is on preventive care and the management of chronic illnesses. The law creating Sustinet also established task forces to address the problems of obesity, tobacco use, and the healthcare workforce shortage.

LOCAL GOVERNMENT STRUCTURE

Local US governments typically fall into one of two levels: county or municipality (e.g., cities, towns, villages). Counties—called *boroughs* in Alaska and *parishes* in Louisiana—may be further divided into townships. Service districts, such as school districts and police and fire protection districts, may be congruent with county or municipal boundaries or set their own borders.

The structures of county and municipal governments vary greatly, but they all follow the democratic model. States assign powers to the local governments rather than to individuals; however, mayors, city council members, and members of other governing bodies are usually elected directly by the local residents. Laws are typically passed by majority votes at local council sessions.

The powers granted to a given municipality or county often depend on the size of its population. New York City, for example, has millions of residents and controls its own fire, police, and emergency medical services as well as its own libraries, parks and recreation, public transportation, and public works services. Smaller communities, on the other hand, may rely on county or state governments to provide these services.

POLICYMAKING PROCESS AT THE LOCAL GOVERNMENT LEVEL

As with state policymaking, the legislative process can vary significantly between counties and cities or towns (see, e.g., Erie County Legislature 2011; Monroe County 2011; Metropolitan Government of Nashville and Davidson County 2011). However, in general, these local government structures follow the same democratic process to make laws as federal and state legislatures. The exception is that local legislatures and councils typically have only one chamber, unlike the federal and state legislatures, which also have an upper chamber. Proposals for new laws are written into resolutions, also referred to as referrals, ordinances, or bills. They are brought in front of the county legislature, city council, or other local governing body to be considered.

Resolutions can be introduced by the local government or elected representatives. In some counties, concerned citizens can write a resolution for presentation at the local government meeting. Resolutions are usually reviewed by committees in larger counties or cities and by the entire council or legislature in smaller local governments. The resolution then proceeds through multiple readings—amendments to the legislation are often introduced after each reading—and its merits debated before being voted on by the elected representatives. Some types of resolutions, such as tax laws, may require a greater than 50 percent majority vote to pass.

After the resolution has passed, it may need to be signed into law by the mayor or council executive. Once they become law, resolutions may continue to be called resolutions or become known as bylaws, local laws, or ordinances.

EXAMPLES OF LOCAL HEALTHCARE LEGISLATION

The public health departments of county and city governments enforce laws that complement state-level healthcare legislation. One of the most common areas for health legislation at the local level is the regulation of tobacco products and smoking in public environments. In Monroe County, New York, for example, the local government has instituted a general smoking code and a law intended to prevent adolescent tobacco use (Monroe County Department of Public Health 2011; Monroe County 2005). Monroe County's smoking laws are part of a wider public health campaign in the state of New York to curb tobacco use and reduce nonsmokers' exposure to second-hand and environmental smoke.

Public health campaigns in many US municipalities have also begun to urge adults and children to be more active and engage in outdoor activities to curb obesity. Examples of recent measures include offering healthy lunches and limiting soft drinks in schools and providing portion-control and nutrition information in restaurants (mandatory in some states).

PRIVATE HEALTH RESEARCH INSTITUTES

As with federal, state, and local government, the private sector has contributed to health policy development. Here, the role of private research institutes—also known as think tanks—in influencing health policy is demonstrated through the work of the RAND Corporation.

RAND Corporation

The RAND Corporation conducts research and analysis to improve and inform policymaking in the areas of health, education, and national security. RAND, located in Santa Monica, California, strives to provide objective analysis and operates independently of commercial or partisan ties (RAND 2011).

The RAND Health division conducts studies on public policy issues related to healthcare reform, health insurance coverage, and the use of information technology in healthcare. Obesity, post-traumatic stress disorder, and complementary and alternative medicine are RAND's public health focus areas. As a well-regarded participant in policymaking circles, RAND is highly influential through its studies and reports. See the Research from the Field box for an example of health policy research conducted by RAND.

Research from the Field
RAND Health Policy Research: An Assessment of High-Deductible Health Plans

High-deductible health plans (HDHPs), also known as consumer-directed health plans (CDHPs), have increased in popularity in recent years as methods for controlling healthcare costs. By shifting a larger portion of the cost to the patient through increased deductibles, some believe, consumers will use less care, especially unnecessary care. Approximately 20 percent of Americans covered under employer-sponsored health plans were enrolled in an HDHP or a CDHP in 2009, and more than 54 percent of employers offered at least one such plan in 2010.

In 2011, researchers at RAND Corporation conducted a cost-related assessment of HDHPs (Beeuwkes Buntin et al. 2011). The researchers for this retrospective study looked at data previously collected from the healthcare plan claims and enrollment information reported for 808,707 households by 53 major employers in the United States. Of these employers, 28 offered HDHPs or CDHPs to their employees. The increase in healthcare costs for those who enrolled in one of these types of plans for the first time from 2004 to 2005 was compared to the cost increases for those enrolled in traditional healthcare plans during the same period. Similar comparisons were made for the rates of use of preventive care services between the two groups.

Overall, through the duration of the study, the RAND researchers found that healthcare costs increased for both those with high-deductible plans and those with

(continued)

(continued from previous page)

traditional plans. However, costs grew at a lower rate for those in the HDHP group. Similarly, expenditures for those families with HDHPs were lower for inpatient and outpatient care and for prescription drugs than for those enrolled in traditional health plans; spending on urgent care did not differ between the two groups.

The RAND study also found that families who enrolled in HDHPs reduced their use of preventive care services. These included childhood immunizations, the rates of which increased among traditional plan users; mammography; cervical cancer screening; and colorectal cancer screening.

The popularity of HDHPs is expected to increase further with the advent of healthcare reform in the United States. They will be among the featured health plans offered by the insurance exchanges being established in many states to assist those without health coverage to find insurance. Studies such as that conducted by RAND can guide policymakers when assessing the effectiveness of government health programs. Under the Affordable Care Act (ACA), for example, deductibles must be waived for preventive healthcare services. Thus, one implication of the RAND study is that clearly communicating information to families enrolled in HDHPs and the employers that offer these plans about this provision of the ACA must be a priority if the goal of increasing preventive care is to be met.

SOURCE: Beeuwkes Buntin et al. (2011).

PRIVATE HEALTH FOUNDATIONS

In addition to conducting health policy research, private health foundations work to advance policy through grant programs that fund promising social experiments. The Pew Charitable Trusts comprise one such foundation.

PEW CHARITABLE TRUSTS

The Pew Charitable Trusts conduct research and public policy work to address the challenges facing the United States and global community. Areas of study include the environment, early education, and public health. The trusts also conduct public opinion polls to study trends in specific issues relevant to Americans. Pew's mission is to advance solutions to these issues (Pew Charitable Trusts 2011).

The Pew trusts support health research in four policy areas: consumer product safety, emerging science, food and health, and medical safety. Within these four topics, the Pew Health group focuses on identifying and reducing potential risks and hazards with everyday items such as foodstuffs, financial products, household items, and prescription drugs. Solutions are policy oriented, such as supporting mandatory food safety standards and organizing informational campaigns to curb the overuse of antibiotics in livestock (Pew Charitable Trusts 2011). The Research from the Field box presents an example of Pew Charitable Trusts' work to ensure that children have access to safe and nutritious food.

PRIVATE INDUSTRY

Corporate America influences health and health policy primarily through the services or products it provides and through its lobbying activities. The fast-food and tobacco industries, for example, have extensive business interests in the United States and around the world, and their products are key influencers of the population's health status.

FAST-FOOD INDUSTRY

More than 25 percent of American adults eat fast food every day. In 2000, Americans spent approximately $110 billion on fast food, whereas in 1970, they spent only $6 billion. In addition to those with drive-through access, fast-food restaurants can be found in airports, hospitals, schools and universities, stadiums, cruise ships, and many other locations where people gather (CBS News 2009; Schlosser 2001; Walker 2001).

In general, fast food is inexpensive, convenient, filling, and prepared quickly for the consumer. The food does not require dishes or utensils for eating, is mostly deep-fat fried, and comes in large portions with uniform specifications. Few vegetables are used because they are difficult to store long term.

The fast-food industry consists mainly of multimillion-dollar national restaurant chains. McDonald's Corporation alone franchised 32,737 restaurants worldwide in 2010 and continues to expand each year (*NASDAQ.com News* 2011). It hires more people per year than does any other American organization and is the country's largest purchaser of beef, pork, and potatoes. McDonald's is also the largest owner of retail property in the world and spends the most money of any brand on marketing (Schlosser 2001).

In addition to its vast marketing campaigns, the fast-food industry and its suppliers spend large sums lobbying the US government to promote or oppose legislation according to their interests. Worker safety, food safety, and minimum wage laws have historically been opposed by the fast-food industry.

The consumption of fast food contributes to obesity among American adults and children (CBS News 2009; WHO 2011a). In addition to the commonly cited factors linking fast-food consumption to obesity (e.g., large amounts of fat, highly processed ingredients), studies have shown that proximity to fast-food outlets is a factor (e.g., Currie et al.

2009; Rabin 2009). Currie and colleagues (2009) found that when a fast-food restaurant was located within a tenth of a mile of a school, the obesity rates for children attending the school increased 5.2 percent more than for children who attended a school with a fast-food restaurant a quarter of a mile or farther away.

In 2002, a group of obese and overweight children filed a class-action lawsuit against McDonald's, asking the court to award compensation for their obesity-related health problems and requesting that it force McDonald's to improve its nutritional labeling and provide funding for a health education campaign on the dangers of fast food. The lawsuit was dismissed a year later, but it raised important questions about legal accountability for the poor nutritional standards of most fast-food menu items. Mello, Rimm, and Studdert (2003) draw parallels between the fast-food industry's intention to process and manufacture food to be addictive and the tobacco industry's aim to manufacture addictive cigarettes. However, observers generally agree that eating fast food is a consumer choice.

Research from the Field
An Example of Pew Health Policy Research: The Kids' Safe and Healthful Foods Project

The Kids' Safe and Healthful Foods Project, funded by the Pew Health Group in partnership with other private foundations, aims to improve the food choices available in schools to curb the rate of childhood obesity and to reform food safety policies in schools to stop the spread of foodborne illnesses. As part of the project, the Pew Health Group works with the US Department of Agriculture (USDA) by providing the agency with evidence-based analysis and policy recommendations.

The three major goals of the Kids' Safe and Healthful Foods Project are to (1) ensure that the nutrition standards established by the USDA for foods and beverages available in schools are based on scientific evidence, (2) make sure schools have sufficient resources to properly train cafeteria employees and keep cafeteria equipment in good working order, and (3) help the USDA to establish and enforce stringent food safety policies for use in schools. (Prior to the launch of the Kids' Safe and Healthful Foods Project, the USDA nutritional standards for school meals had not been updated in more than 15 years.)

As a result of the project, which also is closely aligned with the White House Task Force on Childhood Obesity, food safety has improved. Under the new school food safety policies, which arose from the Healthy, Hunger-Free Kids Act and was guided by

(continued)

> *(continued from previous page)*
>
> the Kids' Safe and Healthful Foods Project, the USDA is required to enhance its communication with other government agencies, including its hold and recall procedures, so that notifications of food recalls are disseminated to schools in a timely manner. The agency must also ensure that food served outside the cafeteria—in classrooms or elsewhere—meets the same safety standards. These additional requirements will help schools to avoid outbreaks of foodborne illness, such as in 2009 when schools may have served students peanut products contaminated with Salmonella because they did not receive the recall notices in time (Kids' Safe and Healthful Foods Project 2013).
>
> SOURCE: Kids' Safe and Healthful Foods Project (2011).

CIGARETTE AND TOBACCO INDUSTRY

The tobacco industry is composed mainly of large, multinational corporate tobacco growers and cigarette manufacturers. The industry represents historical significance in the United States, as it was an important commodity in colonial times. Tobacco is the seventh largest cash crop in the country; in 2009, the industry reported $614 billion in revenue (American Lung Association in Washington 2011; IRS 2011; Lepore 2011).

Tobacco products are the most heavily taxed consumer product in the United States when measured by percentage of retail price. The industry is also highly regulated, with quotas set for each farmer's land and the end product graded by US Department of Agriculture (USDA) inspectors. The sale of tobacco to dealers and warehouses is monitored by the USDA's Agricultural Stabilization and Conservation Service.

The five largest cigarette manufacturers in the country spent a total of $12.5 billion on advertising in 2006, the last year in which data were available. Most promotional efforts came in the form of price discounts to wholesalers and retailers (American Lung Association 2011b). It has been shown that lowering the price of cigarettes increases youth consumption; conversely, with each 10 percent increase in the price of cigarettes, youth consumption drops by 6 to 7 percent (Boonn 2012).

According to the American Lung Association (2011a), smoking cigarettes is the number one preventable cause of morbidity and mortality worldwide. Nearly 450,000 Americans die from tobacco smoking–related diseases annually (CDC 2011; Cummings, Morley, and Hyland 2002; WHO 2011b). The smoke from one cigarette contains more than 4,800 different chemicals—69 of which are known to be carcinogenic (cancer causing). Chronic lung disease, including lung cancer and chronic obstructive pulmonary disease, accounts for about three-quarters of smoking-related morbidity in current smokers and half of smoking-related morbidity in former smokers.

In 2004, smoking-related deaths and diseases cost the United States $193 billion, including $96 billion from direct healthcare expenditures and $97 billion from lost productivity.

ATTRIBUTES OF HEALTH POLICY DEVELOPMENT IN NONFEDERAL SECTORS

Health policymaking in nonfederal sectors—state and local governments and the private sector—is characterized by several factors:

◆ The constraints imposed by the broader policy landscape

◆ The relationship between politics and policy

◆ The level of public health funding

◆ The ways in which the private sector shapes policy direction

◆ Policy entrepreneurship at the grassroots level

◆ The lack of integration and coordination among policymaking groups in creating policy initiatives

CONSTRAINTS UNDER FEDERAL POLICY

Policymaking at the state and local levels is limited by broader federal policy. Although regulation is primarily the states' responsibility, federal laws can preempt state legislation. For example, states cannot require firms to offer insurance to their employees because federal law, in the form of the Employee Retirement Income Security Act, would override any attempt by the state to do so.

The private sector is also influenced and constrained by federal regulations, in areas such as practitioner licensing, security and privacy of patient information, and reimbursement. For example, the Medicare and Medicaid programs periodically adjust their reimbursement methodologies—the methods by which they calculate how much money to pay providers for services rendered—which prompts healthcare organizations to make changes in the way services are delivered.

RELATIONSHIP BETWEEN POLITICS AND POLICY

Legislation is most likely to pass if the governor and the majority of the legislature carry the same political party affiliation. Similarly, legislation often is stalled or diluted when the policymakers considering it represent different parties.

Another link between politics and policy, which applies to all sectors involved in policymaking, is the election cycle. In the time preceding an election, politicians running for reelection often emphasize legislation that is expected to garner immediate results, thus benefiting their reelection bids. Difficult problems that take a long time to solve are frequently left for future congressional sessions. As a result, many problems facing US residents are cumulative, but the policies meant to address those problems are symptomatic— not addressing the root cause but rather its symptoms—and piecemeal. The underlying problems, left unresolved, tend to worsen over time and exact an even heavier toll on all those affected than an earlier, more comprehensive solution would have.

LEVEL OF PUBLIC FUNDING

The market-oriented economy in the United States attracts private entrepreneurs to carry out key healthcare delivery functions at a profit, leaving the public sector to assume a secondary role when the market alone cannot address all healthcare needs (particularly for members of vulnerable populations who cannot afford expensive care). The resulting healthcare system is functionally fragmented, with little standardization, resulting in duplication of certain services and inadequacy of others.

Funding for public health in the United States is relatively low, at less than $150 per capita, or less than 2.5 percent of the overall healthcare spending (Salinsky and Gursky 2006), compared to that in Canada, which spent 5.5 percent of its total health expenditure

---

For Your Consideration
Traditional Republican and Democratic Stances

The 2012 election cycle highlighted a number of policy positions (known as planks in their platform) favored by each major party. While Republicans traditionally have sought small government (government that practices limited use of regulation, as opposed to "big," centralized government) and limited taxation and supported business interests, Democrats have historically favored social programs, assistance for vulnerable populations, and a larger tax share from the wealthy than from the middle and lower classes.

How do you view these positions in light of comments made by party leaders during the 2012 presidential and congressional elections as reported by the mainstream media? Do the comments consistently reflect these traditional stances? Why or why not?

on public health (Canadian Institute for Health Information 2005). Little public investment is made in health technology, workforce training and recruitment, or facility construction or renovation. In addition, the fact that spending on public health varies widely across communities raises concerns about whether and how these differences might affect the availability of essential public health services.

SHAPING POLICY DIRECTION

The private sector shapes policy direction more than state and local governments do. As described earlier in this chapter, the research topics addressed by private research institutes and the projects funded by private foundations lead to findings that contribute to better understanding of the health problems studied, their underlying causes, and potential solutions to them, thus paving the way for policy development. Another way private research institutes and foundations drive policy is in their evaluations of existing policies, the results of which are often incorporated in policy modifications or new policies.

POLICY ENTREPRENEURSHIP AT THE GRASSROOTS LEVEL

Grassroots efforts by policy entrepreneurs involve community stakeholders and may be funded by private foundations. Such efforts are critical to adapting successful experiences to other environments and identfying innovative approaches to solving health-related issues.

Typically, community-based projects stress participation and empowerment; deeply involving community members leads to acceptance of the initiative and helps promote sustainability of the intervention. Community members plan and manage initiatives, and through community mobilization, skill building, and resource sharing, communities are empowered to identify and meet their own needs, making them stronger advocates for the vulnerable populations within and across their community boundaries.

KEY POINTS

◆ Although the policymaking process can vary substantially from state to state, states generally apply the same legislative system as the federal government does.

◆ Local government structures follow the same democratic process for making laws as federal and state legislatures do, with the exception that local legislatures and councils typically have only one legislative chamber.

◆ The private sector, including private research institutes, foundations, and industry, contributes to health policy development.

◆ The major attributes of health policymaking in the public nonfederal sector include the constraints imposed by the broader federal policy landscape, influence of politics, availability of funding, level of entrepreneurship at the local level, and lack of integration and coordination among policymaking groups.

REFERENCES

Alabama State Legislature. 2011. "Alabama's Legislative Process." Accessed July 23, 2012. www.legislature.state.al.us/misc/legislativeprocess/legislativeprocess_ml.html.

American Lung Association. 2011a. "Smoking." Accessed July 21, 2012. www.lungusa.org/stop-smoking/about-smoking/health-effects/smoking.html.

———. 2011b. "Tobacco Industry Marketing." Accessed July 21, 2012. www.lungusa.org/stop-smoking/about-smoking/facts-figures/tobacco-industry-marketing.html.

American Lung Association in Washington. 2011. "Facts About Tobacco." Accessed July 21, 2012. www.alaw.org/tobacco_control/facts_about_tobacco/index.html.

Beeuwkes Buntin, M., A. M. Haviland, R. McDevitt, and N. Sood. 2011. "Healthcare Spending and Preventive Care in High-Deductible and Consumer-Directed Health Plans." *American Journal of Managed Care* 17 (3): 222–30.

Boonn, A. 2012. "Raising Cigarette Taxes Reduces Smoking, Especially Among Kids (and the Cigarette Companies Know It)." Campaign for Tobacco-Free Kids. Published October 11. www.tobaccofreekids.org/research/factsheets/pdf/0146.pdf.

Canadian Institute for Health Information. 2005. *National Health Expenditure Trends 1975–2005*, Table C.1.2.7. Ottawa, Ontario: Canadian Institute for Health Information.

CBS News. 2009. "Americans Are Obsessed with Fast Food: The Dark Side of the All-American Meal." Published February 11. www.cbsnews.com/stories/2002/01/31/health/main326858.shtml.

Centers for Disease Control and Prevention (CDC). 2011. "Health Effects of Cigarette Smoking." Accessed July 21, 2012. www.cdc.gov/tobacco/data_statistics/fact_sheets/health_effects/effects_cig_smoking/.

Cummings, K. M., C. P. Morley, and A. Hyland. 2002. "Failed Promises of the Cigarette Industry and Its Effect on Consumer Misperceptions About the Health Risks of Smoking." *Tobacco Control* 11 (Suppl. 1): 110–17.

Currie, J., S. Della Vigna, E. Moretti, and V. Pathania. 2009. "The Effect of Fast Food Restaurants on Obesity." Published in April. http://elsa.berkeley.edu/~sdellavi/wp/fastfoodApr09.pdf.

Erie County (New York) Legislature. 2011. "How the Legislature Takes Action." Accessed July 29, 2012. www2.erie.gov/legislature/index.php?q=how-legislature-takes-action.

Health Care for All Oregon. 2011. "Oregon Legislation." Accessed July 24, 2012. www.healthcareforalloregon.org/oregon/.

House Democrats of Connecticut. 2011a. "House Passes Healthcare Pooling, Sustinet." Published May 27. www.housedems.ct.gov/healthcare/PR11.asp#a052711.

———. 2011b. "Speaker Donovan Statement on Senate Passage of Health Care Reforms." Published June 6. www.housedems.ct.gov/healthcare/PR11.asp#a060611.

Internal Revenue Service (IRS). 2011. "Market Segment Specialization Program: Tobacco Industry." Accessed July 21, 2012. www.irs.gov/pub/irs-mssp/tobacco.pdf.

Johnson, A. 2009. "Connecticut Pushes Ahead on Health Care." *Wall Street Journal.* Published July 22. http://online.wsj.com/article/SB124822088310970327.html.

Kaiser Family Foundation. 2012. "Massachusetts Health Care Reform: Six Years Later." Focus on Health Reform. Published in May. www.kff.org/healthreform/upload/8311.pdf.

Kids' Safe and Healthful Foods Project. 2013. "School Food Safety." Accessed February 6. www.healthyschoolfoodsnow.org/policy/improving-school-food-safety/.

———. 2011. Home page. Accessed January 3 2013. www.healthyschoolfoodsnow.org.

Lepore, M. 2011. "15 Facts About the Cigarette Industry That Will Blow Your Mind." *Business Insider.* Published April 8. www.businessinsider.com/facts-about-tobacco-industry-2011-4.

Longest, B. 2010. *Health Policymaking in the United States*, 5th ed. Chicago: Health Administration Press.

Maryland General Assembly. 2006. "The Legislative Process: How a Bill Becomes a Law." Published in June. www.msa.md.gov/msa/mdmanual/07leg/html/proc.html.

Mello, M., E. B. Rimm, and D. M. Studdert. 2003. "The McLawsuit: The Fast-Food Industry and Legal Accountability for Obesity." *Health Affairs* 22 (6): 207–16.

Metropolitan Government of Nashville and Davidson County, Tennessee. 2011. "Overview of Metropolitan Council." Accessed July 29, 2012. www.nashville.gov/mc/council/legislative_process.htm.

Miller, D. 2012. "Medicaid Spending." Council of State Governments. Accessed February 6, 2013. http://knowledgecenter.csg.org/drupal/content/medicaid-spending.

Monroe County, New York. 2011. "Legislature." Accessed January 3, 2013. www2.monroe county.gov/legislature-index.php.

———. 2005. "Public Health Law—Article 13-F: Regulation of Tobacco Products and Herbal Cigarettes; Distribution to Minors." Published December 1. www.monroecounty.gov/File/Health/ATUPA/13F_05.pdf.

Monroe County, New York, Department of Public Health. 2011. "Smoking Code/Adolescent Tobacco Use Prevention Act." Accessed July 30, 2012. www.monroecounty.gov/eh-smoking.php.

NASDAQ.com News. 2011. "Subway Tops McDonald's for Number of Stores in World." Published March 21. www.nasdaq.com/article/subway-tops-mcdonalds-for-number-of-stores-in-world-cm63138#.URIvUlrFT_l.

Oregon Health Authority. 2011. "U.S. House Health Reform Vote." Accessed February 6, 2013. www.oregon.gov/oha/pages/features/feature_federal_intersect_ore.aspx.

Oregon State Legislature. 2011. "Citizen's Guide to the Oregon Legislative Process." Accessed July 23. www.leg.state.or.us/citizenguide/.

Oregon.gov. 2011. Press Release: June 30, 2011. Accessed July 24, 2012. www.oregon.gov/gov/media_room/pages/press_releasesp2011/press_063011.aspx.

Pew Charitable Trusts. 2011. Home page. Accessed January 3, 2013. www.pewtrusts.org.

Rabin, R. C. 2009. "Proximity to Fast Food a Factor in Student Obesity." *New York Times*. Published March 25. www.nytimes.com/2009/03/26/health/nutrition/26obese.html.

RAND Corporation. 2011. "History and Mission." Accessed June 29, 2012. www.rand.org/about/history.html.

Salinsky, E., and E. A. Gursky. 2006. "The Case for Transforming Governmental Public Health." *Health Affairs* 25: 1017–28.

Schlosser, E. 2001. "Fast Food Nation: The Dark Side of the All-American Meal" [book review]. *New York Times*. Published January 21. www.nytimes.com/books/first/s/schlosser-fast.html.

State of Connecticut. 2011. "Sustinet: About Us." Published April 8. www.ct.gov/sustinet/cwp/view.asp?a=3826&q=450132.

State Legislature of Alaska. 2011. "Legislative Process in Alaska." Accessed July 23, 2012. http://w3.legis.state.ak.us/docs/pdf/legprocess.pdf.

Walker, R. 2001. "No Accounting for Mouthfeel." *New York Times*. Published January 21. www.nytimes.com/books/01/01/21/reviews/010121.21walkert.html.

West Virginia Legislature. 2011. "How a Bill Becomes Law." Accessed July 23, 2012. www.legis.state.wv.us/Educational/Bill_Becomes_Law/Bill_Becomes_Law.cfm.

World Health Organization (WHO). 2011a. "Obesity and Overweight." Published in March. www.who.int/mediacentre/factsheets/fs311/en/index.html.

———. 2011b. "Tobacco." Published in July. www.who.int/mediacentre/factsheets/fs339/en/index.html.

CHAPTER 10

THE FUTURE

The healthcare reform journey will continue because every year, Congress (and each state legislature) revises existing laws to meet the current environment. Healthcare reform is never finished.

Laws usually change because of:

◆ legislation that works poorly or is difficult to implement,

◆ new policies that are working in pilots and demonstrations that can be applied more broadly,

◆ funding availability or lack thereof,

◆ changes in the legislative majority party or the executive branch that bring a new governing philosophy, or

◆ system changes in the healthcare system that are independent of current legislation.

This chapter explores the processes of change and identifies which sections of the Affordable Care Act (ACA) might be modified and which are likely to remain. In addition, major changes that may occur in the healthcare delivery system are also identified, as they may affect future health policy.

MAKING CHANGES: THE PROCESS

Because the enactment of the ACA was controversial and partisan, some changes to the law are likely. Congressional majorities will change, as will the president in 2016. During these transitions a number of strategies and tools will be used to modify existing law.

LAWSUITS

The most direct method to change legislation is with a lawsuit. States and interested parties continue to challenge aspects of the law. However the US Supreme Court has ruled on the major policy aspects of the law—the individual mandate and the Medicaid expansion (see **Reading 2A**). Any additional litigation will likely have substantially less impact.

OVERSIGHT HEARINGS BY CONGRESS

Another possible way to change legislation is through congressional hearings and oversight. Administration officials can be called on to testify, and modifications may be made to regulations. Congress can threaten to reduce a federal agency's budget if it does not respond to recommendations from a committee.

NEW LEGISLATION AND BUDGET CHANGES

The most likely vehicle for change is new legislation. However, all changes must be negotiated with the president, and during his term of office President Obama would likely veto any radical change to the ACA. More likely, legislation will be created that corrects perceived errors in the ACA and reduces funding for some aspects of the law.

Because the House of Representatives proposes all appropriations, some key elements of the ACA might not receive funding.

The Appendix provides a list of changes to the ACA that have already been made via congressional or administrative action.

POTENTIAL TARGETS FOR CHANGE

INSURANCE MANDATE

The section of the ACA that is most often seen as inconsistent with American values is the insurance mandate. This mandate will be subject to the change strategies outlined in the previous section. If this mandate is repealed, the ACA begins to unravel.

The most likely individuals to resist having coverage are the healthiest. If the healthy no longer buy insurance, rates for those left in the health insurance exchanges will increase, fewer individuals will be able to afford health insurance, and eventually the system will collapse. (This is sometimes called the risk-pool death spiral.) In response to this inflation, health insurers will attempt to use preexisting conditions to deny individuals coverage again. Doctors and hospitals will provide higher levels of uncompensated care and rightfully demand that the reductions in Medicare payments be restored. Without the insurance mandate, creative new legislation will be required to maintain balance within the ACA.

A potential substitute for the insurance mandate is a late enrollment penalty. Medicare has had an insurance mandate for Medicare Part D (the drug benefit) since 2005, which seems to have been readily accepted by Medicare beneficiaries. Here is how it works. When an individual is eligible for Medicare, he must enroll in Part D or pay a penalty. This penalty applies when he does obtain Part D coverage and includes additional payment of 1 percent of the average cost of coverage for those months he does not have Part D. However, if he continues to work and can demonstrate "creditable coverage" for drug coverage through his employer-based insurance, the penalty does not apply (CMS 2013).

For example, assume a participant was on Medicare for two years without a drug plan, and this year she wants to enroll. The penalty is 1 percent of the average of all drug plans per month, which amounts to around 30 cents. The penalty is permanent, which can add up, as two years' (or 24 months') worth of penalties can raise the premium by more than $7 a month, perpetually. Because the cheapest Part D plans run between $15 and $18 per month, most experts recommend that even if an individual is on few or no medications, she should enroll in the least expensive plan.

If the insurance mandate is changed, it will likely be replaced with alternatives such as the Medicare Part D penalty.

Standard Benefits

Although a standard benefit set in the exchanges levels the playing field for health plan competition, it also creates other challenges. For example, providers of services not included in the standard benefit set will lobby for inclusion; if more services are included, the cost of insurance will increase.

Another problem with standard benefits is that they are standard. They prevent health plans from developing creative policies that are less expensive or customized for unique markets. The standard benefit regulations will be a battleground for special interests; this fight may force changes in the ACA.

Some legislators have proposed a "copper plan" that would have reduced benefits and would be less expensive than the current four levels available in the health exchanges (platinum, gold, silver, and bronze).

Medicaid Funding Requirement of States

The ACA provides 100 percent funding for the increased state portion of Medicaid, but only from 2014 to 2016. After that time, federal support gradually declines. For states that have low income-eligibility levels before 2014, this change will be expensive over the long term. Although increased levels of income eligibility are a key way the ACA increases insurance coverage in the United States, state pressure may change this policy.

For this reason, some states have declined to expand their Medicaid programs. However provider pressure may be enough to move these states to expand their Medicaid programs in spite of this concern.

TAXES

The ACA contains many new taxes on individuals, health plans, device manufacturers, tanning salons, and more. The political makeup of Congress and the presidency will affect the level of interest in changing these revenue-raising policies. However, these taxes are important for funding the subsidies in the exchanges and Medicaid. If they are repealed, the funds will need to be replaced through other sources.

COMPARATIVE EFFECTIVENESS RESEARCH

Evidence-based practice was once derided as "cookbook medicine." However the Agency for Healthcare Quality and Research (2014) defines it as "Applying the best available research results (evidence) when making decisions about health care. Health care professionals who perform evidence-based practice use research evidence along with clinical expertise and patient preferences. Systematic reviews (summaries of health care research results) provide information that aids in the process of evidence-based practice."

Although that attitude has changed significantly, some providers still resist—particularly those that provide care that may be of limited benefit. Although research funded by the ACA is not supposed to be used for payment policy, Medicare and Medicaid will not continue to pay for services found to be ineffective. Providers and suppliers will realize the effect on their incomes, which may lead to an attack on this segment of the ACA.

INDEPENDENT PAYMENT ADVISORY BOARD

The addition of this board was resisted by providers during the legislative debate but finally included as a blunt tool to control healthcare inflation. If the many cost-saving policies in the ACA work well, it will not be needed. However, if they do not, this board will be given more flexibility to devise payment solutions beyond reducing fee-for-service rates.

A more flexible solution that is effective in controlling costs is to use global budgets for hospitals and caps for physician salaries. If this strategy sounds familiar, it is—look north to Canada.

MALPRACTICE

The ACA contains state demonstration projects to reduce malpractice expense (§10607). During the debate surrounding the ACA, Republicans pushed for much stronger policies; these new policies may be enacted as part of a bargain to retain other segments of the law.

THE PUBLIC OPTION

The concept of including a government-run health plan (probably Medicare) as part of the exchanges was highly controversial during the legislative process and was dropped from the final bill. However, if healthcare inflation appears to be increasing rapidly, the public option might make a comeback.

GOOD IDEAS LIKELY TO REMAIN

HEALTH INSURANCE EXCHANGES

Although many conservatives do not like the insurance mandate, they do support health plan competition as a markets solution to healthcare costs. The exchanges provide a useful and contemporary system to foster competition. However, the standard benefit feature might be modified to provide for a wider range of products, which would allow for different benefits, deductibles, and coinsurance. In addition, subsidy levels may be modified if the ACA funding sources (taxes) are reduced or eliminated.

The challenge of running a state-based exchange was clearly demonstrated during the 2013–2014 enrollment period, when many websites had trouble responding to the sudden increase in traffic. Although most states prefer local control, it is unclear whether all states will eventually operate state-based exchanges. Because of the challenge to some state exchanges, these states may close their exchanges and let the federal government operate them.

Another interesting possible evolution of exchanges would be for them to function as public utilities. In this model all health plans would use one organization and website to compete for all the various health insurance markets—ACA individual and small group, Medicaid, Medicare Advantage, and private employer exchanges.

QUALITY, WORKFORCE, FRAUD, AND INNOVATION

The goals of increasing quality, increasing the supply of primary care practitioners, and fighting fraud have never been controversial. However, funding for these activities might be reduced based on general federal budget concerns.

The Center for Medicare & Medicaid Innovation had broad support in the policy community but may be modified, as it has taken some authority away from Congress.

Accountable Care Organizations, Bundled Payments, Readmissions, and Hospital-Acquired Conditions

These financial incentives and penalties for accountable care organizations (ACOs), bundled payments, readmissions, and hospital-acquired conditions are built on years of research and demonstration projects and would probably have been enacted without the ACA. These initiatives will likely continue but be modified as results become available.

What About a Repeal?

The House of Representatives voted more than 50 times to repeal the ACA since its enactment. However, during President Obama's term a total repeal would not likely be passed by Congress and signed by the president.

In addition, as long as the exchanges continue to meet enrollment targets, a substantial number of Americans will benefit from this new program. The federal government has never repealed a program that affected so many individuals (except Prohibition, perhaps). Therefore the ACA is likely to continue with the changes and improvements previously discussed.

System Changes

Health policy does not operate in a vacuum. It is strongly influenced by trends and strategies that occur in the healthcare system that are independent of current law. Some trends that may affect future health policy include:

◆ *Chronic disease management*: The greatest costs in a system are for care for patients with chronic disease. Effective systems of care need to be implemented, and the ACA rewards this behavior.

◆ *Primary care:* The increase in the number of individuals with insurance will put pressure on primary care providers. However new models of primary care (e.g., nurse practitioners, retail clinics, Internet services) will change the structure of primary care delivery.

◆ *Greater use of health information technology (HIT)*: Automation holds great promise to improve care delivery and reduce cost. Funding for these new systems is available from the American Recovery and Reinvestment Act of 2009. Many healthcare providers have traversed the difficult path of converting from paper records to HIT, and they are now beginning to reap some of the rewards of advanced analytics and increase automation of routine processes.

◆ *Community and population health:* Providers are making the transition away from episodes of acute care to systems that improve the health of a community. The ACA encourages a population view of healthcare, and this will grow in the future.

◆ *Financial incentives for quality and efficiency:* All payers are moving from payment for the quantity of service to payment for value. Public reporting of quality will increase, and providers that deliver high-quality services will be rewarded.

◆ *New price-based systems:* Price competition is not directly addressed in the ACA. However, the use of centers of excellence and reference pricing is increasing, which is reducing costs to large employers and payers.

◆ *Closer integration with all parts of the system, particularly physicians:* Integrated systems have been shown to deliver high-quality, low-cost care. The ACA supports and rewards systems-based care, and consolidation of providers continues to increase. This trend will concentrate markets in some areas of the country and effective price competition may not occur. This may prompt a different form of government intervention, perhaps similar to the energy utilities model of regulation.

◆ *New relationships with health plans:* Health insurance exchanges and ACOs allow providers and health plans to work together in innovative care delivery systems. New relationships can reduce the amount of overhead of a system and provide price-effective health plans to be offered in exchanges.

◆ *Expanded use of health insurance exchanges:* Because the ACA exchanges have been effective, some private employers may move their employees to these exchanges—particularly firms with many low-wage workers. In addition large firms are viewing private exchanges as effective models to provide health insurance, and their use will expand. The exchange models will encourage narrow networks of highly efficient providers.

SUMMARY

All laws are modified by future legislatures, and the ACA will be as well. Policies in the law that have high probability of change include the insurance mandate, standard benefits, funding for expanded Medicaid, taxes, comparative effectiveness research, the Independent Payment Advisory Board, and malpractice reform. If healthcare inflation grows unreasonably, the public option might again receive serious consideration.

Key policies in the ACA unlikely to be significantly changed include health insurance exchanges; quality improvement and reporting; workforce enhancements; incentives for ACOs and bundled payments; penalties for readmissions and hospital-acquired conditions; and the Center for Medicare & Medicaid Innovation.

Future changes to US health policy will be influenced by trends in the healthcare system. These trends include improved chronic disease management, new models of primary care, the use of HIT, community and population health, financial incentives for quality and efficiency, price-based systems, integration of the system, relationships between providers and health plans, and the expanded use of health insurance exchanges.

CONCLUSION

The Affordable Care Act of 2010 is a remarkable legislative achievement. However, it will only serve the country well if healthcare leaders make the many needed changes supported by the law. Energetic healthcare leadership can ensure that the US healthcare system will lead the world in quality and effectiveness for many years.

APPLICATIONS: DISCUSSION AND RESEARCH

1. What changes to the ACA would be most strongly supported by
   - Partisan elected officials?
   - The general public?
   - Healthcare providers?
   - Health plans?

2. Pick a future industry trend. What health policy could be enacted to support this trend?

REFERENCES

Agency for Healthcare Quality and Research. 2014. "Glossary of Terms." Accessed August 6. http://effectivehealthcare.ahrq.gov/index.cfm/glossary-of-terms/?pageaction=showte rm&termid=24.

Centers for Medicare & Medicaid Services (CMS). 2013. "Creditable Coverage and Late Enrollment Penalty." Accessed August 1, 2014. www.cms.gov/Medicare/Eligibility-and-Enrollment/MedicarePresDrugEligEnrol/CreditableCoverageLateEnrollmentPenalty.html.

APPENDIX

SIGNIFICANT CHANGES TO THE AFFORDABLE CARE ACT (ACA) SINCE ENACTMENT IN 2010

SUPREME COURT

◆ The provision in the ACA that mandated that states expand Medicaid eligibility to 133 percent of the poverty level was made voluntary.

◆ The court determined that the penalty for individuals not purchasing health insurance was a tax and therefore legal under the Constitution.

CONGRESS

◆ Congress made it clear that TRICARE and VA benefits qualified as meeting the essential health benefit coverage standard of the ACA and clarified that children of TRICARE beneficiaries could be covered to age 26.

◆ The 1099 mandate to report to the IRS all transactions with vendors more than $600 per year was repealed.

◆ The CLASS act was repealed.

◆ Congress reduced or eliminated funding for a number of ACA programs:

- Co-ops

- Independent Payment Advisory Board

- IRS enforcement of ACA rules

- Special funding for Louisiana

- Prevention and public health

- Community-Based Transition Program

◆ The cap on deductibles for small groups was eliminated in order to allow high-deductible plans paired with health savings accounts.

FEDERAL AGENCIES

Federal agencies, primarily the Centers for Medicare & Medicaid Services (CMS) and the Internal Revenue Service (IRS), issue numerous rules and regulations throughout the year. The following lists of administrative decisions are highlighted, as they have significant policy or political impact on the ACA.

◆ CMS and IRS delayed a number of deadlines in the original ACA

- Employer reporting on the W2 of insurance costs

- Small business employer mandate

- Low-income plan availability

- SHOP (Small-Employer Health Option Plan) availability on the health exchanges

◆ Provided that insurance companies can reoffer plans that had been cancelled as not meeting the ACA regulations

◆ Extended federal subsidies to plans that are not offered on the exchanges

SOURCE: The Galen Institute. 2014. "42 Changes to Obamacare. . . So Far. Posted July 18. www.galen.org/newsletters/changes-to-obamacare-so-far.

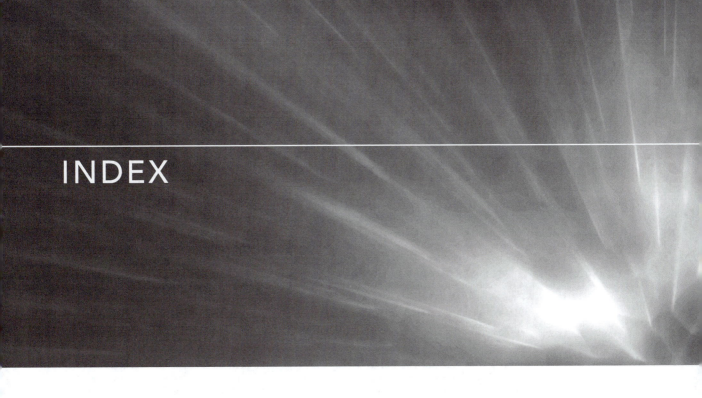

INDEX

Note: Italicized page locators refer to figures or tables in exhibits.

ACA. *See* Affordable Care Act

Access: ACO model and, 249; American Academy of Family Physicians PCMH model and, 154, 155; enhanced, patient-centered medical home and, 107; Medicare beneficiaries and issues around, 283–84; National Committee for Quality Assurance PCMH model and, 156; National Demonstration Project PCMH model and, 156; population health management and, 45, 46–47, 53; to primary care, 162–63, 165

Accountable care organizations, 57, 60, 62, 91, 182, 185, 283, 286, 287, 295; ACA, chronic care, and, 105; acknowledging paradox within, 269; Affordable Care Act and, 17, 132, 240, 287; antitrust issues related to, 265; care integration and, *255,* 256; challenges to be met by, 250–51; CMMI initiatives, *74, 75, 199*; CMS definition of, 206–7; CMS strategy and, 242–43; core competencies of, 254–57; culture and, 255, *255*; defining, 240–41, 244, 291; demand for transparency and, 278; edge of chaos concept applied to, 258; effectiveness and, 248, 249; efficiency and, 248; elements and attributes common to, 258–59; equitability and, 248, 250; HHS and partial capitation to, 229; history behind, 252; implementing, challenges in, 229; implementing, overview of early stages of, 244–45; leadership and, 254–55, *255*;

long-term *vs.* short-term solutions and, 265–66; measuring effectiveness and efficiency in, 253–54; network theory, and less likelihood of vertical integration between acute and post-acute care following implementation of, 293–94; operational excellence and, *255,* 256; organization of, 257–67; patient-centeredness and, 248, 249–50; payment incentives and, 228–30, 235; payment models within, 261–64; for pediatric Medicaid patients, 228; physician alignment and, *255,* 256–57; physician employment *vs.* physician alignment and, 260–61; possible future modifications for, 411; post-acute care sector and, 290–91; potential legal impediments with, 262–65; ACA's basic requirements for, *246*; provisions in ACA, 247; quality and, 248–49; readiness for, steps in building, 267–69, *268*; requirements for, 228–29, 245–46; six goals of, 248–50; TCE, increased vertical integration between acute and post-acute care, uncertainty, asset specificity, and implementation of, 292, 293; technology enablement and, *255,* 257; timeliness and, 248, 249; transforming current healthcare nonsystem and, 243; Tucson Medical Center pilot site, 266–67; various perspectives and interpretations of, 241–43

Accreditation: quality measures and, 204; reviews, 51

Accreditors: as drivers of quality, 201

Acquaviva, Kimberly D., 194

Actuarial costs: "medals levels" in health insurance exchanges and, 334, 335, *335*

Acute care organizations: accelerated patient discharges and, 289; asset specificity and transactions between post-acute care organizations and, 292; bundled payments and, 290, 291; critically ill patients and, 281; network embeddedness, ACA reforms, and less likelihood of vertical integration between post-acute care organizations and, 293–94; question of vertical integration with post-acute care organizations and, 287, 288; transaction cost economics, ACA reforms, and increased likelihood of vertical integration between post-acute care and, 291–93

Acute care services: US medical care system and, 35

Acute myocardial infarction, 171; Hospital Compare measure set for timely and effective care of, *209*

Administrative costs: estimated, for Alabama exchange, *340*; global payment systems and reduction in, 304; health insurance exchanges and, 322, 323; vertical integration and, 288

Administrative Simplification provisions: of HIPAA, 118, *119*

Admission rates: declining, trend in, 279; population health management and, 62

Advanceable, refundable tax credits: health insurance exchanges and, 336–37

Advanced Payment Accountable Care Organization Model, *199*

Advanced practice registered nurses: PCMH quality improvement and, 213

Adverse effects: drug-related, 52; pay-for-performance and, 206

Adverse events: hospital-based, Medicare enrollees and, 205

Adverse selection, 317; risk adjustment, exchanges, and, 338; state-based exchanges and enhancement of, 331

Affordability: achieving, ACA and, 234–35; quest for, in healthcare, 277–82

Affordable Care Act, 57, 117, 133, 134, 137, 177, 191, 216, 261, 266, 286; accountable care organizations and, 241, 244, 287; ACO program requirements of, *246*; ACO provisions in, 247; affordability and, 11, 234–35; aggregate funding for, 10; bundled payments and, 230, 287, 290; Center for Medicare & Medicaid Innovation and, 196; chronic disease policy initiatives and, 102; clinical prevention and, 22–23, 28; community benefit by nonprofit healthcare organizations and, 26, 28; community transformation grants and, 26, *27*, 28; coordination and, 23–24; demand management and, 22; education and, 24, 28; employer-based coverage and provisions of, 17; enactment of, 5, 16–17, 349; essential health benefits for

exchanges required by, 333–35; estimates of under age 65 enrollment before and after implementation of, in millions, *342*; fraud and Title V of, 233; fundamental theories of, 5, 6–13, 14; future improvements in, 233–34; goals of, 1, 4, 113; good ideas likely to remain in, 410–11, 413; groundwork laid for, 5–6; healthcare cost deflation and, 235; healthcare disparities and, 305–6; health insurance exchanges and, 316–20; Health Plan Identifier required by, 125; health plan quality rating system in, 175–76; information privacy and confidentiality protection and, 135; integration and, 76; key legislative features of importance to AHA's constituents, 132; legal challenges to, 13, 18–21; lifestyle management and, 22; lowest cost site of care, incentives, and, *10*; making changes to: process in, 406–7; markets theory of, 315, 321, 323; Medicaid and provisions of, 17; Medicaid expansion under, 302; Medicaid quality measures and, 175; Medicare and provisions of, 17; Medicare PPS update and, 283; Multi-Payer Advanced Primary Care Practice Demonstration, 213; National Quality Strategy and, 211–12; network theory and reforms of, 291, 293–94; objectives in understanding of, 3–4; Oregon healthcare reform and, 391; organization of text and examination of, 3; payment incentives and, *9*, 226; payment reform activities introduced by, 181; penalties and, 231–32; perfect market competition and, *13*; policies to support chronic care in, 104–9; political storm surrounding enactment of, 1, 16; population health approach and, 144; potential targets for change to, 407–10; prevention activities and Title IV of, 24; primary care physicians and Title V of, 108; programs, 73–76; quality improvement and, 205; quality measures and, 173–74; quality reporting and, 173; recovery audit contractors and, 272; regulations on operations of healthcare exchanges, 320; as remarkable legislative achievement, 413; repeal question and, 411; rural and safety-net hospital demonstrations in, 304–5; safety-net organizations and, 301; Section 3022 of, 290, 291; Section 3023 of, 290; signed into law, 16, 131; significant changes to, since 2010 enactment, 415–16; states' activities related to, 350; subsidies within exchanges and, 335–37, *336*; systems-based care rewarded by, 412; transaction cost economics and reforms of, 291–93; value-based approach of Title III in, 170, 171; value-based purchasing and, 205; virtual marketplaces and, 326; waiver of deductibles for preventive services under, 395; wellness promotion through, 25–26, 28

Age: annual number of physician visits by, 2006, 165, *166*; dental visits in past year by, 2006, 165, *166*; number of annual visits to physicians by, 2006,

163, *164*; premium costs in exchanges and, 344, 346, *346*

Agency for Healthcare Research and Quality, 67, 106, 204, 207, 212; consumer information and, 209; evidence-based medicine defined by, 409; healthcare disparities reports and, 305; home health care quality improvement and, 216; quality and mission of, *197*; quality and productivity improvement and, 176, 177; quality measure development and, 203

Aging population: population health management and, 33; spending policies and issues related to, 361

Ambulatory care: outpatient care settings and, 281; primary care and, 162; quality improvement and, 212–13

American Academy of Family Physicians, 204, 377; patient-centered medical home model and, 107, 151, 152, 153, 154–55

American Academy of Pediatrics: patient-centered medical home and, 106, 107, 152, 154, 184, 213

American College of Healthcare Executives, 134; healthcare disparities Call to Action and, 311

American College of Physicians, 204; patient-centered medical home and, 107, 154; policy battles over Medicare and, 377

American Hospital Association, 134, 145, 285, 350; healthcare disparities Call to Action and, 311, 314; policy battles over Medicare and, 377; quality measure approval and, 203

American Medical Association, 350; policy battles over Medicare and, 377; quality improvement and, 202; quality measure development and, 203

American Nurses Association: National Database of Nursing Quality Indicators, 201–2; quality measure development and, 203

American Osteopathic Association: patient-centered medical home and, 107, 154

American Recovery and Reinvestment Act (2009), 104, 106, 109, 137, 205, 411; Health Information Technology for Economic and Clinical Health Act, 113; provisions of, 125

Americans: deaths of, at younger ages than those in less prosperous nations, 57, 63

Annual Survey of Hospitals (2012), 145

Antibiotics: hospital-acquired infections and resistance to, 232; Pew Charitable Trusts campaign to curb overuse of, in livestock, 396

Antitrust issues: accountable care organizations and, 265

"Any willing provider" statutes: state policymaking and, 350

Appeals: levels of, 274–75; lodging valid, theories invoked in, 274

AQA Alliance: quality and mission of, *198*; quality measure approval and, 204

Assessment and analysis: ACO readiness and, 267–68, *268*

Asset specificity, 295; defined, 292; embeddedness and, 293–94; transactions between acute and post-acute care and, 292

Association of American Medical Colleges: healthcare disparities Call to Action and, 311; quality and mission of, *198*; quality measure approval and, 203

Association of Departments of Family Medicine: medical home concept and, 152

Association of Family Medicine Residency Directors: medical home concept and, 152

Asthma care for children: Hospital Compare measure set for timely and effective care, *210–11*

Attachment points: transitional reinsurance, health insurance exchanges and, 338

Balanced Budget Act (1997), 289

Bard, Marc, 240

Barton, Phoebe Lindsey, 161

Bed days per thousand patients: for PCMH *vs.* non-PCMH patients, *185*

Behaviors: individual, health and, 40

Benchmarking data: quality assessment and, 51

Benefit design: health insurance exchanges and, covered categories in, 320–21

Berwick, Donald M., 84, 265

Bilingual workforce: equity in care and, 314

Billing: code assignments and, 273; Medicare and discouragement of errors in, 284–85

Bills. *See also* Law(s): local government and, 393; policymaking process at state level and drafting of, 389–390

Biometric wellness programs: employer-based, cost-effectiveness concerns with, 25

Blood clot prevention and treatment: Hospital Compare measure set for timely and effective care, *211*

Blood pressure levels: employer-based biometric programs and, 25

Body mass index: employer-based biometric programs and, 25

Bonuses: ACO participants in MSSP and, 291; NCQA PCMH model and, 157; patient, Medicare ACE project and, 230; pay-for-performance programs and, 183–84

Breast cancer: Community Guide interventions related to prevention and control of, *68*; early-stage, shared decision making, surgery, and, 109; race, healthcare disparities, and, 309

Bridges to Excellence, 180, 187; case study: pay-for-performance model, 183–84

Bronze plans: estimated enrollment in, 341, *342*; in health insurance exchanges, 334, *335,* 408

Budget changes: Affordable Care Act, new legislation, and, 407

Budget neutrality: CMMI and lack of need for, 234

Budgets: population health management and, 45

Bundled payments, 185, 230–31, 278, 283, 286, 287, 295; acute care facilities and, 290, 291; bending the cost curve and integration of P4P, shared savings, and, *264*; defined, 190; driving forces behind, 190–91; network theory, and less likelihood of vertical integration between acute and post-acute care following implementation of, 293–94; payment incentives and, 235; possible future modifications for, 411; post-acute care services and, 290; risk tolerance and, *263*; TCE, increased vertical integration between acute and post-acute care, uncertainty, asset specificity, and implementation of, 292, 293

Bundled Payments for Care Improvement Initiative: CMS Innovation Initiatives, *74,* 75, *199*

Bureaucrats: as suppliers of health policies, 370–71

Businesses and business groups: quality improvement and, 196, *197*

Business practice: government intervention and, 117

Buyers: in political marketplace, 359, *359*

California: Medicare expenditures in, 272

California Endowment, 93; Building Healthy Communities program, 97

California HealthCare Foundation, 202; privacy policy study by, 124; quality and mission of, *198*

California Public Employees Retirement System: managed competition and, 49; reference pricing and, 226–227

Canada: funding for public health in, 400–1; healthcare cost controls in, 409

Cancer prevention and control: Community Guide interventions related to, *68*

Capitation, 244; expenditures controlled under systems of, 48–49; global, 261, 264; partial, to select accountable care organizations, 229; risk tolerance and, *263*; value-based purchasing and, 181, *181,* 183

Care integration: ACOs and core competency of, *255,* 256

Care management: National Committee for Quality Assurance PCMH model and, 156, 157

Case studies: Bridges to Excellence, 183–84; Massachusetts healthcare reform, 387–88; PROMETHEUS Payment model, 187–91

Cash assistance programs: Medicaid system and, 302

Catastrophic care: population health management and, 22, 32, 36, *37,* 45

Catastrophic plans: estimated enrollment in, 341; "medals levels" of coverage in, 334, 335

Center for Medicare & Medicaid Innovation, 73, 181, 191, 228, 233–34, 242, 304, 351, 353; Health Care Innovation Awards program, 91; initiatives of, *74,* 74–76, *199–200*; possible future modifications for, 410; quality and mission of, *197*; quality improvement mandate of, 196

Centers for Disease Control and Prevention, 69; Community Guide, 67; "Guide to Community Preventive Services," 95; as leading public health agency, 66; public health functions identified by, 64, *65*

Centers for Medicare & Medicaid Services, 84, 120, 138, 179, 182, 203, 229, 248, 253, 261, 265; accountable care organizations and strategy of, 242–43; accountable care organizations defined by, 206–7; ACO enrollment and, 259; ACO implementation and, 244, 245; Acute Care Episode Demonstration, 187; administration of Medicare RACs and, 273; clinical quality measures for meaningful use standards of, 128, *129–30*; core measures for meaningful use standards for eligible professionals, *128*; DRG payments and clinical quality targets defined by, 170–71; Hierarchical Condition Categories, 339; Hospital Compare website, 208; hospitals, quality improvement, and, 214; integrated delivery systems and, 240–41; meaningful use incentive payment schedule for Medicare-eligible professionals, 126, *127*; medical home testing and, 108; Medicare ACO regulations, 230; Medicare PPS update and, 283; menu objectives for meaningful use standards of, 128, *129*; network sufficiency issues and, 318; Nursing Home Compare website, 208; Nursing Home Quality Initiative, 214; Physician Quality Reporting System, 213; Pioneer ACO Model program, 207; policy impacts on ACA and administrative decisions by, 416; Premier Hospital Quality Incentive Demonstration, 206; public reporting and, 205; quality and mission of, *197*; quality improvement and, 196; quality improvement organizations and, 202; Quality Indicator Survey project, 215; quality measure approval and, 204; Recovery Audit Contractors program and, 233, 272; regulatory force of, 201; Rural Community Hospital Demonstration and, 304; Shared Savings Program, 207; Stark provision enforcement and, 265; wage index calculations by, 306n3

Cervical cancer screening: Community Guide interventions and, *68*; high-deductible health plans and reduced use of, 395

Charitable hospitals: tax-exempt, ACA community benefit plan and, 28

Chief executive officers: education on HIT-related legislative matters and, 134; population health management and, 145

Children: fast food consumption and obesity rates in, 396–97; Hospital Compare measure set and asthma care for, *210–11*; uninsured, in United States, 46

Children's Health Insurance Program, 10, 306; expansion of, 302; health insurance exchanges and eligibility determination for, 331; health insurance exchanges and enrollment in, 331; health insurance exchanges as point of entry in, 326; Massachusetts healthcare reform and, 387; navigators and help with, 303; states as purchasers of services under, 356; state's responsibility for health policy and, *390*

Child survival to age 5, 45

Cholera: Snow's epidemiological work and London epidemic of (1854), 66

Cholesterol levels: elevated, insurance status and, 316; employer-based biometric programs and, 25

Chronic care. *See also* Chronic disease: Affordable Care Act and policies in support of, 104–9; comparative effectiveness research and, 105, *105,* 106, 109; medical homes and, 105, *105,* 106–8, 109; shared decision making and, 105, 108–9

Chronic care model, 102, 109; patient-centered medical home and, 153

Chronic disease. *See also* Chronic care: ACA and policy initiatives for, 102; cost of, 34; HITECH Act, meaningful use, and management of, 104; as important cost driver, 109; insurance status and, 316; Medicare and costs of care for beneficiaries with, *103*; Medicare spending for, *103*; population health management and, 33, 34–35; preventing, 145

Chronic disease management: future health policy and, 411, 413; universal coverage and, 316

Chronic obstructive pulmonary disease: cigarette smoking and, 398; Medicare beneficiaries and costs of care for, *103*

Cigarette industry: healthcare policymaking and, 398–99

Civil restitution and settlements: Medicare and Medicaid fraud/abuse and, 233

CLASS Act, repeal of, 415

Clinical documentation: federal power over healthcare and, 273

Clinical information systems: ensuring security of, 122

Clinical prevention: Affordable Care Act and, 22–23, 28; definition of, 22; savings accrued from, 23

Clinical quality: measures for CMS meaningful use standards, 128, *129–30*; monitoring, 51

Clinton, Bill, 203

Coding rules: billing and, 273–74

Coinsurance and coinsurance rates: cost-sharing subsidies for exchanges and, 337; financial risk and, 49; health insurance exchanges and, 321, 410; "medals levels" in health insurance exchanges and, 334

Colorectal cancer screening: Community Guide interventions and, *68*; high-deductible health plans and reduced use of, 395; physicians and practice guidelines for, 23

Commerce Clause: Constitution, ACA supporters, and, 20

Commissioners: state, 388, *389*

Common purpose: community health business model and, 83

Commonwealth Care program (Massachusetts), 387

Commonwealth Fund, 202; quality and mission of, *198*

Commonwealth of Massachusetts Health Care Quality and Cost Council, 228

Communicable disease control: states and, 356

Communication standards: government, business practice, and, 117

Community and Migrant Health Center Program, 162

Community-Based Care Transitions program, 416; CMS Innovation initiative, 2012, *74,* 74–75

Community-based organizations: CMS-specified criteria for, 74–75

Community-based providers: states as safety net providers and, 357

Community benefit: ACA, tax-exempt charitable hospitals and, 28; definition of, 64

Community building: definition of, 22

Community Guide (CDC), 67; excerpt from: interventions related to cancer prevention and control, *68*

Community health: actions by healthcare executives for, 70–72; definitions in, 64–66; epidemiology and, 66–67; free national data sources that include local data on, 69, *69*; future health policy and, 412, 413; implementation plans in, 73; measures of status for, 67–70; needs assessments, 73; public health and, 64; realistic expectations for, 70

Community health activities: definition of, 64

Community health business model: collective multisectoral response and, 96–97; defining, 82–84; elements of, in design and implementation in communities across the country, 83–84; organizations involved in development of, 88–90; reaching beyond core mission: a healthcare example, 86–88

Community health centers, 301; in Massachusetts, 387

Community health improvement: bottom line and, 93

Community health teams: healthcare homes and, 108

Community Need Index, 70

Community partners: integration and, 77, 78

Community partnership business model: incentives for, 90–91; resources for, 91–93

Community partnerships: hospitals and, 148

Community Preventive Services Task Force: public education and, 24

Community residents: integration and, 78

Community Services Task Force, 24

Community social service agencies: population health improvement and, 93

Community transformation grants (ACA): examples of, *27*; purpose of, 26

Community-wide initiatives, 44

Comparative effectiveness research: ACA, chronic care, and, 105, *105,* 106, 109; as potential target of change, 409, 412

Competition: health insurance exchanges and fostering of, 410

Competitive negotiating strategies: best situations for, 360

Competitive (win/lose) strategy: in economic exchanges, 359

Complementary and alternative medicine: RAND Health division and studies on, 394

Complementary states: interest group strength in, *364*

Complementary/subordinate states: interest group strength in, *364*

Comprehensive Primary Care: CMS Innovation initiative, *74, 76, 199*

Computerized physician order entry: specification for measure of, 128

Confidentiality: information privacy and, 135–36, 137

Congress, 368; Affordable Care Act and oversight hearings by, 407; Affordable Care Act enacted by, 16–17; debate over health reform, constitutionality of ACA, and, 19–20; Innovation Center established by, 196; significant changes to Affordable Care Act since 2010 enactment and, 415–416

Congressional Budget Office, 179, 182, 290, 295n1; on ACA's coverage provisions, 10–11; on Medicare and Medicaid projected expenditures, 360, 361

Connecticut: healthcare reform in, 391–92

Conservative legal analysis: Supreme Court on constitutionality of ACA and, 19, 20

Consolidated Omnibus Budget Reconciliation Act (1985), 357

Consortia: quality measure approval and, 203–4

Consumer Assessment of Healthcare Providers and Systems, 61, 203

Consumer assistance: health insurance exchanges and, 332–33

Consumer-directed health plans, 394

Consumer information: quality improvement and, 208–9

Continuous patient-physician relationship: National Demonstration Project PCMH model and, 156

Continuum of care: formal mechanisms to coordinate across, 148; paradigm shift toward population health management across, 149–50; population health and degree of control across, 145

Contraceptives: ACA and employer-based insurance coverage for, 18

Coordinated care: American Academy of Family Physicians PCMH model and, 154

Coordination: clinical prevention and, 23–24

Coordination of care: community resources and, 282; dual-eligible beneficiaries and, 303; EMR technology and, 281; patient-centered medical home and, 107

Copayments: consumer value consciousness and, 208; cost-sharing subsidies for exchanges and, 337; financial risk and, 49; health insurance exchanges and, 321; "medals levels" in health insurance exchanges and, 334; premium calculators for

health insurance exchanges and, 333; state-based exchanges and, 328

Core competencies: of accountable care organizations, 254–57

Corporate America: health policy and influence of, 396–99

Corporate business leaders: population health improvement and engagement of, 93

Cost-based reimbursement: rural hospitals and, 304

Cost containment methods: capitation systems, 48–49; fee-for-service systems, 48; healthcare home, 108; shared decision making, 109

Cost reduction reform: accountable care organizations and, 291

Cost(s): of chronic illness, 34; consumer sensitivity to, 208; disability-related, 34–35; electronic medical record implementation and, 158; of market exchanges, 359; population health management and, 45, 47–50, 53; private exchange model and control on, 319

Cost sharing: "medals levels" in health insurance exchanges and, 334; subsidies, health insurance exchanges, and, 337

County governments: public health departments of, 393

County Health Rankings Model, 2012: University of Wisconsin Population Health Institute, *81,* 81–82

Courts. *See also* US Supreme Court: health policymaking and role of, 371–74; public policymaking process and, 378; state, 389

"Creditable coverage": waiver of Medicare Part D penalty and demonstration of, 408

Critical access hospitals: Medicare cost reimbursement for, 304

Crossing the Quality Chasm (IOM), 52–53, 152, 153, 180, 184, 250

Cultural competency: building in delivery of care, 311; hospitals, equity in care, and, 313–14

Culture: ACOs and core competency of, 255, *255*

Databases: community health and, 69, *69*

Data security: essential elements of, 134–35

"Death panel" concern: critics of IPAB and, 17

Deductibles: consumer value consciousness and, 208; cost-sharing subsidies for exchanges and, 337; financial risk and, 49; health insurance exchanges and, 410; "medals levels" in health insurance exchanges and, 334, 335; premium calculators for health insurance exchanges and, 333; preventive services and waiver of, under ACA, 395; state-based exchanges and, 328

Default exchanges: availability of individual subsidies and, 337

Defined contribution plans: private exchanges and, 319

Demanders: of health policies, 362–63, 382; in operation of political markets, *362*; in political marketplace,

359, *359*; political marketplace and interplay among suppliers and, 374–76

Demand management: population health management and, 31–32, 36, *37*

Demand management programs: cost containment and, 48; population health management and, 44, 45

Demographics: population health management and shifts in, 33–34

Dental visits: in past year, by race/ethnicity and age, 2006, 165, *166*; in past year by gender, 2006, 163, *165*

Design and deliver: ACO readiness and, 268, *268*

Device makers: ACA and taxes on, 409

Diabetes + COPD: Medicare beneficiaries and costs of care for, *103*

Diabetes/diabetes mellitus: disease management program development for, 33–34; Hispanics, healthcare disparities, and, 309; insurance status and, 316; multiple disabling conditions related to, 35

Diabetes + heart failure: Medicare beneficiaries and costs of care for, *103*

Diagnosis-related groups, 48, 153; Medicare, value-based purchasing, and, 170–71; Medicare savings and, 10; Medicare wage index and payments related to, 304–5; RAC audits, discovery of miscoding, and, 273

Diagnostic and therapeutic laboratory staff: primary care and, 162

Dietitians: ambulatory care, value-based purchasing, and, 213

Disability: population health management and, 22, 34–35

Disability-adjusted life expectancy, 45; need for system improvement on basis of, 35

Disability management: population health management and, 32, 36, *37*

Disaster preparedness and recovery planning: HIT leadership roles and, 135

Disease. *See also* Chronic disease: population health management and, 22; smoking-related, 398–99

Disease management programs, 46; cost containment and, 48; population health management and, 32, 36, *37,* 44; uninsured population and, 47

Disparities in healthcare: Call to Action and, 311–312; *Futurescan* survey results, 312–13; Healthy People 2010 and elimination of, 41–42; hospital leaders and, 313–14; racial and ethnic minorities and, 309; REAL challenge and, 309, 311; safety-net providers and, 305–6

Disproportionate-share hospital payments, 303

Diverse patient population: equity of care and, 312–13, 314

"Double blind" methodology: ACO enrollment and, 259

"Doughnut hole": ACA, Medicare, and eventual elimination of, 17

DSH formula: Medicare hospital payment update and, 285

Dual-eligible beneficiaries: of Medicaid and Medicare, 303

Durable medical equipment: competitive bidding and suppliers of, 13; fraud and abuse policies and, 233

Economic incentives: community health business model and, 84

Economic markets: influence in, 375; political markets and, 359, 362

Education: ACO readiness and, 267, *268*; health and, 40, *41*; preventive services and, 24, 28; US healthcare system and, 7, *8*

Effectiveness: ACO model and, 248, 249; ACOs and measurement of, 253–54; Institute of Medicine quality agenda and, 53

Efficiency: ACO model and, 248; ACOs and measurement of, 253–54; future health policy and financial incentives for, 412, 413; Institute of Medicine quality agenda and, 53; MedPac and, 284

Electronic Data Interchange, 120; workgroup for, 139

Electronic health records, 125; ambulatory care and uptake of, 213; benefits of meaningful use and, 126; evidence of impact for hospitals and physicians and adoption of, 131; HITECH, meaningful use, and, 104, 137; integrated care and, 76; Mayo Clinic confidentiality policy and, 136; NCQA PCMH model and, 158; quality improvement and, 207–8; reduced cost of care and hospital investment in, 281; robust, accountability care organizations and, 257

Electronic record keeping: HIPAA and, 118

Eligibility: ACA Medicaid expansion and, 302; health insurance exchanges and determination of, 331

Eligible professionals: reporting of quality information by, 172

Elitist perspective: on role of interest groups in policy-making, 366–68

Employee Retirement Income Security Act, 357, 399; Supreme Court and hospital rates ruling, 372–73

Employees: private exchanges and, 319; provider choices and, 12

Employer-based health insurance: Affordable Care Act and provisions for, 17

Employer-based wellness programs, 25, 28

Employers: health insurance purchasing and, 12, 179; health management programs and, 47; private exchanges and, 319

Employment-based healthcare system: Affordable Care Act and, 16, 17; market perspective on, *11,* 12

Enrollment: in health insurance exchanges, estimates of, 341–43, *342*; health insurance exchanges and, 331–32

Environmental scanning and organizational education: HIT leadership roles and, 133–34

Epidemiology, 66–67

Equitability: ACO model and, 248, 250

Equitable care: planning for and improving, 311

Equity of care: *Futurescan* survey results and, 310–11, 312–13; hospital leaders and, 313–14

Equity of Care: platform, 313; website, 312

Ethics: in political marketplace, 377–78

Ethnicity: annual number of physician visits by, 2006, 165, *166*; dental visits in past year by, 2006, 165, *166*

Evashwick, Connie J., 64, 73

Everett Clinic: Physician Group Practice Demonstration and, 252

Evidence-based interventions: community health business model and, 83–84

Evidence-based knowledge: population health management and, 53

Evidence-based medicine, 170, 282; early criticism of, 409

Ewing, Michael, 151

Executive branch: policy implementation and, 380; in state government, 355, 388, *389*

Executives: as suppliers of health policies, 370–71

Fast-food industry: health policymaking and, 396–97

FBI: healthcare fraud cases investigated by, 232–33

Federal agencies: role of, in quality improvement, *197*; significant changes to Affordable Care Act since 2010 enactment and, 416

Federal default exchanges, *327*, 347; availability of individual subsidies and, 337; benchmark plan and, 334; state-based exchanges *vs.*, 326–328

Federal deficit: financial crisis of 2008 and, 361

Federal government: health policymaking and, 355; state governments modeled after, 388, 401

Federally Qualified Health Center: Advanced Primary Care Practice, CMS Innovation initiative, *74, 76, 199*

Federally qualified health centers, 305; states as safety net providers and, 357

Federal poverty level: cost-sharing subsidies for exchanges and, 337; exchanges with no state Medicaid expansion and, 338; MassHealth and, 387; tax credits for exchanges and, 335, *336*

Federal Tax Relief and Healthcare Act (2006): section 302 of, 272

Federal Trade Commission, 265; clinical integration standard, 249

Fee-for-service model: shifting to provider capitation model from, 278–79

Fee-for-service payments, 181, 191

Fee-for-service systems, 236; groups within, 48; value-based purchasing and, 181, *181*, 182

Fees: financing state-based exchanges and, 339, 341

Females: premium costs in exchanges and, 344–45, *346*

Financial crisis of 2007–2009: executive branch and responsibility for, 370; federal deficit and, 361;

Health Information Technology for Economic and Clinical Health Act and, 113

Financial incentives, 90; integrated care and, 76; physicians and, 9; for quality and efficiency, 412, 413; quality improvement and, 196

Financial risk: population health management programs and, 49–50

Food choices: Kids' Safe and Healthful Foods Project and, 397–98

Food safety: fast-food industry's opposition to, 396; Pew Charitable Trusts and health research on, 395, 396

For-profit hospitals: policy debates and, 377

Foundations, 262; healthcare policymaking and, 402; policy direction shaped by, 401; quality improvement and role of, *198*

Fragmentation. *See also* Integration: of healthcare system, 235, 400; population health management and, 35–36; in post-acute care sector, 289, 290

Fraud: fighting, ACA changes and reduced funding for, 410; Medicare, incentives, and, 228; Medicare and Medicaid, 232–33, 236; Medicare and prevention of, 284; Medicare's recovery audit contractor program in battle against, 272

Fraud-and-abuse regulations: government intervention and, 117

Frontier states: DRG system, wage index, and, 304–5, 306n3

Full-risk bundles: value-based purchasing and, *181,* 182

Funding: for public health, 400–1

Funds flow and incentives theory: in Affordable Care Act, 5, *6,* 8–11, 14

Future of Family of Medicine Project: formation of, 152

Futurescan surveys: on equity of care, 310–311; implications for hospital leaders and results of, 149; on population health, 58–59, 60, 145; on reimbursement and cost management, 280–281

Gawande, Atul, 133, 243, 249

Geisinger Health System, 248, 249, 261, 268; Physician Group Practice Demonstration and, 252

Gender. *See also* Females; Males; Men; Women: dental visits in past year by, 2006, 163, *165*; number of annual visits to physicians by, 2006, 163, *164*; premium costs in exchanges and, 344–345, *346*

Glandon, Gerald L., 112

Global budgets, 48; for hospitals, 409

Global capitation, 261, 264

Global Payment System demonstration project (Medicaid), 304

Goldberg, Alan J., 272

Gold plans: estimated enrollment in, 341, *342*; in health insurance exchanges, 334, *335, 408*

Governing boards: equitable care and makeup of, 313

Government: healthcare information technology and role of, 113–14

Governmental funding: for population health improvement, strengthening, 92–93

Government intervention: business practice and, 117; in healthcare field, 115–16; justification for, 114–15; types of, *115*

Government regulation: health insurance exchanges and, 321

Governors: state government, 388, *389*; as suppliers of health policies, 370

Graduate medical education: states as educators and, 357–58

Gross domestic product: healthcare cost increases relative to, 116; healthcare spending in US as percentage of, 45, 151, 277

Group theory of politics: central tenets of, 365–66

Health: definitions of, 39–40; multiple determinants in, 40–41, *41*, 354

Health-adjusted life expectancy, 41, 57; need for system improvement on basis of, 35

Healthcare: ACO model and access to, 249; federal power over, 273; government intervention and, 115–16; quest for affordability in, 277–82; rural, 304–5

Health Care and Education Reconciliation Act (2010), 16, 131–32

Healthcare associations: lobbying and, 350–51

"Health care choice" interstate compacts: Affordable Care Act and, 319

Healthcare complexity industry, 285–86

Healthcare costs: containment of, 48; escalating, 116, 151; high-deductible health plans and, 394; projected increases in, 196; reducing, 50; unsustainability of, 277

Healthcare coverage: employer-based, 179

Healthcare Effectiveness Data and Information Set: quality measure development and, 201; quality measures use and, 204

Healthcare executives: community health and actions for, 70–72; fostering of community health business partnerships and, 80; integration and actions by, 79

Healthcare expenditures. *See also* Cost containment methods: eliminating healthcare disparities and, 313; finite healthcare resources and, 45; per person, in US, 151; quality and, 50; real per capita growth in, *236*; for services considered to be ineffective, 91; smoking-related disease and, 398–99; in United States, 45, 47, 159

HealthCare.gov, 138, 228

Healthcare home, 106; components for success of, 107

Healthcare industry: vertical integration in, 286, 287

Healthcare legislation: Health Information Technology for Economic and Clinical Health Act, 125–31; Health Insurance Portability and Accountability Act, 118–25; local, examples of, 393; Patient Protection and Affordable Care Act, 131–33

Healthcare organizations: impact of privacy rules on, 123; prices and consolidation of, 288

Healthcare policymaking: fast-food industry and, 396–97; foundations and, 402; in nonfederal sectors,

attributes of, 399–402; private health foundations and, 395–96; private industry and, 396–99; private research institutes and, 393, 402; private sector and, 402; system changes and future trends in, 411–12

Healthcare reform. *See also* Affordable Care Act: in Connecticut, 391–92; continuing journey in, 406; criticism of, 273; debate over constitutionality of ACA and, 19; edge of chaos concept applied to, 257; elements needed for, in US, 6; evaluation of vertical integration within, 288–89; federally-led efforts in early 1990s, 355; as journey not as destination, 1; in Massachusetts, 387–88; in Oregon, 391; population health and, 57, 60; in states, 358; in United States, 1

Healthcare system in US: core elements of, *7*; fragmentation of, 35–36; high cost of, two major causes of, 28; lessons learned about integration in, 76–78; rising costs and average quality care in, 151; second-level model of, *8*; Title III in ACA and solving problems in, 170

Healthcare systems: equity of care and meaning for, 313; specificity around appropriate admissions to, 279

Health information technology, 23–24, 112, 114, 115, 131, 235; administrative simplification, ACA exchanges, and, 322; coordinated care and, 154; future health policy and greater use of, 411, 413; government funding for research in, 115; government intervention and, 117; government's role in, 113–14; leadership roles and, 113; Marshfield Clinic and, 230; National Quality Strategy and meaningful use of, 212

Health Information Technology for Economic and Clinical Health Act, 113, 117, 125–31, 133, 134, 137, 205; electronic health records and, 126, 207; information privacy and confidentiality protection and, 135; meaningful use and, 104, 109, 126–28, 131; NCQA PCMH model and, 158; PQRS program and meaningful use policies of, 172

Health insurance, 7; access to, in United States, 46; access to primary care and, 162; benefit design in, controversy over, 320

Health insurance benefits: quality improvement and, 196

Health insurance coverage: healthcare disparities and, 309

Health insurance exchanges, 12, 18, 175, 316–20; administrative simplification and, 322, 323; essential health benefits required by ACA and, 333–35, 347; estimated enrollment in, 341–43, *342*; functions of, 331–33, 347; future health policy and expanded use of, 412, 413; governance of, 329–30; increased government regulation and, 321–22; "medals levels" of coverage in, 326, 334, *335*, *408*; Medicaid expansion and, 318, 323; Medicare exchanges, 320; narrow networks and, 317–18; with no state Medicaid expansion, 337–38,

347; possible evolution of, 410; premium costs in, 343–46; private exchanges, 319–20; problematic roll out of, 316; purchasing across state lines and, 319; rate increases and, 322, 323; risk adjustment and, 338–39, 347; risk management and, 317; role and structure of, 328–29; standard benefits and, 320–21; state decisions on creation of, *327*; state *vs.* federal, 326–28; subsidies and, 317, 335–37, *336*; surprises from, 318–19; true marketplace question and, 323; as virtual marketplaces, 326

Health insurance industry: states as regulators and, 357

Health insurance plans: aggregate funding for ACA and, taxes on, 10; population health management initiatives and, 44

Health Insurance Portability and Accountability Act, 113, 114, 117, 133, 134, 137, 322; enhanced privacy regulation with, 117; information privacy and confidentiality protection and, 135; information privacy and security and, 120–25; Information Series for Providers, *121*; overview of, 118, 120; states as regulators and, 357; Summary of Administrative Simplification provisions of, 118, *119*; transactional and code set standards and, 120

Health insurance reform, 315–25; health insurance exchanges, 315, 316–20; increased government regulation in, 315, 321–23; standard benefits and, 315, 320–21; universal coverage and, 315–16

Health maintenance organizations, 46, 228; accountable care organizations and, 252; capitation-based cost control and, 48–49; choice, systemness, and demise of, 260; public backlash against, 278–279; underutilization and, 253

HealthPartners (Minnesota): Health Driver Program, *88*; multisectoral community business model partnership and, 87, 88, 96

Health plans: ACA, Medicaid, and, 175; ACA and taxes on, 409; future health policy and new relationships with, 412, 413; insured members of, 43; NCQA and accreditation for, 204; quality improvement and, 196

Health policy: advocacy and, 350–52, 353; healthcare associations and lobbying, 350–51; innovations in care delivery, 351–52; policy expertise, 352, 353; broad domain of, 354; demanders of, *362*, 362–63, 382; overlapping domains in, 354–55; politics and, 399–400; states' responsibilities through, examples of, *390*; suppliers of, 368–74

Health policy development: states' involvement in, illustrations of, 391–92

Health policymaking: ethics and, 377–78; federal-state responsibility for, 355–58; as highly political process, 381–82; at local government level, 392–93; major activities in, 349; political marketplace and, 358–62

"Health Policymaking at the State and Local Levels and in the Private Sector" (Shi), 386

Health policy research: RAND Corporation and, 394–95

Health Privacy Stories (Health Privacy Project): examples from, 121–22

Health-related technology: US as world's major producer and consumer of, 380

Health savings accounts, 12, 335, 416

Health systems: formal care coordination structures and, 148; *Futurescan* survey results: population health, 146–47; population health management and, 61

Healthy Communities Institute (California), 70

Healthy Community movement (1980s), 82

Healthy People initiatives, 41; goals and objectives of, 68–69

Healthy People 2000: goals of, 41

Healthy People 2010: goals of, 41–42, *42*; health indicators for, 42, *42*

Healthy People 2020: Leading Health Indicators and, 61

Heart failure, 171; Hospital Compare measure set for timely and effective care of, *209*

Heart failure + COPD: Medicare beneficiaries and costs of care for, *103*

High-deductible health plans, 416; healthcare cost deflation and, 235; increase in, 12; RAND Corporation cost-related assessment of, 394–95

"High utilizers": ACO enrollment methodology and, 259, 260

HIT leadership roles, 133–36, 137; disaster preparedness and recovery planning, 135; environmental scanning and organizational education, 133–34; information privacy and confidentiality protection, 135–36; information security policies and procedures, 134–35

Home Health Quality Improvement: National Campaign, 216; potentially avoidable events measures, *217*

Home health services: fraud and abuse policies and, 233

Hospital-acquired conditions: ACA penalties and, 232, 236; possible future modifications and initiatives for, 411; preventable, CMS and nonpayment of, 214

Hospital Compare: measure set for timely and effective care, *209–11*; numeric rating scores, 209; website, 172, 205, 208

Hospital Consumer Assessment of Healthcare Providers and Systems, 214

Hospital leaders: accountable care organizations and needs of, 250; aggregate *Futurescan* survey results and, 149; creativity and resourcefulness in quality care and, 282; equity of care and implications for, 313–14; focus on wellness and prevention by, 279; payment continuum, risk, and implications for, 281–82; population health management and implications for, 61–63

Hospitals: accountable care organizations and, 246–47; alternative sites of care delivery and investment by, 279, 281; appeal statistics and, 274; community partnerships and, 148; competition and, 9; degree of control across continuum of care and, 145; diversity training and, 314; EHR adoption and evidence of impact for, 131; epidemiology, community health, and, 66–67; equity of care and meaning for, 313; equity of care promotion by, 312–13; faith-based, *149*; formal care coordination structures and, 148; for-profit, 377; *Futurescan* survey results: population health, 146–47; global budgets for, 409; healthcare disparities and, 306; investment in electronic medical records systems, 281; Joint Commission and accreditation for, 204; markets model and, 12; meaningful use standards and, 126; medical errors and adverse effects in, 52; Medicare beneficiaries and, 284; network adequacy concerns and, 318; population health advancement considerations by type of, *149*, 149–50; population health management and, 61; presumptive eligibility determinations for Medicaid and, 302; public, 301, 306n1, 377; quality improvement and, 213; quality scores and low- *vs.* high-performing, 207; rural, *149*, 301, 304, 306; safety-net, 303–4, 387; specificity around appropriate admissions to, 279; teaching, 358, 377; technology, affordability, and, 235

Hospital staff: integration and, 78

Hospital value-based purchasing program: Title III of ACA and, 170

Humana, 288; PCMH program, 157

ICD-9: codes and, 106; description of, 110n1

ICD-9-CM Official Guidelines for Coding and Reporting, 273

Illness burden: US healthcare system and, *7, 8*

Incentives. *See also* Financial incentives; Payment incentives: ACA, lowest cost site of care, and, *10*; ambulatory care, value-based purchasing, and, 213; for community partnership business model, 90–91; HITECH Act, meaningful use provision, and, 126–28, 137; for hospital quality measures reporting and, 214; meaningful, pay-for-performance and, 183–84; moral, 90; NCQA PCMH model and, 157–58; patient-centered medical homes and, 185; payment policies and, 228; as primary ACA tool, 10; in PROMETHEUS Payment model, 188; quality measures and, 204–5; quality-related, 194; for recovery audit contractors, 272; regulatory, 90; remunerative, 90; state-based, healthcare goals, and, 358; Value-Based Payment Modifier program and, 172; wellness, 25

Independence at Home Demonstration: CMS Innovation initiative, *74, 75, 199*

Independent Payment Advisory Board, 10, 228, 236, 416; Medicare spending, ACA, and, 17; as potential target of change, 409, 412; purpose of, 234

Independent practice associations, 262; risk tolerance and, *262*

Individual health insurance exchanges, 330

Individual insurance coverage: employer-based coverage and provisions of, 18

Individual mandate: Supreme Court, ACA, and dispute over, 20; Supreme Court ruling on, 407

Ineffective healthcare spending: capturing funding from reduction of, 91

Infant mortality: OECD nations and US lag in, 151

Infections: healthcare-associated, 171; hospital-acquired, penalties and, 232

Inflation: healthcare, 235

Influence: of interest groups, 376–78; in political markets, 375–76

Information management systems: integration and, 77–78

Information privacy and confidentiality protection: HIT leadership roles and, 135–36

Information privacy and security: components of, *136*; HIPAA and, 120–25

Information security policies and procedures: HIT leadership roles and, 134–35

Information system managers: security, privacy standards, and, 117

Information technology: "exoskeletons" or "umbrellas," 257; meaningful use criteria and use of, 208; NCQA PCMH model and, 158; population health management and, 53

Informed consent: shared decision making and, 109

Innovations: ACA changes and reduced funding for, 410; in care delivery, 351–52; CMMI initiatives and capacity of, *200*; universal coverage and, 316

Institute for Healthcare Improvement, 84, 96, 202; call for primary care models by, 213; quality and mission of, *198*; Triple Aim of, 61, 62

Institute of Medicine, 82, 83, 115, 187; comparative effectiveness research prioritization report, 24; *Crossing the Quality Chasm*, 52–53, 152, 153, 180, 184, 250; future of primary care report, 213; on medical home, 152; patient-centered care defined by, 153; population health improvement report, 92; *Primary Care, America's Health in a New Era*, 162; primary care defined by, 161–62; public health defined by, 64; quality and mission of, *197*; quality measures for population health report, 61; quality of care defined by, 50; Roundtable on Population Health Improvement, 86; *To Err Is Human*, 51, 153

Institutions of Purely Public Charity Act (Act 55): in Pennsylvania, 373

Insurance mandate, 410; ACA, as potential target for change, 407–8, 412

Integrated delivery systems, 240, 241, 244, 248, 251, 252; population health management paradigm shift and, *149*; risk tolerance and, 262, *262*; vertical integration and, 288

Integration: ACO model, quality, and, 248–49; future health policy and trends in, 412, 413; lessons learned about, US healthcare system, 76–78; risk tolerance and levels of, 262, *263*

Intermountain Healthcare Medical Group, 248; NCQA model-based PCMHs and, 157

Internal Revenue Service: community benefit resources and, 64, 91; health insurance premium tax credits under ACA and, 18; policy impacts on ACA and administrative decisions by, 416

Internal transaction costs: vertical integration and, 288

Interstate commerce: ACA, Supreme Court, and Congressional regulation of, 19

IRM International: disaster recovery program, 135, 138

Iron triangles: breaking, 376–77; defined, 376

Isham, George, 80

Jacobson v. Massachusetts, 372

Job lock: universal coverage and elimination of, 316

Joint Commission, The, 201; accreditation for hospitals and, 204; ORYX system, 203; public reporting and, 205; quality and mission of, *197*; quality measure development and, 203

Joint Commission International, 204

Jorna, Heather, 144

Judicial branch: state government, 388, *389*

Judiciary: independence of, 374; as supplier of health policies, 371–74

Kaiser Family Foundation, 151

Kaiser Permanente, 76, 248, 261

Kids' Safe and Healthful Foods Project: goals of, 397–98

Kindig, David A., 80

Knowledge: US healthcare system and, 7, *7, 8*

Law(s): continuing healthcare reform journey and, 406; interpretative role of courts and, 372–74; legislators as suppliers of health policies and, 369; local government and passage of, 392–93; policymaking process at state level and, 389–90

Leadership: ACOs and core competency of, 254–55, *255*

Leading Health Indicators, 61, 62

Leapfrog Group, 180; public reporting and, 205; quality and mission of, *197*; quality and patient safety practices identified by, 201

Legal system (US): outline of, provided by Department of State, 374; public policymaking process and, 378

Legislative branch: implementing policies formulated in, 380; in state government, 355, 388, *389*

Legislators: policy expertise and, 352; as suppliers of health policies, 368–69

Licensing of health professionals: policymaking constraints under federal policy and, 399; states as regulators and, 357

Life expectancy: extension of, 33; need for system improvement on basis of, 35; OECD nations and US lag in, 151

Lifestyle management: population health management and, 22, 31, 36, *37*

Lobbying: by Corporate America, 396; healthcare associations and, 350–51

Local governments: community health data sources and, 69; policymaking process at level of, 392–93; structure of, 392–93, 401

Logic models: framework for, *66*; public health experts and use of, 66

Longest, Beaufort B., Jr., 349, 352, 354

Long-term care programs: computer-assisted surveying and, 215

"Make or buy" arrangements: vertical integration and, 287, 291

Males: premium costs in exchanges and, 344–45, *346*

Malpractice reform: ACA-related debate around, 409, 412

Mammography: high-deductible health plans and reduced use of, 395

Managed care, 32; consumer rejection of restrictions imposed on, 260; reimbursement for primary care physicians and, 167; underutilization and, 253; vertical integration and, 288

Managed care organizations: population health management strategies and, 32; value-based purchasing movement and, 180

Managed competition: capitation-based cost control and, 48, 49

Market competition: perfect, Affordable Care Act and, *13*; perfect, characteristics of, 12

Market facilitator model: state-based exchanges and, 328, 329, *329*

Market failure: government intervention and, 114, 117

Markets theory: in Affordable Care Act, 5, *6*, 11–13, 14, 315, 321, 323

Marshfield Clinic, 229–30; Physician Group Practice Demonstration and, 252

Martin, Stephen A., Jr., 144

Massachusetts, 332; estimated exchange-related premium increases in, 344; federal healthcare exchanges based on pioneering model in, 350; healthcare reform in, 249; medical underwriting eliminated in, 344; RAC audits in, 272; retention of monthly premiums for exchanges in, 341

Massachusetts healthcare reform (case study), 387–88

MATCH models: Triple Aim compared with, 85–86, *86*

Mayo Clinic, 261, 268; confidentiality policy of, 136

McAlearney, A. S., 22, 31, 39

McLaughlin, Daniel B., 283

Meaningful use: clinical quality measures for CMS standards of, 128, *129–30*; CMS incentive payment schedule for Medicare-eligible professionals, *127*; core measures for CMS standards for eligible professionals, *128*; HITECH Act, electronic health records, and, 126–28, 131, 137; information technology, quality improvement, and, 208; menu objectives for CMS standards of, 128, *129*; PQRS program and, 172

Measure and monitor: ACO readiness and, *268, 269*

"Medals level" of coverage: in health insurance exchanges, 326, 334, *335,* 408

Medicaid, 1, 10, 14, 16, 133, 235, 301, 306, 355, 410; ACA, states and, 13; access to primary care and, 163; ACOs for pediatric patients and, 228; adjustments in reimbursement methodologies by, 399; Affordable Care Act and provisions for, 17; CMS innovation demonstrations and, 79; CMS quality improvement process and, 196; Commonwealth Care program (Massachusetts), 387; disease management programs and, 46; dual-eligible beneficiaries and, 303; EHR Incentive Programs, 208; enrollees, CMMI initiatives and, *200*; estimates of private coverage with and without full expansion of, 343, *343*; expansion of, under ACA, 302; federally qualified health centers and, 357; fraud and abuse and, 232–33, 236; Global Payment System demonstration project, 304; graduate medical education subsidies and, 357–58; healthcare homes and, 108; health insurance exchanges and eligibility determination for, 331; health insurance exchanges and enrollment in, 331; health insurance exchanges and expansion of, 318; health insurance exchanges as point of entry in, 326; health insurance exchanges with no state expansion of, 337–38, 347; HITECH Act, meaningful use, and eligible professionals for incentive program for, 126–27; HITECH Act and, 104, 137; hospital-acquired infections, prohibited payments, and, 232; integration and, 76; iron triangle and, 377; Oregon program, 391; payment incentives and, 226; percent of personal health expenditures paid by, 116; preventive services for recipients of, 24; primary care services and payments through, 108; quality measures, creation and reporting of, 175; RACs, 273; reduce avoidable hospitalizations among nursing facility residents initiative, 75; reviews, appeal management process, and, 275; rural healthcare and, 304; state funding and, 356; state funding requirement of ACA, as potential target of change, 408–9; state policymaking and, 350; states and expansion of, 316; Supreme Court ruling on expansion of, 407; Welfare Reform Act and eligibility for, 354–55; wellness incentives and, 25–26

Medicaid Incentives for Prevention of Chronic Diseases Program, *74, 200*

Medical care services: Americans and unaffordability of, 47–48; financial risk in payment systems for, 49

Medical care system: health and, 40, *41*

Medical devices: aggregate funding for ACA and taxes on, 10

Medical education: state subsidization of, 357–58

Medical errors, 50; devastating impact of, 51; disparities in health care and, 309; reducing, Institute for Healthcare Improvement and, 202

Medical Expenditure Panel Survey, 341, 344

Medical homes. *See also* Patient-centered medical homes: ACA, chronic care, and, 105, *105,* 106–8, 109; introduction of concept, 152; key components needed for success of, 107; principles for, 107

Medical loss ratios, 321–22, 323

Medicare, 1, 14, 16, 20, 46, 133, 180, 187, 235, 261, 306; ACO enrollment process and, 245, 259; Acute Care Episode Demonstration, 230; adjustments in reimbursement methodologies by, 399; Affordable Care Act and provisions for, 17; balancing newly insured with reductions in payments, 9, *9*; beneficiaries with multiple chronic conditions and costs of care for, *103*; bundled payment system and, 290; chronic conditions spending and, *103*; CMS innovation demonstrations and, 79; CMS quality improvement process and, 196; decreased reimbursements and adaptations made by, 153; DRG payment reductions, value-based purchasing pool, and, 284; dual-eligible beneficiaries and, 303; EHR Incentive Programs, 208; enrollees, CMMI initiatives and, *200*; federally qualified health centers and, 357; fee-for-service model and, 182; fraud and abuse and, 228, 232–33, 236; fraud prevention and, 284–85; Group Practice Demonstration Project, 228; HITECH Act, meaningful use, and eligible professionals for incentive program for, 126–27, *127*; HITECH Act and, 104, 137; hospital-acquired infections, reduced payments, and, 232; integration and, 76; iron triangle and, 376–77; Part A, 245; Part B, 245; Part D, 10, 226, 285, 303, 320, 408; payment incentives, 226; percent of personal health expenditures paid by, 116; Physician Group Practice Demonstration, 252; political marketplace and, 361; post-acute care sector and payment system reform in, 290; Premier Hospital Quality Incentive Demonstration, 207; primary care services and increased payments through, 108; prospective payment system and, 10; prospective payment system update, 283–85; quality comparison websites, 172; quality reporting for, 175; recovery audit contractors employed by, 272; reduce avoidable hospitalizations among nursing facility residents initiative,

75; reductions in all-cause 30-day readmission rate, 231–32; resource-based relative value scale system of, 184; right to rebill for Part B services, 274; rural healthcare and, 304; shared savings program for, 228; spending with and without reform, *227*; Utilization and Quality Control Peer Review Program, 202; value-based purchasing and, 170, 177, 179, 181; Volume Performance Standards, 48; wage index, 304, 306n3; wellness visit and, 24

Medicare Advantage, 10, 320, 410

Medicare Modernization Act of 2003: section 935 of, 272

Medicare Payment Advisory Commission (MedPac), 231, 283; hospital margins and, 284

Medicare Shared Savings Program: ACO participants in, 290, 291

Men: premium costs in exchanges and, 344–345, *346*

Mental health providers: network adequacy concerns and, 318; primary care and, 162

Methicillin-resistant *Staphylococcus aureus:* hospital-acquired infections and, 232

Mick, Stephen S., 286

Minority population: physicians, pay-for-performance concerns, and service for, 206; population health management programs for, 33; US population and, 309

Modified adjusted gross income level: for subsidies, ACA and, 306n2

Morbidity: CDC analysis of factors affecting, 67; drug-related adverse effects and, 52; preventable, uninsured population and, 116; smoking cigarettes as number one preventable cause of, 398

Morrisey, Michael A., 326

Mortality: CDC analysis of factors affecting, 67; drug-related adverse effects and, 52; preventable, uninsured population and, 116; smoking cigarettes as number one preventable cause of, 398

Multi-Payer Advanced Primary Care Practice Demonstration, *74, 199,* 213

Multisectoral partnerships: community health business model and, 82, 83, 96–97

Municipalities, 392; public health campaigns in, 393

Narrow provider networks: health insurance exchanges and, 317–18; price competitiveness and, 227

Nash, David, 57

National Business Coalition on Health, 93, 196; quality and mission of, *197*

National Business Group on Health, 201; quality and mission of, *197*

National Call to Action to Eliminate Health Care Disparities, 311, 312, 313, 314

National Committee for Quality Assurance, 76, 152, 180, 185; accreditation for health plans and, 204; patient-centered medical home model and, 151, 153, 156–57, 158; PPC-PCMH Recognition Program, 156; public reporting and, 205; quality

and mission of, *197*; quality measure development and, 203; quality-measure recommendations of, 251

National Database of Nursing Quality Indicators, 201–2, 203

National Demonstration Project, 158, 213; PCMH model of, 151, 153, 155–56

National Federation of Independent Business v. Sebelius, 19

National Health Care Quality Strategy and Plan: quality requirements of, 211–12

National Institutes of Health, 69, 106

National Library of Medicine: primary functions of, 115, *116*

National Patient Safety Foundation, 202; quality and mission of, *198*

National Provider Identifiers, 118, 119

National Quality Forum, 96, 186, 188; quality and mission of, *198*; quality measure endorsement and, 203

Navigators: Affordable Care Act and, 302–3; health insurance exchanges and, 332

Network embeddedness, 295; ACA reforms and less likelihood of vertical integration between acute and post-acute care with, 293–94

Network theory: organizational decision factors for vertical integration with post-acute providers and predicted responses with, *296*

New York: estimated exchange-related premium increases in, 344; medical underwriting eliminated in, 344; Medicare expenditures in, 272; Supreme Court in, 389

Nonfederal sectors: attributes of health policy development in, 399–402

Nonprofit organizations: health insurance exchanges and, *329, 330*

North Carolina: bundled payment initiative in, 191; Medicare "646" Demonstration in, 252

Nugent, Mike, 240

Nurse practitioners: ambulatory care, value-based purchasing, and, 213; primary care and, 162

Nursing Alliance for Quality Care: quality and mission of, *198*

Nursing facility residents: reducing avoidable hospitalizations among, CMS initiative, *74,* 75

Nursing Home Compare, 172; quality rating system, 209; website, 205, 208

Nursing homes: quality improvement and, 214–16, *215*

Obama, Barack, 19, 407, 411; American Recovery and Reinvestment Act signed by, 125; Patient Protection and Affordable Care Act signed into law by, 16; on recovery audit contractors, 272

Obama administration: healthcare cost deflation and, 235

"Obamacare." *See* Affordable Care Act

Obesity: ACA, school-based interventions and, 24; fast food consumption and, 396–97; Kids' Safe and Healthful Foods Project and curbing rate of,

397–98; public health campaigns on, 393; RAND Health division and studies on, 394

Office of the National Coordinator for Health Information Technology, 205; responsibilities of, 125–26, 137

Operational excellence: ACOs and core competency of, *255,* 256

Opportunistic behavior: embeddedness and, 294; vertical integration, transaction costs, and limits on, 292

Oregon: Family Health Insurance Program, 356; health policy development in, 391; overriding governor's veto in, 390

Out-of-pocket cost sharing: health insurance exchanges and, 334, 335

Overpayments: minimizing, Medicare payment system update and, 285; RAC audits and, 272

Overutilization of services, 262; healthcare disparities and, 309; peer accountability and, 254

Pacific Business Group on Health, 201; quality and mission of, *197*

Park Nicollet Health Services: Physician Group Practice Demonstration and, 252

Partnership exchanges, *327;* benchmark plan and, 334

Partnership for Patients: CMS Innovation initiative, 2012, 74, *74, 200*

Patient-centered care: IOM definition of, 153; National Demonstration Project PCMH model and, 156

Patient-centered medical homes, 57, 60; American Academy of Family Physicians model, 151, 153, 154–55; background on, 152–53; bed days per thousand patients, *185;* benefits of, 213; chronic care model and, 153; Comprehensive Primary Care initiative and, 76; costs and benefits for primary care with, 158; history behind, 184; lessons learned about, 185–87; mixed financial impact of, 185–86; most prevalent models for, 151; National Committee for Quality Assurance model, 151, 153, 156–57, 158; National Demonstration Project model, 151, 153, 155–56; principles for, 107; quality measure development and, 203; success of NCQA approach to, 157–58; sustainable funding model search and practices of, 186–87

Patient-centeredness: ACO model and, 248, 249–50

Patient-Centered Outcomes Research Institute: chronic disease management and, 106

Patient-Centered Primary Care Collaborative, 180, 184

Patient Protection and Affordable Care Act. *See* Affordable Care Act

Patient-provider relationship: systems view of US healthcare and, 6–7

Patients: as active participants in own healthcare, 148; bringing value to, 282; in US healthcare system, 6, *7,* 8

Payers: as drivers of quality, 196

Pay-for-performance (P4P) strategy, 185; ACA and, 132; bending the cost curve and integration of bundled

payments, shared savings, and, *264;* Bridges to Excellence case study, 183–84; complications and concerns related to, 206; demand for transparency and, 278; mixed quality and efficiency improvements with, 262; natural limits with, 187; risk tolerance and, *263;* value-based purchasing and, *181,* 182

Payment errors: Medicare and discouragement of, 284–85; RAC audits and, 272

Payment incentives, 226–36; accountable care organizations and, 228–30, 235; Affordable Care Act and, 226; balancing in ACA, *9;* bundled payments and, 230–31, 235

Payment models: within accountable care organizations, 261–64

Payment reform: Affordable Care Act and, 181; American Academy of Family Physicians PCMH model and, 154, 155

Pediatrics: primary care, medical home, and, 152, 213

Penalties: Affordable Care Act and, 231–32; for failure to have health insurance, 18, 19; hospital-acquired conditions and, 232, 236; Medicare Part D enrollment and, 408; payment policies and, 228; reducing rate of unnecessary readmissions with, 231, 235–36, 284

Pennsylvania: AdultBasic plan in, 356; Institutions of Purely Public Charity Act (Act 55) in, 373; tax-exempt status of healthcare organizations case in, 373

Perfect market competition: Affordable Care Act and, *13;* characteristics of, 12

Personal physicians: American Academy of Family Physicians PCMH model and, 154; patient-centered medical home and, 107

Personal Responsibility and Work Opportunity Reconciliation Act (1996), 354, 355

Pew Charitable Trusts: health research in policy areas supported by, 395–96

Pew Health Group: Kids' Safe and Healthful Foods Project, 397–98

Physical therapists: ambulatory care, value-based purchasing, and, 213; primary care and, 162

Physician alignment, 260; ACOs and core competency of, *255,* 256–57

Physician assistants: ambulatory care, value-based purchasing, and, 213; primary care and, 162

Physician Compare website, 172

Physician Consortium for Performance Improvement, 202, 203; quality and mission of, *198*

Physician-directed medical practice: American Academy of Family Physicians PCMH model and, 154; patient-centered medical home and, 107

Physician employment, 260

Physician group practices: accountable care organizations and, 246–47

Physician Group Practice Transition Demonstration, 182, *199,* 229, 230, 252

Physician–hospital alignment, 260, 261

Physician hospital organizations, 228, 262; risk tolerance and, *262*

Physician organizations, 262; risk tolerance and, *262*

Physician–physician alignment, 261

Physician Quality Reporting System, 171, 172, 213

Physicians. *See also* Primary care physicians; Providers: accountable care organizations and needs of, 250; annual number of visits to, by age and race/ethnicity, 2006, 165, *166*; Bridges to Excellence and, 183; colorectal cancer screening test practice guidelines and, 23; discretionary surgery, shared decision making, and, 109; EHR adoption and evidence of impact for, 131; fee for service and, 181; fee schedules and, 9; fraud and abuse policies and, 233; incentives, Value-Based Payment Modifier program, and, 172–73; number of annual visits to, by age and gender, 2006, 163, *164*; pay-for-performance concerns and, 206; primary care and, 162; procedural-based, technology advances and competition between, 257; successful hospitals and empowerment of, 282; value-based purchasing approach and, 171–72

Pioneer Accountable Care Organization (ACO) Model, *199,* 207

Plan management: health insurance exchanges and, 332

Platinum plans: estimated enrollment in, 341, *342*; in health insurance exchanges, 334, *335,* 408

Pluralist perspective: critics of, 366; on role of interest groups in policymaking, 365–66, 368

Pneumonia, 171; hospital-acquired, 232; Hospital Compare measure set for timely and effective care of, *209–10*

Policy communities: battles over Medicare and participants in, 377; policy domain and, 376

Policy(ies): shaping direction of, 401; as valued commodities in political marketplace, 362

Political marketplace: ethics in, 377–78; health policymaking and, 358–62; interest groups in, 363–68; interplay among demanders and suppliers in, 374–76; relationships in, 359, *359*

Political markets: economic markets and, 359, 362; operation of, 360–62; power and influence in, 375–76

Population health, 22; community partnerships and, 148; defining, 57, 65; degree of control across care continuum and, 145; future health policy and, 412, 413; *Futurescan* survey results, 58–59, 60, 146–47; reform and, 57, 60; state funding and expertise for, 358; Triple Aim and definition of, 84–86

Population health improvement: better return on investment from policies and programs outside of healthcare, 92; capture funding from reducing ineffective healthcare spending, 91; corporate business leaders and, 93; governmental funding

strengthened for, 92–93; informing cost-effective investment in, 94–96; philanthropy and, 93

Population health management: access and, 45, 46–47, 53; accountable care organizations and, 257; business model concept and, 83; capitation systems and, 48–49; catastrophic care management and, 32, 36, *37,* 45; characteristics of target population and, 31; checklist for, 62; chronic disease and disability and, 34–35; cost(s) and, 45, 47–50, 53; demand management strategies/programs and, 31–32, 36, *37,* 44, 45; demographics and, 33–34; disability management strategies/programs and, 32, 36, *37;* disease management strategies/programs and, 32, 36, *37,* 44; fee-for-service systems and, 48; financial risk and, 49–50; fragmentation and, 35–36; framework for, 22, 36, *37; Futurescan* survey results and paradigm shift toward, 149; healthcare cost reduction and, 50; hospital leaders and, 61–63; initiatives within strategies for, 31–32; IOM quality agenda and, 53; lifestyle management approaches and, 31, 36, *37;* medical errors and adverse effects reduced with, 52; National Committee for Quality Assurance PCMH model and, 156, 157; need for, reasons behind, 39, 45–53; public health principles integrated with, 145; quality and, 45, 46, 50–53; quality assessment and, 51; robust health information technology and, 148; what is to be managed in, 39–42; where it occurs, 39, 44–45; who is to be managed in, 39, 42–44

Populations: defining, 40, 43, 44

Post-acute care organizations, 286; accountable care organizations and, 290–91; asset specificity and transactions between acute care organizations and, 292; bundled payments and, 290; network embeddedness, ACA reforms, and less likelihood of vertical integration between acute care organizations and, 293–94; question of vertical integration with acute care organizations, 287, 288; transaction cost economics, ACA reforms, and increased likelihood of vertical integration between acute care organizations and, 291–93

Post-acute care services: outpatient care settings and, 281; substitutability of, 289

Potentially avoidable complications: per thousand patients with chronic conditions by type of practice, 186, *186*; PROMETHEUS Payment model and, 188; rates of, among commercially insured patients with certain chronic conditions, 188 *188*; regional health plan's total episode costs, split between typical costs and costs related to, *189*; regional health plan's total episode costs, split between typical costs and costs related to, as percentage of total, 190, *190*

ACA. *See* Patient Protection and Affordable Care Act

Preexisting medical conditions: Affordable Care Act and, 18, 28; universal coverage and, 316

Premier Hospital Quality Incentive Demonstration, 206, 207

Premiums: age and costs of, in exchanges, 344, 346, *346*; average forecast increases in non-group market—national average and stages with largest and smallest increases, 2017, *345*; estimated costs in exchanges, 343–46; exchanges and ACA allowance for, 338; financial risk and, 49; gender and costs of, in exchanges, 343–45, *346*; health insurance exchanges and, 321, 333; regional cost differences in ACA exchanges, 318–19; rise of healthcare costs and, 179; state-based exchanges and, 328

Preventing Chronic Disease, 88, 90

Prevention, 23; healthcare in United States and, 22; Healthy People initiatives and, 41–42; hospital leaders and focus on, 279; school-based clinics and, 24; systems view of, *23*; universal coverage and, 316

Preventive care: Hospital Compare measure set for timely and effective care, *210*

Price-based systems: new, 412, 413

Price competition: ACA, careful purchasing, and, 12; health insurance exchanges and, 317

Price controls: examples of, 48

Primary care: access to and utilization of, 162–63, 165; accountable care organizations and, 245; ambulatory care and, 162; defining, 161–62; future health policy and, 411, 413; future of, 167–68; PCMH and costs and benefits for, 158; WHO details benefits of medical home and, 152

Primary care issues in US health services system, 165; access to primary care, 165; availability of primary care providers, 167; future of primary care, 167–68; reimbursement for primary care physicians, 167

Primary care physicians, 162. *See also* Physicians; availability of, 167; medical homes and, 108; network adequacy concerns and, 318; number of annual visits to, 1987–2006, *164*; reimbursement for, 167; visits to, by age group, 2006, *163*

Prioritizing and planning: ACO readiness and, 268, *268*

Privacy: federal power over healthcare and, 273; HIPAA and, 117, 120–125

Privacy of patient information: policymaking constraints under federal policy and, 399

Private employer exchanges, 410

Private exchange model, 319–20

Private healthcare market: changes in, independent of ACA, 319

Private health foundations: healthcare policymaking and, 395–96

Private health insurance plans, 16; formularies and, 226

Private health research institutes, 393–95

Private industry: healthcare policymaking and, 396–99

Private insurance coverage: access and, 46; estimates of, with and without full Medicaid expansion, 343, *343*; premium costs and drop-off in, 343

Private research institutes: healthcare policymaking and, 402; policy direction shaped by, 401

Private sector: healthcare policymaking and, 402; policy direction shaped by, 401

Productivity, 170–73; AHRQ and support for improvement in, 176; total health system model and, *171*; value-based purchasing and, 170–73

Professional organizations: as drivers of quality, 201–2; quality improvement and role of, *198*

PROMETHEUS Payment case study: new frontier in value-based purchasing, 187–91

Prospective DRG payments, 263

Prospective payment systems: Medicare and, 10; post-acute care expenses and, 289; update of, 283–86

Prostate cancer: early-stage, shared decision making, surgery, and, 109

Provider capitation model: shifting from fee-for-service model, 278–79

Provider payment models: in value-based purchasing, *181*

Providers. *See also* Physicians; Primary care physicians: fraudulent, new screening rules for, 233; health insurance exchanges and narrow network of, 317–18; interoperability among, 117; MedPac surveys and, 283–84; post-acute, growth and development of, 289; primary care, 162; safety-net, 301; uncoordinated service provision and, 36; in US healthcare system, 6, 7, *7*, 8; vertical integration and consolidation of, 288

Public health: academic graduate training in, 65; community health and, 64; definition of, 64; funding for, 400–1; police powers and, 372; state healthcare legislation and focus on, 390; states as guardians of, 356; ten essential functions of, *65*; Title IV of ACA and, 24

Public health departments: broad prevention activities of, 23; of county and city governments, 393

Public hospitals, 301, 306n1; policy debates and, 377

Public interest: executives as suppliers of health policies and, 370; federal judges and, 374; maximizing, legislators as suppliers of health policies and, 369; political nature of policymaking and, 382

Public option: excluding from ACA exchanges, 318; as potential target of change, 409, 412

Public policymaking process: conceptual model of, 378–82; external factors influencing policymaking, 378–80; highly political nature of, 381–82; interdependent components of, *379*, 380–81; model of, in United States, *379*; policy formulation phase in, *379*, 380, 383; policy implementation phase in, *379*, 380, 383; policymaking as cyclical process, 378; policy modification phase in, *379,* 380, 381, 383; power elite and dominance of, 367; at state level, 389–90

Public reporting, 228; of quality, increase in, 412; quality measures and, 204, 205

Purchasers: as drivers of quality, 196–201

Qualified health plans, 175; exchanges and certification of, 332

Quality: ACA and reduced funding for activities related to, 410; ACO model and, 248–49; advocacy and technical support organizations and, 202; AHRQ and support for improvement in, 176; American Academy of Family Physicians PCMH model and, 154, 155; assessment of, 51; drivers of, 196, 201–2; future health policy and financial incentives for, 412, 413; health plans, Medicaid, and, 175; measurements of, 50; organizations with major role in, by type, *197–98*; patient-centered medical home and, 107; payers and, 196; population health management and, 45, 46, 50–53; professional organizations and, 201–2; purchasers and, 196, 201; regulators, certifiers, accreditors, and, 201; reporting, 173–75; total health system model and, *171*; universal coverage and, 316; value-based purchasing and, 284

Quality improvement: ambulatory care and, 212–13; consumer information and, 208–9; electronic health records and, 207–8; equity in care and, 313; federal legislation and impact on, 205; home health care and, 216; hospitals and, 213; National Quality Strategy and, 211–12; nursing homes and, 213–16, *215*; trends in, 205–12; in United States, future direction of, 194; value-based purchasing and, 205–7

Quality improvement landscape: complexity of, 194; dynamic nature of, 194

Quality improvement process: organizational roles in, *195,* 195–96

Quality measure development process, 203–5; measure approval, 203–4; measure development, 203; measure endorsement, 203; measure use, 204–5

Quality measures, 194; primary uses of, 204

Quasi-governmental agency: health insurance exchanges and, *329,* 330, 347

Race: annual number of physician visits by, 2006, 165, *166*; dental visits in past year by, 2006, 165, *166*

Race, ethnicity, and language preference (REAL) data: healthcare disparities and, 309, 311, 312, 313

RAND Corporation: health policy research and, 393–95

Rate increases: health insurance exchanges and, 322

Rationing concerns: quality reporting and, 228

Readmissions to hospitals: penalties related to, 231, 235–36, 284; possible future modifications and initiatives for, 411

Recovery Audit Contractor program: payment denial categories and, 273; Review Results Letter and, 274; "two midnight" rule and, 284–85

Recovery Audit Contractors, 233, 236

Reduce avoidable hospitalizations among nursing facility residents: CMS Innovation initiative, 2012, *74, 75*

Reelections: executives, policy-related decisions, and desire for, 370; federal judges free of concerns related to, 374; legislators, policy-related decisions, and desire for, 369; politics and policy in bids for, 400

Reference pricing: CalPERS members and, 226–27

Refundable tax credits: health insurance exchanges and, 336

Regional cost differences: health insurance exchanges and, 318–19

Regional Extension Centers: HITECH grants and, 207

Regional health information organizations: developing security policies for, 124

Regulations, 10; on ACA exchanges, 320; of health insurance companies, ACA and, 18; states' role in, 357; of tobacco industry, 398

Regulators: as drivers of quality, 201

Reimbursement: accountable care organizations and, 244; activities-based, 269; bundled payments and, 290; *Futurescan* survey on, 280–281; policymaking constraints under federal policy and, 399; post-acute care facilities and, 289; for primary care physicians, 167; risk tolerance and, *263*; rural healthcare and, 304

Reinsurance: health insurance exchanges and, 317

Reporting programs: voluntary, additional Medicare payments and, 196

Research project subjects: HIPAA compliance and, 123

Resignation: dissonance in organizational values and, 255

Resolutions: local government and, 393

Resource-based relative value scale system: of Medicare, 184

Resources: community health business model and, 83; integration and adjudication of, 78

Retail clinics: consumer information and, 208

Revenues: aggregate funding for ACA as complex set of, 10; medical loss ratios and, 321–22; quality services and, 9

Revenue sharing: accountable care organizations and, 207

Risk: integrated delivery systems and, 262; payment continuum, hospital leaders, and, 281–82; probability, 181, 182; technical, 181, 182

Risk adjustment: health insurance exchanges and, 317, 338–39, 347

Risk corridors: health insurance exchanges and, 317, 339

Risk management: health insurance exchanges and, 317

Risk pools: medical underwriting, premium costs, and, 344; number of state-based exchanges and, 330–31

Risk tolerance: practice type and, *262*; reimbursement strategy and, *263*

Robert Wood Johnson Foundation, 34, 93; PRO-METHEUS Payment model and, 191; quality and mission of, *198*; Rewarding Results program and, 202; Roadmaps to Health Prize, 96–97; Transforming Care at the Bedside initiative, 202

Roundtable on Population Health Improvement (IOM): population health defined by, 86

Rural healthcare, 304–5

Rural hospitals, 301, 304, 306; population health management paradigm shift and, *149*

Safety: American Academy of Family Physicians PCMH model and, 154, 155; IOM quality agenda and, 53; patient-centered medical home and, 107

Safety-net organizations, 301–6; community clinics, 301, 305; dual-eligible beneficiaries and, 303; eligibility issues and, 302; healthcare disparities and, 305–6; hospitals and, 303–4; navigators and, 302–3; public hospitals, 301; roles provided by, 301; rural healthcare and, 304–5; rural hospitals, 301

School-based healthy lifestyles initiatives: state funding and expertise for, 358

Screenings: high-deductible health plans and reduced use of, 395; measures of community health status and, 67

Security: HIPAA and, 120–25

Security of healthcare information: government, business practice, and, 117

Selective contractor model: state-based exchanges and, 328, *329*

Self-care support: National Committee for Quality Assurance PCMH model and, 156

Self-employed population: universal coverage and, 316

Self-insured employer health plans: states' regulation of, 357

Self-interest: demanders and suppliers in political market-place and, 374; executives as suppliers of health policies and, 370; legislators as suppliers of health policies and, 369; political nature of policymaking and, 382

Self-referrals, 167, 264

Sellers: in political marketplace, 359, *359*

Senate chamber: state government, 388, *389*

Serious reportable events, 214

Shadow pricing, 321

Shared decision making: ACA, chronic care, and, 105, 108–9

Shared governance: accountable care organizations and mechanism for, *246*, *247*

Shared savings, 185; bending the cost curve and integration of P4P, bundles, and, *264*; Medicare and, 228; risk tolerance and, *263*

Shared-savings pool: ACOs, CMS "bending the trend" downward, and, 253, *254*

Shared Savings Program, 207, 290; accountable care organizations and, 245; in Medicare, 17

Shared value principle: business model concept and, 83

Shay, Patrick D., 286

Shi, Leiyu, 386

SHOP exchanges, 330, 332, 341, 416; Alabama exchange and, *340*

Silver plans: estimated enrollment in, 341, *342*; in health insurance exchanges, 334, *335*, 408

Skilled nursing facilities: post-acute sector and, 289

Slovensky, Donna J., 112

Smaltz, Detlev H., 112

Smoking cessation programs, 25, 44

Social entrepreneurship, 90; business models and, 82

Social Security, 20; closing projected outlays/revenues gap in, 361

Social workers: ambulatory care, value-based purchasing and, 213; primary care and, 162

Society of Actuaries: ACA and estimated premium costs in exchanges report by, 344–46, *345*, *346*

Socioeconomic status: health and, 40, *41*

South Carolina: bundled payment initiative in, 191; RAC audits in, 272

Specialty hospitals: population health management paradigm shift and, *149*

St. John's Health System: Physician Group Practice Demonstration and, 252

St. Margaret Seneca Place v. Board of Property Assessment Appeals and Review, County of Allegheny, PA, 373

Stakeholders: community health business model and, 83; in policy community, 376

Stand-alone hospitals: population health management paradigm shift and, *149*

Standard benefit set: ACA, as potential target for change, 408, 412

Standardization: health insurance exchanges and, 320–21

Stark law, 264, 265

State agencies: health insurance exchanges and, *329*, 329–30

State-based exchanges, *327*, 347; benchmark plan and, 334; challenges in running, 410; characteristics of, *329*; federal exchanges *vs.*, 326–28; financing, 339–41; options for, 328–29

State-federal partnership model: health insurance exchanges, 326, *327*

State governmental structure, 388–90; policymaking at state level, 389–90; political system, 388–89, *389*; state healthcare legislation, examples of, 390

State governments: community health data sources and, 69; health policymaking and, 355; police powers and, 19

States: constitutions and bills of rights for, 355, 388; as educators, 357–58; as guardians of public health, 356; healthcare homes, Medicaid systems, and, 108; health insurance benefits to state employees, 356; health policy and role of, 356–58; interest group strength across, *364*; as laboratories, 358; Medicaid, ACA, and, 17; Medicaid expansion and, 302, 316; Medicaid funding requirement for, as potential target for change, 408–9; Medicaid RACs and, 273; Medicaid wellness incentives and, 25–26; nursing home quality and, 214; police powers granted to, 372; as purchasers of healthcare services, 356; quality reporting organizations in, 228; rate increase reviews for health insurance exchanges in, 322; as regulators, 357; as safety net providers, 357; TANF block grants and, 354–55

Stroke: diabetes and, 35; Hospital Compare measure set for timely and effective care, *211*

Subsidies in health insurance exchanges, 317, 326, 335–37, *336*; Commonwealth Care program (Massachusetts), 387; cost-sharing subsidies, 337; eligibility determination for, 331; federal default exchanges and, 337; IRS, ACA, and, 18; limited fraud potential with, 346n1; modified adjusted gross income level for, 306n2; potential changes in, 410; small-employer subsidies, 337; tax credits, 335–37, *336*; for un-reimbursed care, 46

Suppliers: in operation of political markets, *362*; in political marketplace, 359, *359*; political marketplace and interplay among demanders and, 374–76

Suppliers of health policies, 368–74, 382; executives and bureaucrats as, 370–71; judiciary as, 371–74; legislators as, 368–69

Surgery, 171; discretionary, shared decision making and, 108–9

Systems of care: disputable assumption about, 252–53

Systems theory: in Affordable Care Act, 5, *6*, 6–8, 14

Tax credits: health insurance exchanges and, 335–37; IRS and, 18

Taxes: ACA-related, as potential target of change, 409, 412; aggregate funding for ACA and, 10; on tobacco products, 398

Taxing power of Congress: Supreme Court, constitutionality of ACA, and, 20

Tax laws: local government and, 393

Tax policy: health policy and, 354

Tax Relief and Health Care Act (2006), 213

Teaching hospitals: policy debates and, 377; states as educators and, 358

Technical support organizations: as drivers of quality, 202

Technology, 250, 278; hospitals, affordability, and, 235; mobile healthcare and, 279; policymaking process and, 380

Technology enablement: ACOs and core competency of, *255*, 257

Third-party vendors to Medicare: Medicare payment system update and, 285–86

Timeliness: ACO model and, 248, *249*; Institute of Medicine quality agenda and, 53

Tobacco industry, 397; healthcare policymaking and, 398–99

Total cost of care shared-savings models: value-based purchasing and, *181*, 182

Total health system model: productivity and quality portion of, *171*

Tracking and coordinating care: National Committee for Quality Assurance PCMH model and, 156, 157

Transaction cost economics: organizational decision factors for vertical integration with post-acute providers and predicted responses with, *296*; resource dependence theory and, 295n2; vertical integration between acute and post-acute care organizations and, 291–93

Transitional reinsurance: health insurance exchanges and, 338–39

Transparency: accountable care organizations and, with regard to quality, *246*; rise of ACOs and P4P and demand for, 278

Triple Aim, 80; of Institute for Healthcare Improvement, 61, 62; MATCH models compared with, 85–86, *86*; population health defined and, 84–86

"Two midnight" rule: Recovery Audit Contractor program and, 284–85

Tyson, Bernard J., 277

Umbdenstock, Richard J., 309

Uncompensated care, 301; ACA and reduction in, 9, *9*; Medicaid provisions in ACA and, 303; minimizing burden of, under healthcare reform, 91; Pennsylvania court ruling on tax-exempt status and, 373

Underinsured population, 115; access to primary care and, 162

Underutilization of services, 262; healthcare disparities and, 309; preventing in accountable care organizations, 253–54

Uninsured population, 115, 116. *See also* Safety-net organizations; access issues and, 46–47; access to primary care and, 162; Massachusetts healthcare reform and, 387

United States: access to healthcare in, 46; anticipating future direction of quality improvement in, 194; average health spending per person in, 45; burden of disease in, 57; chronic illness as major problem in, 34; fragmentation of medical care services in, 35–36; funding for public health in, 400–1; healthcare expenditures in, 45, 47, 159; healthcare reform elements for, 6; healthcare waste in, 256; ineffective healthcare spending in, 91; lack of universal coverage in, 46; market-oriented economy in, 400; per capita healthcare spending in, 248; political nature of policymaking in, 382; population health management strategies needed in, 53; public policymaking process in, *379*; relative proportion of non-healthcare social services spending to health services spending in, 95; state of health in, 57, 63; state political system in, *389*; total resident population of, 304; ubiquity of interest groups in, 363–65; WHO health ranking for, 151

Universal coverage: Affordable Care Act and, 315–16; lack of, in United States, 46

US Constitution, 371; ACA supporters and interpreting Commerce Clause of, 20; First Amendment, interest groups, and, 363; government branches created by, 374; police powers granted to states by, 372; state healthcare legislation and, 390

US Department of Health and Human Services, 69, 106; benefit design in health insurance exchanges and, 320; bundled payment system and, 290; HealthCare.gov, 138; National Quality Strategy and priority areas identified by, 212; Office of Civil Rights, 138; Office of Inspector General, 205; partial capitation to ACOs and, 229; policy implementation and, 380

US Preventive Services Task Force, 24; primary care practices and recommendations of, 23; public education and, 24; quality and mission of, *197*

US Supreme Court: ERISA and hospital rates ruling, 372–73; *Jacobson v. Massachusetts* ruling by, 372; legal challenges to Affordable Care Act and, 13, 18–21; Medicaid expansion ruling, 302, 341; OSHA benzene case ruling, 371; ruling on health insurance exchanges with no state Medicaid expansion, 337–38; rulings on major policy aspects of ACA by, 407; significant changes to Affordable Care Act since 2010 enactment and rulings by, 414; state's judiciary and, 389; state supreme court decisions appealed in, 389

Utilization and Quality Control Peer Review Program (Medicare), 202

Utilization review programs, 48

Vaccination: compulsory, police powers, public health, and, 372

Vaccination rates: community health and, 70

Value: bringing to patients, 282; definition of, 205

Value-based payment models: successful design of, key principles for, 191–92

Value-Based Payment Modifier (VM) program, 172

Value-based purchasing, 191, 201, 283; accountable care organizations and, 206–7, 242; ambulatory care and, 213; background and terminology related to, 181–83; evolution of, 180; for hospitals, 214; Medicare and, 170, 177, 179, 181; mixed picture of, 206; productivity and, 170–73; PROMETHEUS Payment case study, 187–91; provider payment models in, *181*; quality and, 284; quality improvement and, 205–7

Vertical integration, 286; advocates and critics of, 288; defining, 287; healthcare reform and careful evaluation of, 288–89; "make or buy" arrangements and, 287, 291; post-acute care providers and organizational decision factors for, *296*; potential costs of, 288; resource dependence theory and, 295n2; transaction cost economics and, 291–93

"Virtual" delivery systems, 252–53

Wellness: hospital leaders and focus on, 279; key elements of, 25; outpatient care settings and, 281; population health management programs and, 32; school-based clinics and, 24; systems view of, *23*

Wellness programs: healthcare in United States and, 22; for women, 33

White House Task Force on Childhood Obesity, 397

Whole-person orientation: American Academy of Family Physicians PCMH model and, 154; National Demonstration Project PCMH model and, 156; patient-centered medical home and, 107

Women: population health management programs for, 33; premium costs in exchanges and, 344–45, *346*; public policymaking process and, 368

World Health Organization, 248; global population and, 40; health defined by, 39–40; primary care benefits detailed by, 152; United States health ranking by, 45, 151

Young, Linda M., 272

ABOUT THE CONTRIBUTORS

Kimberly D. Acquaviva, PhD, MSW, is assistant professor in the Department of Nursing Education and director of the National Collaborative on Aging at George Washington University.

Marc Bard, MD, chief innovation officer in Navigant's Healthcare practice, is a nationally regarded expert on physician leadership effectiveness, change management, and organizational design. Dr. Bard is a board-certified internist who now serves as a strategy and leadership consultant.

Phoebe Lindsey Barton, PhD, is professor emerita at the University of Colorado (UC). During her 18-year tenure at the Health Sciences Center campus, she directed the master of science in public health program, taught courses in health care systems, health services research, and public health administration, the latter at UCLA's School of Public Health.

Francois de Brantes is chief executive officer of the nonprofit Bridges to Excellence and based in Fairfield County, Connecticut.

Connie J. Evashwick, ScD, LFACHE, is credentialed in public health (CPH) and association management (CAE) and is a Life Fellow of the American College of Healthcare Executives. Dr. Evashwick has been vice president of long-term care for two major healthcare systems and has authored more than 112 papers and 12 books.

Michael Ewing attends the University of Alabama, Tuscaloosa. Mr. Ewing is the first-place winner of the undergraduate division of the 2013 ACHE Richard J. Stull Student Essay Competition in Healthcare Management.

Gerald L. Glandon, PhD, is president and CEO of the Association of University Programs in Health Administration (AUPHA). Prior to AUPHA, Dr. Glandon was professor and chair of the Department of Health Services Administration at the University of Alabama at Birmingham.

Alan J. Goldberg, FACHE, is partner and president, Applied Management Systems, Inc., Burlington, Massachusetts.

Dean M. Harris, JD, is a clinical associate professor in the Department of Health Policy and Management, Gillings School of Global Public Health, University of North Carolina (UNC) at Chapel Hill. For more than 20 years, he has taught courses on health law at UNC's Department of Health Policy and Management.

George Isham, MD, is senior advisor, HealthPartners, and senior fellow, HealthPartners Institute for Education and Research, in Bloomington, Minnesota.

Jean E. Johnson, PhD, RN, FAAN, is senior associate dean of health sciences and professor at George Washington University.

Heather Jorna, MHSA, is the vice president of healthcare innovation at the American Hospital Association (AHA). In this role, she is responsible for leading the Hospitals in Pursuit of Excellence (HPOE) initiative, which is the AHA's strategic platform to accelerate performance improvement and support delivery system transformation in the nation's hospitals and health systems.

David A. Kindig, MD, PhD, is professor emeritus, and emeritus vice-chancellor for health sciences at the University of Wisconsin–Madison School of Medicine and Public Health and the UW Population Health Institute.

Beaufort B. Longest Jr., is the M. Allen Pond Professor of Health Policy & Management in the Department of Health Policy & Management of the Graduate School of Public Health at the University of Pittsburgh. He is also the founding director of Pitt's Health Policy Institute.

Stephen A. Martin Jr., PhD, MPH, is the executive director of the Association for Community Health Improvement at the American Hospital Association (AHA). Previously, he served as the chief program officer of the Health Research & Educational Trust of the AHA, the health commissioner and chief operating officer of the Cook County Department of Public Health, and a senior executive member of the Cook County Health & Hospitals System.

Ann Scheck McAlearney, ScD, MS, is professor of family medicine and vice chair for research in the Department of Family Medicine in The Ohio State University College of

Medicine. She also holds courtesy appointments as professor in the Division of Health Services Management and Policy in the College of Public Health and as professor of pediatrics, both at The Ohio State University.

Stephen S. Mick, PhD, FACHE, is a professor in the Department of Health Administration at Virginia Commonwealth University in Richmond.

Michael A. Morrisey, PhD, is a professor in the Department of Health Policy and Management in the School of Public Health at Texas A&M University. Dr. Morrisey is the author of five books, more than 160 peer-reviewed research papers, and nearly 100 other encyclopedia entries, commentaries, and professional reports, many dealing with employer sponsored health insurance and managed care. He is a fellow of the Employee Benefit Research Institute and an adjunct scholar at the American Enterprise Institute.

David B. Nash, MD, MBA, is the founding dean of the Jefferson School of Population Health, which provides innovative educational programming designed to develop healthcare leaders for the future. He has edited 22 books, including *Connecting with the New Healthcare Consumer*, *The Quality Solution*, *Governance for Healthcare Providers*, *Population Health: Creating a Culture of Wellness*, and *Demand Better*.

Michael Nugent is managing director and leader of Navigant's Payment Transformation, Managed Care & Pricing Team. Mr. Nugent is an expert and a nationally recognized writer, speaker, and advisor in the area of pricing, managed care contracting strategy, negotiations, and front-end revenue cycle innovations.

Patrick D. Shay is a doctoral candidate at Virginia Commonwealth University, Richmond.

Leiyu Shi, DrPH, is professor of health policy and health services research at the Johns Hopkins University Bloomberg School of Public Health in the Department of Health Policy and Management. He also serves as director of the Johns Hopkins Primary Care Policy Center. Dr. Shi is the author of nine textbooks and more than 150 scientific journal articles.

Donna J. Slovensky, PhD, RHIA, FAHIMA, is professor and associate dean for student and academic affairs in the School of Health Professions at the University of Alabama at Birmingham (UAB). She holds secondary appointments in the Department of Management in the UAB School of Business and the UAB Graduate School.

Detlev H. (Herb) Smaltz, PhD, FACHE, FHIMSS, is chairman, founder, and former CEO of Health Care DataWorks, Inc., an Ohio State University Technology Commercialization Company. He is a Fellow of the Healthcare Information & Management Systems Society (HIMSS) and a Fellow in the American College of Healthcare Executives (FACHE).

Bernard J. Tyson is CEO of Kaiser Foundation Hospitals and Kaiser Foundation Health Plan, Inc. He serves on the board of directors of the American Heart Association and as chairman of The Executive Leadership Council.

Richard J. Umbdenstock, FACHE, is president and CEO of the American Hospital Association. He is a Fellow of the American College of Healthcare Executives and serves on the boards of the National Quality Forum and Enroll America, cochairs the Council for Affordable Quality Health Care Provider Council, and serves on the National Priorities Partnership and on the Center for Transforming Advanced Care steering committee.

Linda M. Young, JD, RHIA, is a senior consultant and assistant general counsel at Applied Management Systems, Inc., Burlington, Massachusetts.

ABOUT THE EDITOR

Daniel B. McLaughlin, MHA, is the director of the Center for Health and Medical Affairs in the Opus College of Business at the University of St. Thomas in Minneapolis, Minnesota. He is active in teaching, research, and speaking at the university, with a special emphasis on healthcare operations and policy. He is the author of a number of textbooks and management guides published by Health Administration Press, including *Make It Happen: Effective Execution in Healthcare Leadership* and *Responding to Healthcare Operations Management*, second edition.

From 1984 to 1992, Mr. McLaughlin was the administrator and CEO of Hennepin County Medical Center, the Level 1 trauma center in Minneapolis. He served as the chair of the National Association of Public Hospitals and Health Systems and served on President Clinton's Task Force on Health Care Reform in 1993. In 2000, he helped establish and direct the National Institute of Health Policy at St. Thomas. He holds degrees in electrical engineering and healthcare administration from the University of Minnesota.